Third edition

BEAUTY THERAPY

Level 2 NVQ/SVQ Diploma

Judith Ifould
Debbie Forsythe-Conroy
Maxine Whittaker

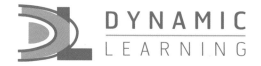

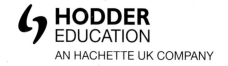

HODDER
EDUCATION
AN HACHETTE UK COMPANY

Orders: please contact Bookpoint Ltd, 130 Milton Park, Abingdon, Oxon OX14 4SB. Telephone: (44) 01235 827720. Fax: (44) 01235 400454. Lines are open 9.00–5.00, Monday to Saturday, with a 24-hour message answering service. Visit our website at www.hoddereducation.co.uk

© Judith Ifould, Debbie Forsythe-Conroy and Maxine Whittaker 2011
First published in 2011 by
Hodder Education, an Hachette UK Company,
338 Euston Road
London NW1 3BH

Impression number   5 4 3 2 1
Year   2015 2014 2013 2012 2011

Cover photo Philippe Regar/Stone/Getty Images
Typeset in Palatino Light 11/13 by Pantek Arts Ltd, Maidstone, Kent
Printed and bound in Italy

A catalogue record for this title is available from the British Library

ISBN 978 1444 135 435

The authors and publishers would like to thank the following for use of photographs in this volume:

p. 9 Maridav – Fotolia; p. 14 Beauty Express; p.17 (top) Photodisc/Getty Images; p.17 (bottom) Photodisc/Getty Images; p. 24 (top) Yuri Arcurs – Fotolia; p. 45 (top) Sebastian Kaulitzki – Fotolia; p. 49 Izzzy – Fotolia; p. 51 © Juice Images/Alamy; p. 57 © Mark Richardson – Fotolia.com; p. 58 Paul Gibbings – Fotolia; p. 64 (bottom) © Philip Harvey/CORBIS; p. 65 © Liquid Light/Alamy; p. 66 © Dennis Hallinan/Alamy; p. 75 Yuri Arcurs – Fotolia; p. 79 (impetigo) © Angela Hampton Picture Library/Alamy; p. 79 (furuncle and carbuncle) DR HAROUT TANIELIAN/SCIENCE PHOTO LIBRARY; p. 79 (conjunctivitis) CMSP/Getty Images; p. 80 (stye) SUE FORD/SCIENCE PHOTO LIBRARY; p. 80 (folliculitis) SCIENCE PHOTO LIBRARY; p. 80 (herpes simplex) SCIENCE SOURCE/SCIENCE PHOTO LIBRARY; p. 80 (Herpes Zoster) © Medical-on-Line/Alamy; p. 80 (warts) DR P. MARAZZI/SCIENCE PHOTO LIBRARY; p. 81 (ringworm or tines) © Medical-on-Line/Alamy; p. 81 (pediculosis) DR. CHRIS HALE/SCIENCE PHOTO LIBRARY; p. 81 (scabies) DR P. MARAZZI/SCIENCE PHOTO LIBRARY; p. 82 Prodakszyn – Fotolia; p. 83 (top) Dimitri Vervitsiotis/Photographer's Choice; p. 83 (middle) David Sacks/ Digital Vision/Getty Images; p. 83 (bottom) DK Stock/Bruce Talbot/Getty Images; p. 86 DR P. MARAZZI/SCIENCE PHOTO LIBRARY; p. 88 (top) Monkey Business – Fotolia; p. 88 (bottom) Yuri Arcurs – Fotolia; p. 89 Beauty Express; p. 90 Beauty Express; p. 91 all Beauty Express; p. 92 all Beauty Express; p. 106 Valua Vitaly – Fotolia; p. 110 yeehaaa – Fotolia; p. 111 DR P. MARAZZI/SCIENCE PHOTO LIBRARY; p. 112 both courtesy of Fake Bake; p. 116 Imagestate Media; p. 122 (automatic tweezers) Beauty Express; p. 122 (manual tweezers) MarkFGD – Fotolia; p. 141 © Asia Images Group Pte Ltd/Alamy; p. 149 Goodshoot RF/Getty Images; p. 150 © Science Photo Library/Alamy; p. 151 © Marka/SuperStock; p. 155 Mat Hayward – Fotolia; p. 159 Karolina Dudys – Fotolia; p. 160 (make-up sponges (Beauty Express); p. 160 (eyelash curlers) Shariff Che'Lah – Fotolia; p. 166 (kabuki brush) College Kits Direct; p. 166 (foundation) Art Deco Cosmetic GmbH; p. 168 Art Deco Cosmetic GmbH; p. 169 Simon Coste – Fotolia; p. 170 (blusher) Art Deco Cosmetic GmbH; p. 170 (eye products Raia – Fotolia; p. 171 Mario Castello/Fancy/photolibrary.com; p. 172 (top) Art Deco Cosmetic GmbH; p. 172 (bottom) mihhailov – Fotolia; p. 187 Louise van Heerden; p. 192 Elisabeth LHOMELET/Photographer's Choice/Getty Images; p. 198 Stanislav Komogorov – Fotolia; p. 200 Andersen Ross/Brand X Pictures/Getty Images; p. 209 (skin type 1) Bernd Fuchs/First Light Associated Photographers/Getty Images; p. 209 (skin type 2) Dimitri Vervitsiotis/Photographer's Choice/Getty Images; p. 209 (skin type 3) Eric Audras/Getty Images; p. 209 (skin type 4) Jann La Pointe/Jann La Pointe/Getty Images; p. 209 (skin type 5) Sherrie Nickol/Citizen Stock/photolibrary.com; p. 209 (skin type 6) Karen Struthers – Fotolia; p. 210 (chloasma) SCIENCE PHOTO LIBRARY; p. 210 (vitiligo) DR HAROUT TANIELIAN/SCIENCE PHOTO LIBRARY; p. 210 (stretch marks) © Medical-on-Line/Alamy; p. 210 (rosacea) CNRI/SCIENCE PHOTO LIBRARY; p. 210 (thread veins) DR P. MARAZZI/SCIENCE PHOTO LIBRARY; p. 219 Steve Mason/Photodisc/Getty Images; p. 221 Lev Olkha – Fotolia; p. 235 all Beauty Express; p. 236 Beauty Express; p. 255 Sandra Gligorijevic – Fotolia; p. 262 Coprid – Fotolia; p. 266 © Science Photo Library/Alamy; p. 268 (ringworm) DR JEREMY BURGESS/SCIENCE PHOTO LIBRARY; p. 268 (whitlow) © Scott Camazine/Alamy; p. 269 (warts) DR P. MARAZZI/SCIENCE PHOTO LIBRARY; p. 269 (scabies) DR P. MARAZZI/SCIENCE PHOTO LIBRARY; p. 269 (eczema); p. 270 (psoriasis) DR P. MARAZZI/SCIENCE PHOTO LIBRARY; p. 270 (nail separation) DR HAROUT TANIELIAN/SCIENCE PHOTO LIBRARY; p. 270 (bruised nail) © Medical-on-Line / Alamy; p. 271 (bitten nails) © Jack Sullivan/Alamy; p. 271 (arthritis) BSIP Medical/photolibrary.com; p. 285 (light unit) Grafton International Ltd; p. 286 Miranda Salia – Fotolia; p. 297 Christoph Hähnel – Fotolia; p. 300 Ellisons; p. 302 Kirill Zdorov – Fotolia; p. 304 Beauty Express; p. 307 Valua Vitaly – Fotolia; p. 209 (verucca plantaris) ERICH SCHREMPP/SCIENCE PHOTO LIBRARY; p. 309 (ringworm) DR P. MARAZZI/SCIENCE PHOTO LIBRARY; p. 309 (ingrowing toe nails) DR P. MARAZZI/SCIENCE PHOTO LIBRARY; p. 310 (corns) BSIP, JOLYOT/SCIENCE PHOTO LIBRARY; p. 310 (bunions) © Bubbles Photolibrary/Alamy; p. 311 Ellisons; p. 324 Paylessimages – Fotolia; p. 327 Beauty Express; p. 328 The Edge; p. 330 (colour wheels) © Mouse in the House/Alamy; p. 330 (nail art design) Mikhail Basov – Fotolia; p. 331 Miranda Salia – Fotolia; p. 332 Beauty Express; p. 333 The Edge; p. 334 Beauty Express; p. 339 altrendo images/Getty Images; p. 341 Ellisons; p. 345 Beauty Express; p. 346 Beauty Express; p. 350 Grafton International Ltd; p. 368 Anne Kitzman – Fotolia; p. 378 Anne Kitzman – Fotolia; p. 379 GIRAND/SCIENCE PHOTO LIBRARY; p. 380 (cultural piercing) © NORMA JOSEPH/Alamy; p. 380 (body piercing) ColorBlind Images/Iconica/Getty Images; p. 384 Skogas – Fotolia; p.386 Antony Nagelmann/Riser/Getty Images; p. 387 Robert Daly/ Stone/Getty Images; p. 388 Adam Gault/OJO Images/Getty Images; p. 392 (top) diego cervo – Fotolia; p. 392 (bottom) anselme – Fotolia; p. 393 © Jack Hollingsworth/Corbis; p. 394 (spa treatment room) aleksandar kamasi – Fotolia; p. 394 (changing area) dextroza – Fotolia; p. 394 (relaxation area) sellingpix – Fotolia; p. 411 Smith Collection/Iconica/Getty Images; p. 419 © O'Brien Productions/Corbis; p. 424 Tandem – Fotolia; p. 425 © Joshua Roper/ Alamy; p. 432 © Kim Kaminski/Alamy; p. 435 ADAM GAULT/SPL/Getty Images; p. 440 Andreas Kuehn/Stone+/Getty Images; p. 441 Andreas Kuehn/ Stone+/Getty Images.

All other photos by Paul Gill/The Rawson Partnership

Illustrations by Simon Tegg Illustration

Every effort has been made to trace and acknowledge ownership of copyright. The publishers will be glad to make suitable arrangements for any copyright holder whom it has not been possible to contact.

Contents

Contributors

Each chapter of this book contains a 'Meet the Professional' case study, in which industry experts give a useful insight into their work.

Daniel Sandler

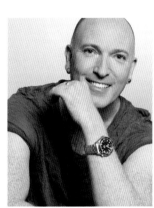

British talent Daniel Sandler has been a make-up artist and leader in his field for over 20 years. Throughout this time Daniel has developed his knowledge and huge talent for creating stunning looks. His multi-award-winning mineral make-up line is now in its 7th successful year.

Over the years, Daniel has worked on both sides of the Atlantic and all over Europe on a number of shoots with high profile fashion photographers for top glossies and with designers backstage at a number of major fashion shows; he is a regular on national TV. Daniel continues to work with high profile celebs getting them ready for red carpet events as well as customers at his Urban Retreat Make-up Studio in the most famous department store in the world, Harrods, London. This year Daniel Sandler Cosmetics celebrate their six-year anniversary of their counter service offering.

Each year Daniel's high profile client list doubles. He has beautified A-list celebrities such as Twiggy, Mylene Klass, Naomi Campbell, Rachel Weisz, Kristen Scott Thomas and Kate Moss.

Daniel has won many accolades for his Colour Cosmetic brand, including two Cosmopolitan Beauty Awards for his Watercolour Fluid Blusher and professional handbag-sized brush range.

Heather Irvine (RGN, INP, HND, CERT ED, BTEC LASER)

Heather Irvine is a leading figure in the medical aesthetic field and is well respected by some of the UK's leading cosmetic surgeons. She is an expert trainer of cosmetic doctors and nurses in the use of Botulinum Toxin and Restylane®. Heather has worked within the medical profession for 25 years and has had her own successful aesthetic clinic for 10 years. Heather has also gained qualifications in nursing, beauty therapy at Levels 4 and 5 and laser therapy. She is a qualified teacher.

Jacqui Bostock (Mphil)

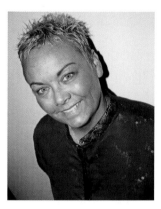

Jacqui Bostock holds City and Guilds in Beauty Therapy, having graduating from Bradford College in 1990. She is a recipient of the prestigious Student of the Year and the City and Guilds Silver Medal for Salon & Business Management. Following a period of employment and working abroad she eventually established her own successful beauty therapy business, Quintessence, in 2004. Her qualifications are extensive, including a degree in Biomedical Sciences, in which she attained a First Class Honours Degree, specialising in Cellular Pathology. She has also successfully completed a Master of Philosophy (MPhil) in Molecular Vascular Medicine at Leeds University and has several published papers. Jackie is a qualified teacher and is currently studying Advanced Aromatherapy. She is a member of the Advisory Committee at Bradford College.

Kirsty Ellis

Kirsty Ellis is a Treatment Manager at Nirvana Spa, Berkshire. After training at Huddersfield Technical College, she began working in a local salon, continuing her professional development and gaining product and skills training. The opportunity to work in a spa on a cruise liner became available to her, and after a month at a training academy she was offered a position as a Spa Therapist and contracted to work for eight months.

Having experienced salon and spa work, Kirsty realised her passion was in the spa and leisure business, so returned to spa work by joining Nirvana Spa. As a Spa Therapist, she has experienced fantastic rewards, perks and ongoing training, as well as sufficient product knowledge to perform treatments to the best of her ability. The company saw her potential and promoted her – first to Senior Therapist and then to Treatment

Supervisor. This has given Kirsty the opportunity to gain more knowledge on how the department operates, for example in relation to understanding department targets, goals and financial figures. With the help and development from her manager she progressed to Assistant and then Treatment Manager.

Kathryn Reeve

Kathryn Reeve has been working for the Studex Corporation for seven years, and involved in the beauty therapy industry for over 10 years, developing and implementing ear piercing procedures and promoting the company's wide range of products and services. With a strong background in business development and language skills, Kathryn works with the worldwide offices on product development and training.

As the world's largest manufacturer of ear piercing equipment and supplies, Studex operates in over 30 countries, guaranteeing high quality products and consistency worldwide, with Kathryn enjoying a wide variety of roles as a Trainer as well as Business Account Manager. The Studex brand is recognised across a wide sector of businesses including salons, pharmacies and jewellers, with tailored training provided to each individual business. There is a strong focus on providing high quality training within educational institutions, with certified training sessions provided throughout the year. All Studex instruments and products are approved and recognised by Local Health Authorities, with Kathryn also dedicating time to co-ordinating presentations to Environmental Health departments nationwide, to educate in ear piercing procedures and instruments available.

Sarah Sheridan

Sarah's passion for the industry started at a very young age, with her mother owning a hair salon, and from then she has never lost interest in this ever-changing industry. Sarah attended a short beauty taster course at her local college after school which soon turned into three years of training in beauty therapy and hairdressing. Her career has taken her from salons into the spa industry, where she has been fortunate to train with some of the leading skin care retail companies. In her current working role she is head of training at a private training academy that specialises in beauty therapy, nail services, holistic therapy and hairdressing training. She finds passing her passion and enthusiasm for this industry to her learners very rewarding and looks forward to new emerging trends popping up within the industry, which continue to inspire us all.

Introduction

Welcome to the new look, third edition of **Beauty Therapy: The Basics for Level 2**.

With the new look comes a new style, improved features and celebrity employer contributions, married with the years of experience and knowledge brought to previous editions.

It would be frightening to add up the accumulated years of experience between the three of us, but what is it that keeps us so interested and fulfilled for this long in the beauty industry? Beauty therapy is a fascinating and ever-changing industry that can engage your interest with new treatments and product developments, and can bring you close to celebrities through employment opportunities in beauty salons, nail bars, health clinics, spas, cosmetic houses, cruise ships and working overseas. We want to share this with you.

The beauty therapy industry is just one of six industries within the 'Hair and Beauty sector' that are controlled by the skills sector professional body called **HABIA**. You will see that we refer and advise you throughout the book to their recommendation for what is considered to be the industry's standards of work and good practice. The six industries are: Beauty therapy, Hairdressing, Nail services, Barbering, Spa, Afro type hairdressing.

Student profiles

Zoe Nichols

Zoe Nichols studied beauty therapy at Basingstoke College of Technology and then trained in Fashion and Editorial Make-up at London College of Fashion. While on work experience she met Daniel Sandler, who was so impressed by her professionalism and skills that he offered her a job with him on leaving college. She then trained with Daniel Sandler, one of the UK's most successful make-up artists, and has worked as part of Team Daniel Sandler on shoots and catwalk shows.

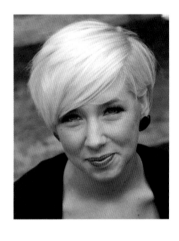

Zoe has recently opened her own salon in Bournemouth – 'Soda' beauty and blow dry bar – offering a range of beauty treatments, but specialising in bridal makeovers; one-to-one make-up lessons, special occasion make-up, photographic/fashion make-up, make-up master classes and group make-up lessons using Daniel's exclusive range of make-up products.

Sophie Steggles

Sophie Steggles studied Beauty Therapy at Bradford College and has worked extensively in the profession, including in a senior position in one of the world's top Mandarin Oriental hotels. Sophie now lives and works in Dubai.

Two of the contributors to this book are also past students of Bradford College – see their biographies for their career journeys in this fast-moving and exciting profession.

About the Book

We are so excited about this new edition of the book as we have covered all the units on the Beauty Therapy General and Make-up routes, as well as those for nail services. We also include threading, meaning this is a 'one-stop shop' of a book.

We have included some useful and interesting features:

Meet the professional

Industry case studies where you can 'meet the professional'.

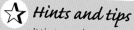 **Hints and tips**
'Hints and tips' boxes to provide important and relevant information.

Equipment checklist

✔ So you know what tools you need to work effectively

'Personal appearance' checklists

 Remember . . .

'Remember to ..' boxes that remind you of key points within the treatment procedure such as link selling

Key term

'Key term' boxes to explain unfamiliar words and terminology.

 Want to know more?

At the end of a chapter you will find 'want to know more' to expand the topic, introduce new technologies and feed your thirst for more as well as a short test to answer to help you with your theory assessment.

Activity

Short 'activities' as checks on your learning

Test yourself

'Test yourself' boxes to answer to help you with your theory assessment

We've also included clear, step-by-step photographs of procedures.

All these and a celebrity make-up artist!

Guide to NVQ/SVQs

Training to a high standard to enable you to access the wide and varied employment opportunities within the Hair and Beauty sector anywhere in the United Kingdom or overseas is essential.

National Vocational Qualifications (NVQs) and **Scottish Vocational Qualifications (SVQs)** are designed to assess your ability to do a particular job according to a set of standards for beauty therapy called the National Occupational Standards (NOS), set by the beauty therapy industry's professional body **HABIA**. This organisation is made up of employers, industry experts and educators and trainers. It is our industry that decides the standards by which we must be trained and perform beauty therapy treatments. When you have successfully completed an NVQ/SVQ and apply for a job, the employer will immediately know what you are capable of doing.

NVQ/SVQs are based on assessment of **practical skills**, **knowledge** and **understanding** at Levels 1, 2, 3 or 4.

An NVQ/SVQ qualification is made up of **units**, which describe a particular treatment or job within the salon, for example B4 'Provide facial skin care treatment'. Each unit is made up of several **outcomes** that break up that treatment into stages and these are broken down further into **performance criteria (PCs)** that reflect our industry's standards. These PCs are what you **must do** to perform the treatment. What you **must know** is a list of **essential knowledge** that supports the practical performance. An NVQ/SVQ requires you to show 'competence' over a period of time so this requires you to perform a treatment more than once to cover a **range** of different circumstances and clients.

To gain an NVQ/SVQ, you will be taught to the national standards by your teacher either in the workplace or at a recognised training centre such as a college of further education, through demonstrations followed by practice on clients in the salon, as well as theory lessons to provide you with the necessary knowledge needed to support the practical activities.

Level	Description
1	An introduction to beauty therapy involving the application of knowledge and skills that are routine and predictable. You might be an assistant helping therapists in a salon.
2	The application of knowledge and skills to varied work activities in a variety of contexts that are non-routine and with some individual responsibility, but also working as part of a team. Basically, performing treatments on clients in the salon.
3	More complex treatments requiring advanced skills and knowledge as well as considerable responsibility and the control or guidance of others such as an assistant manager or supervisor.
4	Knowledge and skills of a broad and complex nature with a high degree of responsibility for self and others as well as resources such as the management of stock, money and people, including training.

It is necessary to make an action plan at the beginning of your course to enable you to watch your progress in both your learning and assessment and to review what you have achieved. Assessment takes place when you and your assessor agree that you have sufficient learning and understanding through practice on clients, written work and collection of supplementary evidence such as client record cards, to perform a treatment to the industry's standard.

Your candidate logbook will help you plan for assessment and your assessor will discuss with you what the assessment process involves.

The assessor will usually be your teacher who will advise you on assessment opportunities such as:

- observation of practical work
- oral questioning
- written tests
- case studies
- assignments or projects.

The assessor will discuss the assessment with you before it takes place and agree how the assessment will be carried out. You will then perform the treatment on a paying client while your assessor watches you work. This is called an **observation** and will be judged against the performance criteria and recorded in your assessment logbook at the time of your assessment, along with the range you have covered performing that treatment.

The assessor will need to be sure that you understand what you are doing and why. This will involve asking you questions. This is called **oral questioning**. As most of your work involves a client this will usually be done after your client has left, unless the assessor wishes to confirm something with you during the treatment.

You will collate evidence of assessment into a **portfolio**. The type of evidence can be divided into **performance evidence** and **knowledge**

evidence. Performance evidence includes items such as client record cards, photographs, case studies and witness testimonies, which help to confirm that you can carry out a task. Knowledge evidence will be such things as written tests and assignments or projects which show that you have gained knowledge of a subject. You are required to provide a guide for your assessor so that the information contained in your portfolio is organised. This is called **referencing**.

To maintain the quality of your work, to ensure that it reaches the standard for our industry, and to ensure that the assessment is fair a process called **verification** is carried out. This involves someone who is trained to observe assessments watching the assessment process and reviewing the marking of written tests, assignments and/or projects. Initially this is carried out by the internal verifier who will sign off units as you complete them and then your portfolio before claiming certification from the awarding body. The training centre will retain your portfolio and assessment logbook for the **external verifier**, who does a further check on behalf of the awarding body.

Awarding bodies offering NVQ/SVQs include City & Guilds, Edexcel and Vocational Training Charitable Trust (VTCT), all of which provide NVQs/SVQs with the same PCs, range, essential knowledge and evidence requirements following the National Occupational Standards (NOS).

There are other qualifications besides the NVQ/SVQ that are recognised by the beauty therapy industry. These qualifications will not have identical information but are written by awarding bodies in line with the NOS; these include Vocational Related Qualifications (VRQs). The information contained in this book will meet the needs of all students of beauty therapy, regardless of which qualification they are working towards.

Progression

Below is a chart indicating NVQ/SVQ in beauty therapy at the different levels:

Note that the NVQ Level 1 Hairdressing and Beauty would also allow entry into NVQ Level 2 Hairdressing or Barbering qualification.

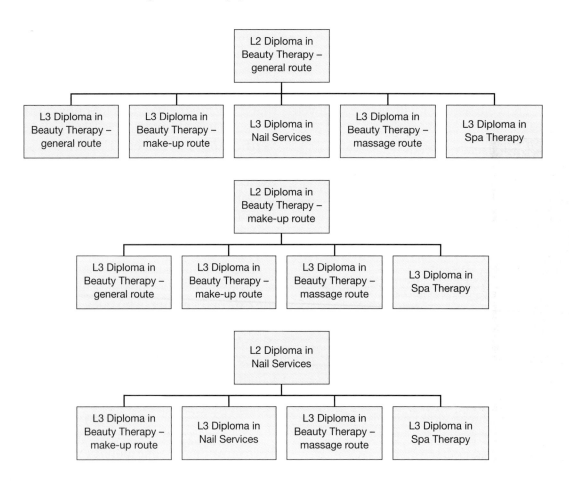

Careers options

A NVQ/SVQ in Level 2 in Beauty Therapy general and make-up routes and Nail Services offers employment opportunities within the hair and beauty sector.

On completion of a Level 2 in Beauty Therapy – general route and Nail Services you can obtain insurance and therefore employment in a salon, spa, clinic or nail bar, performing the treatments in which you are competent while taking NVQ Level 3 as an apprenticeship. Your training can be delivered through a training agency or local further education establishment, or given by your employer with the aid or a peripatetic assessor and/or internal verifier.

This is also true of the Beauty Therapy – make-up route, with employment opportunities being found in department stores for a particular 'cosmetic house' or indeed in salons, clinics or health centres.

We hope that you enjoy your career in beauty therapy as much as we have!

Part 1 : In the salon

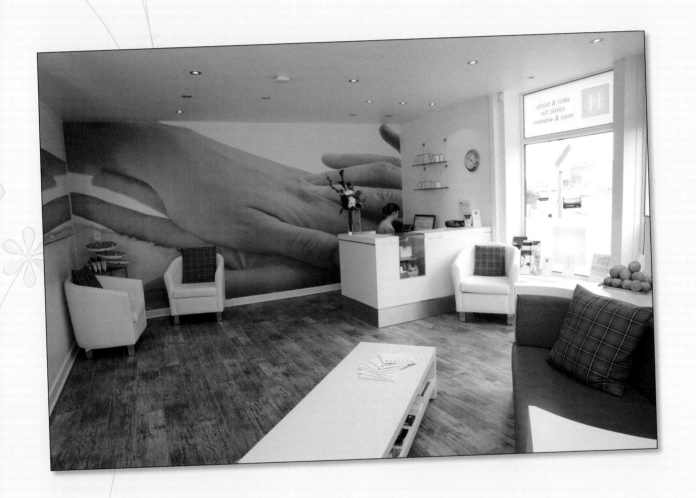

Chapter 1
Professional skills

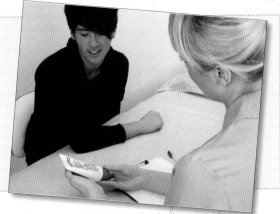

Learning objectives

In this chapter you will learn about:

1 Professional procedures for providing a service, including:
- service standards
- client care
- communicating with clients
- professional codes of practice
- professional practice and behaviour.

2 Personal appearance and hygiene

3 Salon environment, including:
- sterilising and hygiene procedures
- methods of sterilisation and disinfection
- health and safety aspects of performing treatments.
- legal aspects of performing treatments

4 Consultation techniques, including:
- questioning the client
- visual signs
- referral to record cards
- dealing with contraindications
- client referral
- contra-actions
- the treatment plan.

5 Record keeping

6 Client complaints including
- procedure for handling complaints

7 Treatments, including:
- preparing for treatments
- before the start of treatment
- during treatment
- after treatment

Introduction

The customer is at the centre of every business. It is necessary for a business to provide a service of the highest quality to its customers. In beauty therapy, this means the client. The experience the client receives during their visit to the salon will influence whether they return for further treatments and become a regular customer.

The way in which a beauty therapist approaches their job will influence the success of the business. Consideration should be given to the following:

- the technical skills of the therapist to provide efficient and effective treatments
- the salon environment, decor and ambience
- levels of professionalism
- health, safety and security in the salon.

> ⭐ *Hints and tips*
> *Did you know that if a client receives bad service they will tell more people than if they receive good service?*

Professional procedures for providing a service

There are certain procedures that should be followed for each service to maintain high levels of professionalism when working in the beauty therapy industry.

Service standards

The client's perceptions of you and the salon are very important. The image you project should follow the salon policy on standards of appearance and client care. The salon may have a manual or a notice in the staff room that outlines salon practice and procedures and rules and regulations. New members of staff will normally receive information on salon practice during their induction.

The technical skills of the therapist rely on good training through recognised qualifications, the updating of ongoing skills, and experience of working with clients. Treatments should be of the highest quality and should meet the client's needs as closely as possible. All work should be carried out efficiently and should be cost-effective.

Treatments are becoming more advanced, with the use of lasers, injectables and microcurrents being used. After gaining the relevant qualifications, it is the professional duty of a therapist to embark on a programme of Continual Professional Development (CPD). Membership of a professional body will allow you to keep up to date with developments in the industry, as will training courses, trade shows and trade magazines. This will ensure that treatments you perform are to the highest possible standard.

Professional bodies also offer insurance that provides the therapist with financial support should a client take legal action against the therapist for malpractice. Malpractice constitutes adverse reaction or injury to the client from a treatment. However, therapists are only protected if they have followed the relevant professional codes of practice, so it is essential that therapists are qualified and competent to practice.

Client care

Client care is an essential part of the beauty therapist's role, from the moment a client makes an enquiry to the end of the treatment. You will be required to:

- listen carefully
- observe the client
- make appropriate conversation with the client
- offer advice
- provide one-to-one attention throughout the treatment.
- ensure client comfort, warmth and privacy
- protect the client's clothing and hairline if necessary during treatment
- ensure security of the client's possessions

It is important that the therapist is aware of the client's feelings and makes the effort to build good relationships. You can do this by:

- practising good communication skills
- empathising
- caring
- taking responsibility
- showing courtesy and respect.

Practising good communication skills

- Listen carefully to clients, colleagues and others.
- Question appropriately and in a sensitive manner.
- Write clearly, using memos, reports, messages, and so on.
- Use appropriate non-verbal body language and facial expressions.
- Make appropriate conversation with the client.

Empathising

Put yourself in your client's place. Everything you do should be seen from the client's point of view. The client may sometimes feel confused or anxious about their visit to the salon. It could be the first time they have had a treatment and they will naturally feel apprehensive about what it involves. They may feel embarrassed about having to remove clothing or be concerned about whether the treatment will be uncomfortable.

You must make every effort to explain fully what will be involved, and avoid any embarrassment to the client by ensuring privacy and adequate covering to maintain their modesty. The activity on this page will help you to think about your feelings in a range of situations.

Activity

How do you feel when:

- you make a phone call and are left on hold for a long time with no explanation?
- you are kept waiting with no explanation or apology?
- a shop assistant ignores you when you are trying to buy something?
- someone is serving you while they have a conversation with someone else?
- someone looks angry and speaks aggressively to you?
- you arrive for an appointment to find that it has been changed to another time?
- someone promises to do something for you but forgets?
- people are giggling in front of you, as if they are laughing at you?
- you try to explain something but the person does not seem to be listening?

You may be able to think of other situations. Have you ever felt uncomfortable or embarrassed?

Choose two situations and write down or discuss with a partner how the person should have behaved to make you feel more comfortable.

Caring

This is a genuine feeling of wanting to help others. As a therapist, this means:

- being able to recognise when someone needs assistance
- showing a willingness to help clients and others (remember the client will observe how the staff work together)
- showing genuine concern for the well-being of the client
- ensuring that the client is not put at risk
- recognising when clients have special needs and offer assistance.

Communicating with clients

Communication can be seen as an essential part of the therapist's role and is vital for the efficient running of the salon. So, the way in which you communicate with your clients, colleagues and manager will affect the atmosphere and efficiency of the salon.

One of the most daunting tasks when training to be a beauty therapist is meeting clients and knowing what to talk about. For example, a young, inexperienced therapist may find it difficult to relate to an older person.

Conversation with the client is an essential part of the service offered. It plays an important role in:

- making the client feel welcome
- gaining important information during the consultation
- gaining feedback during and after a treatment to ensure that the client is comfortable and satisfied.

 Remember . . .

Some clients see the opportunity to unwind and talk about their problems as part of the treatment. Others prefer to be quiet, without unnecessary talking. It is your job to assess the client's needs and provide conversation or peace and quiet as appropriate.

Starting a conversation

Before you receive your client, find out her name from the appointments book (or ask the receptionist) and also the treatment she is booked for. Then greet the client by using their title and surname. First names are too familiar for a first meeting and should only be used if the client specifically asks you to or if you know them personally.

If the client comes to you regularly, you should try to recall things from her previous visit to start the conversation. For example:

- 'How did you get on with the night cream you bought last time?'
- 'What dress did you decide to wear last Friday night?'

 Hints and tips
'Special needs' is defined as age, disability, race, religion, gender, sexual orientation and gender reassignment by the Equality Act 2010.

The client record card can provide you with information that may help you to start the conversation. For example:

- 'I see you have been using the new product range, Mrs James. How are you getting on with it?'
- 'Has your allergy settled down, Mrs Andrews?'

You will need to have some background information or to remember things about your client to ask these sorts of questions. If you have not met the client before, you could use general topics from the newspaper or television.

 Remember...

You must not gossip.

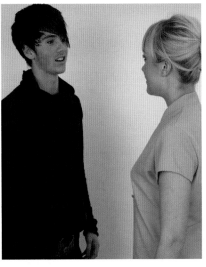

△ Therapist greeting a client

Topics of conversation to avoid include:

- politics
- religion
- other clients
- colleagues
- other salons and their staff.

Professional codes of practice

Codes of practice are written by sector skill councils (SSCs). In the Hair and Beauty sector, the sector skills council is the Hair and Beauty Industry Association (HABIA). At the end of this chapter you will find HABIA's website and those of other professional bodies.

Professional beauty therapy organisations lay down additional standards of practice and ethics for their members.

Codes of ethics are rules of behaviour that aim to protect clients from improper practice. New members of a professional body are usually required to sign an agreement that they will abide by their code of ethics. This includes:

- upholding standards of treatment and not making false claims
- having loyalty to and respect for other beauty therapists by not criticising their work or 'poaching' their clients
- not gossiping or betraying the confidence of the clients.

Professional practices keep the therapist up to date with methods of treatment and procedures for beauty therapy such as hygiene practices, new treatments and findings from research. In beauty therapy, professional practice requires the following:

- Each client has a consultation to establish any contraindications and to find out requirements for treatment.
- Written permission is obtained from the client's doctor for certain treatments where the client's medication or condition requires it.
- The therapist does not make false claims and does not attempt to treat medical conditions.
- The therapist is competent and keeps up to date with the latest treatments.
- Under-age clients are only treated with written permission from a parent or guardian.

Failure to comply with a professional body's codes of ethics and practice can lead to expulsion from the organisation.

Students of beauty therapy can apply for student membership to professional bodies and obtain valuable information about events and new products and treatments, as well as getting insurance that covers the treatment of clients during training.

Professional practice and behaviour

The professionalism of all staff in beauty therapy is important. They all contribute to the image of the salon and the quality of the treatments. The salon will set standards of appearance and behaviour for the therapists to follow, which will be set out in the salon's rules and regulations. The therapist must aim to represent the salon in a positive way and to follow standards of behaviour that comply with the organisation's service standards.

Acceptable standards of behaviour while in the working environment include:

- speaking politely (no slang or bad language)
- courtesy and regard for others
- no smoking, eating or chewing
- appropriate topics of conversation within the salon.

Behaviour is learnt from others and what may be acceptable for one person or within some work or social environments is not always appropriate for the beauty therapist.

You will need to take responsibility within the limits of your authority, which means:

- making decisions or solving problems that affect your client, quickly and effectively
- knowing when to refer your client to a doctor or another practitioner as necessary, without delaying or inconveniencing them
- avoiding passing problems on to others simply because you cannot be bothered to handle the situation
- taking ownership of a problem and resolving it in the best way you can.

Always show courtesy and respect by:

- being polite and showing respect for others (essential in all aspects of life)
- being aware of others
- showing tolerance for differing views and behaviour and for different cultures, religions and backgrounds that influence behaviour
- not judging others or viewing them as inferior because they may appear to be different to you
- recognising that being tolerant and having respect for others does not mean that you have to compromise your own standards and beliefs.

Activity

Observe the way in which senior therapists who are experienced in working with clients in the salon behave. Use the bullet points listed here to check on the appropriateness of their behaviour.

Personal appearance and hygiene

The beauty therapy industry is one where image is very important. To promote a clean and professional image, certain requirements regarding appearance and dress are expected.

- A high level of personal hygiene is expected because of the close proximity with a client a therapist experiences during the course of their work. Bathing or showering every day is expected, as is the use of deodorant/antiperspirant.

- Fresh breath is also expected. Brushing the teeth twice daily and regular visits to the dentist are essential. Also be aware of the foods you eat, especially at lunchtime, and take special precautions if you are a smoker.

- Salon dress or uniform should project an image of cleanliness and professionalism. White uniforms are the traditional dress for beauty therapists, with individual salons using coloured trim or badges as distinguishing features to promote the salon image. Coloured uniforms are also popular, especially in the spa environment.

- Smart, clean shoes that are fully enclosed are required to avoid the possibility of injury to the feet from equipment or products. They should have low heels to avoid fatigue and the development of postural problems.

- Feet and legs should be covered with socks or tights of an appropriate colour to ensure hygiene, to avoid foot odour and also to provide protection.

- Hair should be clean and styled if short, but if long should be secured away from the face and up off the neck. Hair can easily harbour micro-organisms and there is a hygiene issue if the therapist has to continuously touch the hair because it falls in front of the face. Long hair could also easily be trapped or caught by machinery or equipment, which could result in injury.

- Jewellery should be kept to a minimum so as not to offend clients. Hands and arms should be free from jewellery as they will come in contact with the client, may harbour micro-organisms (increasing the risk of infection), and may scratch or injure the client. Plain wedding bands are normally acceptable, but wrist watches should be replaced with a fob watch. Avoiding arm and wrist jewellery will also avoid any unwanted noise (such as the 'clanking' of bracelets) disturbing the client's relaxing treatment.

- Day make-up must be worn at all times when coming into contact with clients. It should be immaculate, with particular attention to skincare. This is often the best way of selling cosmetics to a client. The client will expect to see the therapist following her own advice.

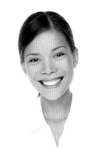

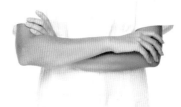

△ A professional therapist

Activity

Look through beauty therapy trade magazines or write to salon wear manufacturers for a brochure and select a uniform for your salon. Briefly describe the reasons for your choice.

⭐ *Hints and tips*

Open shoes and bare feet may be acceptable in the spa environment, especially in the 'wet areas'. Cropped trousers are preferred, reducing the possibility of them becoming wet.

Activity

What are the rules for your salon on dress and appearance?

Ask to see the salon's service standards and make a checklist for your staff notice board on salon rules and regulations. This should be well presented so that it is easy to read. Word process your checklist if possible.

- Nails should be kept short and well manicured but free from nail enamel. Long nails harbour dirt and micro-organisms and can scratch a client inadvertently. Some clients are allergic to nail enamel, so it must be avoided.

- Hands should be clean, soft and warm. Remember that your hands are the primary tools of your trade and you need to look after them. Hand exercises will loosen stiffness and improve strength, which is useful in avoiding repetitive strain injuries. Any open wounds should be covered with a waterproof dressing to prevent cross-infection. Thorough washing of the hands is essential before treating the client, after carrying out treatment and at any time during the day when the hands have come into contact with a possible source of infection, for example after visiting the toilet or carrying out cleaning tasks in the salon. Use hot water and a good liquid detergent in a dispenser, preferably antiseptic, to wash hands. A bar of soap can harbour germs. Wash the front and back of the hands, between the fingers and up over the wrists. Disposable towels should be available for drying and disposed of immediately in a closed bin.

Personal hygiene and appearance checklist

- ❏ Is your salon uniform spotless and neatly ironed?
- ❏ Is your hair clean and in a style that prevents your hair falling over your face during treatment?
- ❏ Are you wearing comfortable, low-heeled shoes that are clean and not scuffed?
- ❏ If you are wearing tights or stockings, are they changed every day and free from holes or ladders?
- ❏ Are you wearing jewellery that may come into contact with equipment or the client, for example rings and bangles?
- ❏ Have you brushed your teeth today?
- ❏ Did you take a bath or shower before starting work today?
- ❏ Are you wearing day make-up?
- ❏ Does your make-up look professionally and carefully applied?
- ❏ Did you wash your hands using hot soapy water and disposable towels to dry them, before and after treating your client?

Salon environment

The salon environment depends largely on the investment in the business by the salon owner(s) and the image they wish to project. Cleanliness is of utmost importance and this is reflected in the decor and care of fixtures, fittings and equipment of the salon.

The ambience of the salon will be very important to the client. Clients will wish to feel relaxed and comfortable in a peaceful and unhurried atmosphere.

Lighting should be considered when planning a therapy room, depending on its usage. If the room is to be used for general treatments it is useful to have lighting that can be varied for the type of treatment being performed, perhaps with a dimmer switch. For example low, subdued lighting may be required for massage or facial treatments, but general areas such as the reception area or stairwells need to be bright in order to be welcoming or for safety reasons. There should be sufficient light in order to perform treatments safely and effectively.

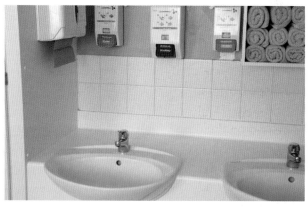

△ Hot water, liquid soap and disposable towels should be available for staff to wash their hands

Temperature is also important for the comfort of clients and therapists: extremes in temperature may be uncomfortable for the client and they may be unable to relax. Extreme heat can cause fatigue and raise blood pressure.

Ventilation can be used to moderate the temperature of a room but extractor devices may also be needed in rooms where products that emit strong fumes are used or dispensed.

Sterilising and hygiene procedures

During your training you will be constantly reminded of the importance of hygiene and the need to carry out thorough hygiene procedures. The nature of beauty therapy requires close contact with the client and it carries the risk of cross-infection. Clients have a right to expect high standards of hygiene throughout the treatment, making cleanliness a priority for the salon. There are new strains of viruses that are resistant to simple cleansing methods. This makes strict hygiene working practices a necessity.

Hygiene procedures

- Cleaning equipment, work surfaces and implements with appropriate cleaning agents should be part of your working routine.
- Fresh laundered towels and bed linen must be available at all times. Therefore, attending to laundry will be an important part of your salon duties.
- Washing hands is the simplest but one of the most effective hygiene procedures. It must become second nature to you to protect yourself from infection and also your clients and all those within the salon environment. Use bactericidal hand wash from a dispenser and have the water as hot as possible, followed by thorough drying with a disposable hand towel.
- Cover cuts or abrasions on your hands, or on the area to be treated on the client, with a waterproof plaster.
- Wear disposable gloves for treatments where there is any possibility of coming into contact with blood or body fluids (depilatory waxing, particularly underarm and bikini-line waxing where blood spots during treatment are common). There have been concerns about the possibility of passing on the HIV virus or hepatitis through some treatments such as electrical epilation, ear-piercing or where the skin can become broken. The risk of spreading these conditions is low but if contracted the consequences are serious so procedures must be in place to minimise the risk of cross-infection from any source.
- Sterilise small implements using an autoclave or sterilising fluid.
- Disposable items, such as paper towels, spatulas, tissues and cotton wool must be used where possible and disposed of immediately after use in a covered waste bin.

Health and safety

The Workplace (Health, Safety and Welfare) Regulations 1992 give guidelines to employers regarding the safe lighting, temperatures and ventilation requirements for a workplace.

Everyone must be aware of the importance of carrying out strict hygiene procedures to protect themselves, other therapists and clients from infection.

The therapist must be able to recognise skin disease and disorders associated with the area of the body being treated and carry out the meticulous hygiene procedures that are outlined in this chapter.

Infection

Infection is caused by micro-organisms that invade the body and cause inflammation. These include:

- bacteria
- fungi
- viruses.

Bacteria

Bacteria that can cause disease are known as pathogenic; those that do not cause disease are known as non-pathogenic. They are categorised by their shape. Bacterial infection can usually be treated with antibiotics. Signs of bacterial infection are redness, swelling, pain and pus.

Health and safety

Guidelines set down by the Local Government (Miscellaneous Provisions) Act and the Codes of Practice outline hygiene procedures that are particularly important when the treatment involves skin piercing.

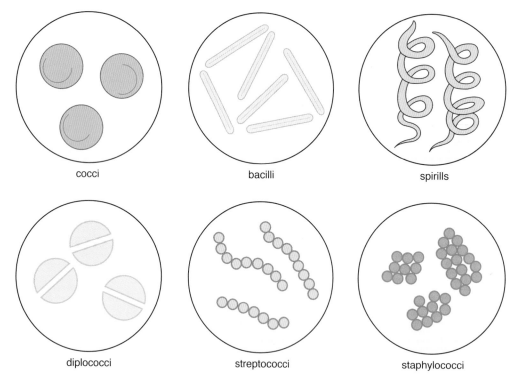

cocci   bacilli   spirills

diplococci   streptococci   staphylococci

△ Types of bacteria that can cause infection

Fungi

Fungi that live on decaying or dead matter are known as saprophytic. Those that live on living matter are known as parasitic. Both types cause disease within the human body. Examples include:

- tinea capitis (ringworm of the scalp)
- athlete's foot (ringworm of the feet)
- onychomycosis (ringworm of the nail).

Viruses

Viruses are smaller than bacteria and infections caused by them are more difficult to control as they are unaffected by antibiotics. Viral diseases are divided into two main groups:

- **Highly infectious diseases**. These are transmitted by direct contact through droplets of moisture or mucus from the nose or mouth. Measles and the common cold are passed on in this way.
- **Infectious diseases**. The method of transmission is not obvious, but can be by direct or indirect contact. Viral infections of the skin fall into this group, such as warts or herpes simplex (cold sores).

There are two serious viral diseases that a beauty therapist should be aware of. They are Acquired Immune Deficiency Syndrome (AIDS) and Hepatitis B.

AIDS

The virus known as the human immunodeficiency virus (HIV) affects the body's natural defence or immune system, leaving it susceptible to attack from other diseases, some of which can be fatal. Acquired immune deficiency syndrome (AIDS) is a disease of the human immune system that is caused by (HIV). As yet, there is no cure.

The HIV virus is transmitted within body fluids, such as blood. An HIV-positive person can remain without any symptoms of AIDS for several years. In fact, in the early stages of infection the virus can be present but remain undetected when tested. It is imperative that strict hygiene precautions are followed during all beauty therapy treatments but especially when performing treatments that may involve contact with body fluids. For example, waxing and eyebrow tweezing may draw blood.

Hepatitis B

Hepatitis B is a viral disease of the liver, which is also transmitted within body fluids. The virus is more infectious than HIV. This is because the virus is more resistant and is able to live outside the body for a considerable time. The disease is very debilitating and can be fatal. The same strict hygiene precautions should be taken with the Hepatitis B virus as with HIV, to avoid cross-infection.

Infestations

This is a term used to describe the transmission of diseases caused by small parasites. The most common infestation is by head lice. These infect the scalp and are common in small children. The condition is spread directly by contact or by the communal use of brushes or towels.

Another condition that the therapist may come across is scabies, where very small mites burrow through and along the epidermis to lay their eggs. The condition can appear red with the presence of swelling and fine lines indicating where the mites have burrowed.

Cross-infection

Micro-organisms that cause disease are usually spread by coming into direct contact with the source. Sources include contaminated blood, body fluids, pus, sores or infected skin cells. Unclean tools, shared towels, dirty work surfaces and unwashed hands can be a source of infection in the salon.

Good hygiene procedures and the use of disposable materials will ensure that risks to yourself and to others can be minimised.

Methods of sterilisation and disinfection

The terms sterilisation and disinfection are sometimes confused.

- Sterilisation destroys all micro-organisms using chemicals or high temperature.
- Disinfectants are usually chemical agents that destroy most disease-causing micro-organisms but not their spores so the disease can reoccur.
- Antiseptics are a dilute disinfectant for use on the skin. They inhibit the spread of disease by slowing the growth of bacteria or fungi.

Sterilisation methods

- The **autoclave** uses high-pressure steaming at a minimum temperature of 126°C. Autoclaves for salon use are small compact units that provide sterilisation for small metal implements. They are safe and easy to use providing the manufacturer's instructions are followed closely.
- The **glass bead steriliser** uses dry heat at a temperature of 200–300°C. These have limited use in the salon due to the small area available at the correct temperature for sterilisation. Because of the risk of burns when the implements are removed, they need to be used with care.
- **Ultraviolet light steriliser** uses ultraviolet rays from a quartz mercury vapour lamp. This method is very limited because of the need to turn the implements over to expose each surface to the rays. The cabinets do, however, provide a germ-free environment to store previously sterilised implements.
- **Gamma radiation** is used to sterilise epilation needles and extraction lances at the point of manufacture. It is used under controlled conditions when large-scale sterilisation is required. It is not used in the salon.

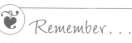

Remember...

Unless items that have been sterilised are stored correctly, they can easily be contaminated by organisms that are carried in the air.

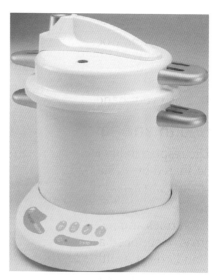

△ Autoclave

- **Chemical agents** are available which, when diluted, can be used as sterilising fluids or disinfectants, depending on the dilution. There are implications for health and safety in the salon due to the very toxic nature of the chemicals. A COSHH (Control of Substances Hazardous to Health) risk assessment would be required to ensure that special safety precautions are followed when preparing sterilising fluid for the salon. Chemicals used are:
  - quaternary ammonium compound (QUATS)
  - gluteraldehyde
  - alcohol or surgical spirit.

Precautions to prevent the spread of infection

1. Cover any cuts or broken skin on the hands with a waterproof dressing.
2. Wear rubber gloves when carrying out any treatment where blood may be drawn to the surface of the skin.

Bleeding may occur during treatments where the skin is pierced or a needle is inserted into the hair follicle, for example ear piercing, electro-epilation.

Blood spots from the hair follicle may also appear during eyebrow shaping or depilatory waxing, particularly if very coarse hair is being removed, such as with underarm or bikini-line waxing. The coarse hairs grow from follicles that are deep within the dermis and surrounded by blood capillaries. It is these capillaries that rupture as the hair is plucked from the follicle.

Dealing with blood spots requires very strict hygiene procedures to ensure that the therapist does not come into contact with the blood, to reduce the risk of infecting the client and to ensure that contaminated materials are disposed of correctly.

Procedure for dealing with blood spots or cuts during treatment

1. Wear disposable gloves
2. Soak cotton wool in antiseptic or surgical spirit and apply pressure.
3. Place contaminated cotton wool in a covered waste bin inside a securely tied bin liner.
4. Wash your hands.

Health and safety aspects of performing treatments

The responsibility for health, safety and security in the salon should be shared by all staff to ensure that clients are never put at risk.

Health and safety legislation demands that employers set out policies on safe working practice. This will usually take the form of salon rules and regulations that are posted on noticeboards in staff areas or supplied as part of the employee's contract of employment. Standards of health and safety are maintained by ensuring that:

- practices and procedures are implemented and monitored
- staff are trained in safety procedures.

You can find out more about the health and safety aspects of performing treatments in Chapter 3.

 Hints and tips
Implements must be thoroughly cleaned to remove skin debris and cosmetics, by washing in hot soapy water, before sterilisation. The effectiveness of disinfectants and sterilising fluid is lowered when debris is left in the container or on the implements.

 Health and safety
Health and safety law requires the therapist to wear Personal Protective Equipment (PPE) such as rubber gloves, plastic apron and overall.

 Hints and tips
The therapist may choose to take added precautions against infection by the hepatitis B virus. It is possible to be vaccinated against this disease by a doctor.

Posture and client positioning

Although the employer has a legal duty to ensure health and safety of their employees and clients, ultimately the therapist must take the responsibility for their own safety during treatments. They should consider the position of the client during the treatment, not only for their comfort but to enable safe and ease of administration of the treatment.

Waste disposal

Each work area should have a pedal bin with a lid for the disposal of cotton wool and other general waste, which should be emptied after each client. However, for waste that is contaminated with body fluids, such as blood, a separate bin with a yellow bin liner should be provided. The yellow liner identifies the waste as contaminated. It must be removed by specialists and incinerated.

Care should be taken when disposing of certain chemicals and the Manufacturer's Safety Data sheet should be consulted for the procedures to follow.

Legal aspects of performing treatments

Other than the health and safety requirements there is the legal age of consent to consider when performing treatments on the general public. The treatment of 'minors' (i.e. those under 18 years of age in England and 17 in Scotland) is against the law unless parental or legal guardian written permission is obtained. When treating clients under the age of 16 years of age the parent or legal guardian should be present during the treatment. Treating minors also require the therapist to be checked by the Criminal Records Bureau (CRB).

Consultation techniques

Consultation requires the therapist to listen carefully and use questioning in a sensitive manner to find out the important information required before the client's treatment. Information is recorded on a client record card or computer database. Client consultation must be part of every treatment to check for contraindications and to establish the needs of the client before carrying out a treatment. The client consultation concerning individual treatments is given at the beginning of each relevant chapter.

To enable you to gain the information you need during the consultation, follow these stages:

1. Questioning – used to ascertain personal information.
2. Visual check – look closely at the area you will be treating and the overall appearance of your client.
3. Manual examination – touching the skin is important as it enables you to feel the texture and elasticity.
4. Referral to records – however, this will not be possible if the client is new to the salon.

Health and safety

The following points will help to reduce fatigue and injury such as lower back pain and repetitive strain disorders:

- Treatment couches and therapist's chairs and stools should have adjustable height mechanisms.
- If bending, do so from the knees rather than from the lower back.
- Perform hand exercises to strengthen the muscles in the hands and wrists, such as squeezing a 'stress ball'.
- Place equipment on a trolley of a convenient height that enables it to be moved close to the work area, preventing stretching and reducing the risk of accidents.

Health and safety

The legislation and directives related to waste disposal are:

- The Environmental Protection Act 1990
- The Control of Pollution (Amendment) Act 1989
- The Waste Management Licensing Regulations 1994 (as amended)
- The Controlled Waste (Registration of Carriers and Seizure of Vehicles) Regulations 1991.

Questioning the client

At the start of every treatment, time must be allowed for client consultation. You should assess whether the treatment is suitable for the client and then prepare a plan of what the treatment involves. Sometimes, a client will be offered a separate consultation to establish whether or not a particular condition can be treated in the salon.

A professional manner requires you to speak clearly, ask only appropriate questions, listen carefully to what the client has to say, and show respect. The way in which the consultation is carried out will give the client confidence and trust in your ability. Allow the client time to ask questions, too. It is important to build the relationship with your client and make them feel relaxed.

Questioning techniques

- Ask appropriate questions that are not intrusive. It is not necessary to pry into your client's private affairs. It should only be necessary to ask general questions that allow the client to tell you as much or as little as they want to.
- Ask questions in a tactful manner.
- Display empathy and understanding.
- Use open questions as much as possible to gain information.
- Only question to gain the minimum appropriate information.

Open and closed questions

With an open question, the client can give you a detailed answer. The answer to a closed question is either 'Yes' or 'No'. Examples of open and closed questions that may be used in consultation are:

Open question: 'Can you tell me about the skincare routine you follow at home?'

Closed question: 'Do you cleanse your skin at home?'

Open question: 'If you are taking any medication, could you explain what condition it is for?'

Closed question: 'Are you taking any medication?'

Body language

We all have days when we feel irritable, upset, confused or anxious. This is part of human nature. What is important is that you can recognise these feelings in yourself and in others and learn how to handle them. The way in which you respond to the client when you recognise expression of feelings can affect the whole experience for the client and may influence whether they return to the salon for treatment in the future. Equally, the way in which you handle your own feelings by presenting a professional image will influence how successful you will be as a beauty therapist. You will be expected to display a calm and efficient manner at all times.

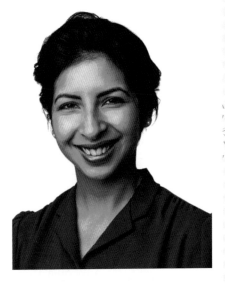

△ A positive expression

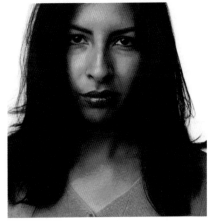

△ A negative expression

Questioning the client about requirements

Making sure that the client has realistic expectations of the treatment and the products is an important part of consultation. The client may have unrealistic expectations of what can be achieved or how they should be caring for themselves. They may have experienced pressure selling, with over-enthusiastic cosmetic sales assistants claiming that a product will do far more than is actually possible, or they may have read exaggerated articles in women's magazines. It is the job of the therapist to produce actual results by either improving the client's home-care regime or by changing their views on the benefits of good salon care.

Where client's expectations are not achievable you should politely make alternative suggestions and give as much explanation as possible.

 Remember . . .

It is against the law to make false claims (The Trades Description Act 1968 and 1972). Truthful and realistic outcomes are what matter if you are to keep your clients. Work together to change bad habits, to keep clients motivated and to keep them informed about best practice.

Questioning the client on their home-care routine

It is important to gather information during the consultation about the way in which the client cares for themselves between salon treatments. It will give an indication of how committed the client is to skincare and health regimes, whether they spend time and money on themselves and recognise the importance of visits to the beauty salon.

Questioning the client about their lifestyle

Selecting appropriate treatment for the client may depend on their needs at a particular time. This can be influenced by a number of factors, such as eating habits, smoking, alcohol intake, exercise and sleeping patterns, how busy they are and whether or not they are happy and contented.

Questioning the client about previous salon treatments

These will be shown on the record card if the client visits your salon regularly. This is one of the reasons why record cards should be completed fully after every treatment and filed correctly for future reference. Any problems, such as adverse reactions to a treatment, can be recorded, enabling you to establish appropriate treatment quickly and efficiently. If the client has had treatment at other salons it will be more difficult to gain information, other than what the client tells you. You can, however, expect the client to be more relaxed if they have experienced salon treatments before.

Discuss the recommendations for treatment

Use your skill and experience to ensure that the treatment relates to the individual needs of each client. For example, the choice of product for treating the skin will depend on the client's skin type and the choice of depilatory wax method will depend on the client's hair growth. Explain your reasoning and provide an opportunity for the client to ask questions.

Visual signs

The therapist should be prepared to look for signs of infection first and foremost, and then observe any abnormalities in the area. Diagnosis of any condition is against the therapists' code of practice. However, you may need to make certain judgements about a skin lesion or unusual swelling, for example. The client may be able to explain the condition and, providing you can establish that it does not amount to a contraindication and that the treatment will not aggravate it in any way, you will be able to perform the treatment.

Your assessment of the client will include on a visual check of the condition of the area you are treating. This will enable you to select appropriate products and treatment. For example, you must establish the client's skin type before beginning a facial.

Observing the client as they arrive at the salon can help with your assessment, by giving you an indication of their temperament and attitude. If you are doing make-up for the first time, it can be useful to look at the client's clothes, the colours they wear and how they do their own make-up.

You should observe your client's body language to see if they are relaxed or uncomfortable.

Manual signs

Assessing the client by touching the area to be treated helps to confirm or provide new information, such as the skin's texture or warmth. It may be necessary to **palpate** the skin to feel muscle tone or to assess the elasticity of the skin. The therapist must be confident when touching the client. Always have freshly washed hands.

Another form of manual assessment is sensitivity testing, which involves the application of a small amount of a product to an area of the body to establish whether or not the client has any adverse reaction to it. (More information on sensitivity or patch testing can be found on page 130.)

> **Key term**
>
> **Palpate** – to feel or touch lightly an area of the skin to determine the size, shape, firmness or location of a blemish, lump or other concern.

Reference to record cards

If a client has had a treatment at the salon before, they should already have a record either as part of a database or a hard copy. It is good practice to refer to this record if one exists in order to check on previous treatment procedures and adaptations and to ensure continuity of service. There may be important medical information, such as permission to treat from a doctor where there is a medical condition that normally contraindicates treatment.

Contraindications

Contraindications are signs or symptoms that are presented by the client at the time of the consultation that will prevent or restrict the treatment.

Those that prevent treatment include medical conditions and skin infections. The former may be a concern as the condition may be made worse if the treatment is performed, or it may affect any medication or treatment being undertaken. Medical conditions should be referred to the appropriate medical practitioner, for example a doctor, consultant or dermatologist. You should also ask about any medication they may be taking. Under no circumstances should the therapist diagnose or make comment on any condition the client presents at the consultation.

Examples of the sort of conditions you may come across include undiagnosed skin lesions, lumps or swelling or where a client is taking medication that causes skin irritation or rash. In all such circumstances, the client should contact their doctor and provide a letter advising you that it is safe to provide the treatment. This will also apply to long-term health problems.

On no account should the therapist make direct contact with the client's doctor by telephone or letter. The responsibility lies with the client. You may wish to write down the details of the treatments or products you would be using for the client to show their medical practitioner.

Conditions that restrict the treatment may mean that the treatment can go ahead with adaptations in place. Adaptations such as avoiding the affected area, reducing pressure and covering the area with a protective dressing are common examples. Many conditions are localised: a verruca on the foot would not prevent you from doing a manicure or facial on the client, for example. Others are temporary – in these cases you can advise the client to wait until the condition has cleared up before having treatment.

Client referral

It may be necessary to refer clients to other services within the salon or to recommend that they seek advice from other professionals, such as their GP or a chiropodist.

For example, during a pedicure a client may ask you to remove hard skin on her toes. On examination you find the client has calluses and a corn, which you are not qualified to treat. The salon may work closely with a chiropodist, in which case you could refer the client by giving them a business card so that they can make contact themselves.

The salon should have a policy on referral to ensure that staff are aware of the procedure. This will usually include the following:

1. A full consultation to check for contraindications must be given prior to every treatment.

2. The therapist must be able to recognise infectious skin conditions, skin diseases and other disorders and establish what constitutes a contraindication to treatment.

3. Clients should be directed clearly towards medical advice where necessary.

Remember . . .

Refusing the client treatment is a sensitive situation, especially when a medical condition is present. Do so quietly and sympathetically and in a private area away from others. Offer another treatment that is not contraindicated to alleviate embarassment.

Activity

Think about how you would handle the following situations.

1. A client arrives at the salon reception where several other clients are waiting. She very loudly announces her dissatisfaction with a recent leg wax treatment. She mentions the therapist by name and complains about her directly. She asks you to make a comment on how good you think she is as a beauty therapist.

2. During a consultation, when you ask your client for information on her general health, she begins to give details of recent major surgery and becomes very upset.

4. Referral must be handled in a sensitive manner and on no account must a diagnosis be made by the therapist.

5. A letter from the client's doctor giving permission for a specific salon treatment may be necessary. This must be attached to the client's record card.

Contra-actions

Contra-actions are unwanted effects that may occur during or after treatment. Examples include erythema, irritation, bruising and allergic reactions. The client should be informed of the possible contra-actions as part of explaining the treatment. In this way the client can decide whether or not to go ahead with the treatment.

It is important to give the client the opportunity to ask questions about the treatment to clarify points and confirm their understanding of what is about to happen during the treatment.

The treatment plan

The information gained throughout the consultation is used to establish the best course of action to meet the needs of the client. This is called a treatment plan.

Each treatment requires specific information and the detail appears in each relevant chapter of this book. However, the general information that needs to be recorded includes:

- client's name, address and telephone number (and email address if appropriate)
- type of treatment and products
- area to be treated
- contraindications – notes on any medical referral
- any known contra-actions
- client's homecare routine and any relevant information on lifestyle
- aftercare advice given and products purchased
- course of treatments – number and advanced payments
- outcome of treatment – results and effects
- client's comments and signature
- therapist's recommendations and signature.

The treatment plan should be ongoing and record progress over a period of time. Looking back over past records and seeing improvements can be very encouraging for the client.

Informing clients about costs and times taken for treatments

Clients will want to know how long they will spend in the salon for treatment and how much it will cost. An up-to-date price list must be available in the salon. If there is a change to the published prices, the client must be informed during the consultation. This will avoid any embarrassment when the client comes to pay. It is not good practice to present the client with an unexpected addition to the treatment when it is complete.

You should give an estimated time for the treatment to be completed. This allows the client to make arrangements and for you to keep to your appointments schedule. The therapist must be aware of time so that treatments are cost-effective. For example, taking an hour to do a treatment that would usually be done in 45 minutes is not making the best use of time and your manager may question your efficiency. If, however, you are able to sell further treatments or products, this would be regarded favourably by your manager, provided that your next client is not kept waiting.

Courses of treatment paid for in advance offer financial benefits to the salon. A special offer for the client of one free treatment or a free skincare product can be an added incentive to attend the salon regularly.

Record keeping

Confidentiality

It is important to ensure that details recorded on the record card are accurate and that the client is aware of what you have written. Give them the opportunity to read the details and to sign the card. This information is confidential and should be stored in a locked filing cabinet or secure computer for access only by the beauty therapy staff. Alternatively, information may be stored on a computer database. Storage of information is governed by the Data Protection Act. You will need to comply with the Data Protection Act to ensure that personal details remain confidential at all times.

It is important that you observe strict rules on confidentiality when dealing with clients. Your discussions with the client should be discreet and, when appropriate, take place in private. You must never repeat what your client has discussed with you in confidence. In some circumstances it may be necessary for you to seek advice, making it necessary to discuss client details with your supervisor. This would be acceptable in a professional context, but you would need to ensure that it was carried out in a professional manner to maintain client confidence.

Junior staff should be instructed on the importance of confidentiality and follow salon rules on approach to clients and appropriate topics of conversation.

Client complaints

Inevitably, there will be occasions when a client makes a complaint. Complaints may include:

- dissatisfaction with a salon treatment (a depilatory wax not completely removing leg hairs, for example)
- being kept waiting
- a mix-up over an appointment.

A more serious complaint would involve injury to the client or damage to the client's clothing. Complaints may be made verbally to the therapist as they happen. Sometimes, the client may request to see the manager or they may complain in writing after the incident. The salon will have a policy on the way in which a complaint should be handled. If so, this must be followed at all times.

Remember...

It is important to provide time for the client to ask questions. This ensures client satisfaction before the treatment begins.

Remember...

It is important to obtain signed, written, informed consent from the client prior to starting treatment. Your insurance provider will expect this as a minimum requirement should any legal action be necessary.

Activity

Using the following list of negative actions to help you, write a list of positive actions you should follow to give a good impression to your client.

Negative actions

- No information available for your client (price list, product information).
- Your client is ignored as they arrive at the salon.
- Telephone is left ringing.
- Promises you make to do something for the client are forgotten.
- Surroundings are dirty or untidy (magazines are old and torn, the plants are dusty and dying due to lack of care).
- Client is left waiting without an explanation.
- You forget to give a message from a client to one of the staff.

You may be able to think of others.

Facial treatment card					Name:							
Address:					Tel:							
Medical history:					Medication:				Date of birth:			

Skin assessment	Date	Date	Date			Date	Date	Date			Date	Date	Date
Seborrhoea					Open pores				Milia				
Comedones					Acne				Scars				
Sensitive					Dry				Dehydrated				
Mature					Flakey				Loss of firmness				
Skin colour					Dilated capillaries				Pigmentation				
Superfluous hair					Skin blemishes				Lines/ageing				
Other													

Treatment	Products used	Advised for home use	Products purchased
Date			

Treatment progress:

Client comments:

Homecare checklist:

Client signature:	Date:
Therapist signature:	Date:

△ Example of a client record card

Procedure for handling complaints

1. Listen attentively to what the client has to say, preferably in a private area. You may need to deal with the client's emotions first if they are angry or distressed. Acknowledge that they are upset and make them feel valued by showing genuine concern.

2. Decide whether it is within the limits of your authority to deal with the complaint following the salon's policy, or whether you should pass it on to a more senior member of staff.

3. A serious complaint carries a threat of litigation and must be referred to the manager, who will make decisions on appropriate recompense or compensation. If the client wishes to take legal action there will need to be a formal record of events with witness statements and physical evidence of the complaint. Fortunately, most complaints are fairly minor and can be handled by offering free treatment or by refunding the cost of the treatment.

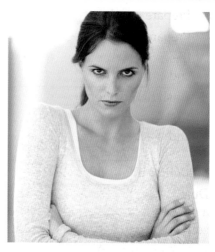

△ Unacceptable expression when dealing with a complaint

Treatments

Careful consideration must be given to the tasks involved in preparing for treatments, as well as during and after treatments.

Preparing for treatments

Preparation before starting any treatment is essential to ensure that hygiene and safety procedures have been carried out. A treatment area must never show signs of the previous client, for example crumpled bed paper, used towels, or used products left on the trolley.

Time must be allowed between treatments to:

- prepare the treatment area
- allow the therapist to check their appearance.

Think ahead

The key to good preparation is to think ahead.

- What do I need to carry out the treatment?
- Will my client be comfortable?
- Is the treatment area clean, tidy and hygienic?
- Have I accounted for likely hazards that may put me or my client at risk?
- Is my appearance immaculate and professional?

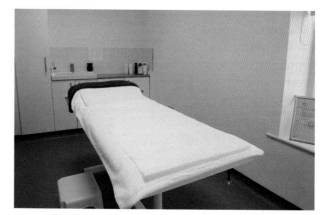

△ A well-prepared treatment room

Before the start of treatment

- Wipe the trolley with disinfectant and cover with disposable paper.
- Tidy bottles and containers on the trolley. Wipe bottle tops and ensure lids and tops are secure.
- Prepare products and materials for the next client by checking the appointment page for treatment required. For example, ensure wax is heated to the correct temperature, prepare make-up pallet, prepare manicure trolley.

- Prepare couch with clean towels and disposable paper.
- Prepare disposable gloves, if used.
- Ensure there are sufficient disposable materials – bed paper, tissues and cotton wool.
- Wash hands thoroughly.
- Collect sterilised tools, for example tweezers, cuticle implements, and place in disinfectant until required.

Preparing the trolley

Dust and spillages on trolleys can harbour infection and will give a very poor impression to the client. Bottle tops should be wiped, containers will need washing and a supply of dry and damp cotton wool and tissues will be required.

> Remember. . .
>
> There should be no sign of the previous client when inviting your client to the treatment area (e.g. used towels, crumpled bed paper on the couch, waste in the bin).

Preparing tools and equipment

Any item that is used on the client's skin has the potential to carry infection. Wherever possible, such items should be disposable and thrown away after use, or be easily washed and sterilised or disinfected. Small tools and equipment such as tweezers should be wiped over or washed as appropriate and placed on the trolley in a jar containing disinfectant. Disposable items such as eyeshadow applicators should be placed in the bin to be thrown away.

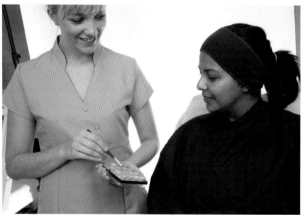

△ A professional beauty therapist prepared and ready for work

Facial sponges and cosmetic brushes can very easily harbour infection when they are left unwashed after use. The damp, warm conditions encourage growth of micro-organisms. Sponges can smell sour if left dirty or placed in plastic bags. While the use of sponges can be economical, saving on cotton wool, the chances of passing on infection is greatly increased.

Sponges and cosmetic brushes must be thoroughly washed in hot soapy water, rinsed in disinfectant solution (such as Milton), allowed to dry naturally and stored in an ultraviolet sterilisation unit or in an airtight container.

During treatment

- Personal hygiene is essential for the therapist when working in confined areas and in such close proximity to the client. Check personal hygiene and appearance regularly throughout the day.

- Prepare the area to be treated as appropriate (see individual treatments for preparation of the area to be treated).

- Wash hands before and after treatment or at any time it is necessary to break away from the treatment, for example, to sneeze, or to answer the telephone.

- Always place tops back on containers immediately after use to prevent micro-organisms contaminating the product.

- Wipe up any spillages immediately.

- Tidy the treatment area and the trolley.

After treatment

- Discuss the results of the treatment with the client and ensure that it is completed according to the client's wishes.

- Provide aftercare advice.

- Dispose of all waste materials (for example contaminated tissues) in a plastic bin liner and tie securely.

- Clean equipment, particularly depilatory wax heaters, immediately after use. The heaters can become unsightly and harbour germs if they are not kept free from wax.

- Make-up pallets should be cleaned and stored until required.

- Nail polish tops must be wiped before replacing the cap. This ensures that the tops do not stick, making opening difficult, and that the solvent does not evaporate, making the polish thick (for further examples of procedures for clearing up after treatments see individual treatment procedures).

- Prepare the couch/manicure table, etc., with clean linen ready for the next client.

- Empty the waste bin.

- Wash your hands.

Remember...

You will come into close contact with your clients. Bad breath from smoking or spicy foods can be very offensive. Good personal hygiene is of the utmost importance to avoid unpleasant body odour.

Want to know more?

To download industry codes of practice, go to www.habia.org
Additional professional bodies are:
www.beautyguild.com
www.babtac.com

Test yourself

1. Client consultation should be carried out:
   a) at the end of the treatment
   b) during the treatment
   c) before beginning every treatment
   d) when requested by the client.

2. Which piece of legislation ensures that information gained from a client during the consultation remains confidential?

3. Give two examples of professional practitioners to which you might refer a client.

4. List six requirements of personal appearance and hygiene before treating a client.

5. List four skills required for effective communication with a client.

6. Give an example of each of the following:
   a) fungal infection
   b) viral infection
   c) bacterial infection.

7. Give two examples of personal protective equipment (PPE) required by the therapist.

8. Explain the difference between a contra-action and a contraindication.

9. Give four important salon hygiene procedures before taking the client to the treatment area.

10. It is important to recycle salon waste:
    a) so that that the salon is not charged by the Council
    b) to prevent the spread of infection
    c) to keep the salon tidy
    d) to help to protect the environment.

Chapter 2
Unit G4: Fulfil salon reception duties

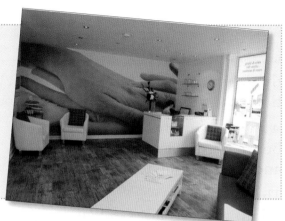

Learning objectives

This chapter covers Unit G4 'Fulfil salon reception duties': the efficient systems of work at a salon reception as well as the skills and knowledge required to be a successful receptionist.

There are four learning outcomes for Unit G4 and they are:
1 Maintain the reception area.
2 Attend to clients and enquiries.
3 Make appointments for salon services.
4 Handle payments from clients.

You will need to achieve all of these outcomes to be a competent receptionist.

Evidence requirements

Your assessor will need to observe you perform salon reception duties successfully on at least three occasions. You must be able to:

1 Handle three out of four of the following types of people:
- those who have different needs and expectations
- those who appear angry
- those who may be confused
- those who have a complaint.

2 Handle two out of three of the following types of enquiry:
- in person
- by telephone
- electronically.

You must, however, prove to your assessor that you have the knowledge and understanding to be competent in any of the above.

3 Make appointments, both:
- in person
- by telephone.

4 Obtain all the following appointment details:
- client's name
- client's contact details
- service required
- estimated price
- date
- time
- member(s) of staff booked for service.

5 Handle all the following methods of payment:
- cash
- cash equivalents
- cheques
- payment cards.

(When naturally occurring performance cannot be obtained, simulated activities to produce performance evidence is possible for cash equivalents, cheque and payment cards.)

6 Deal with all these types of discrepancy:
- invalid currency
- invalid card
- incorrect completion of cheque
- suspected fraudulent use of payment card
- payment disputes.

Introduction

Welcoming and receiving clients and visitors to the salon is an important part of the salon service. The client gets their first impression of the salon from the receptionist, whether the communication is on the telephone or in person.

All visitors and people making enquiries are potential clients. Therefore they must be treated in a polite and helpful manner. Also, keeping the reception area clean and tidy is essential to maintain a good impression of the salon.

The receptionist needs to have an understanding of the treatments offered by the salon and how long each therapist needs to carry out the treatment. It is important to communicate with the therapists to understand treatment timings fully.

The salon will have a system for booking appointments, whether it involves writing in an appointment book or using a computer system for bookings.

This unit appears as a mandatory unit for the Level 2 Nail Services qualification but is an optional unit for the Beauty Therapy General and Make-up routes. It is worth three credits.

Meet the professional

"The only important person in the salon is your client. They dictate the treatments you offer, the hours you open, how busy your salon is, your salary, what new training you need to undertake and how well your reputation spreads. Each and every client is your 'boss'.

As a receptionist your ability to ensure that a client books a treatment will depend upon several key attributes. You must be well presented, polite, genuinely friendly and confident in the degree of background knowledge you have. You can never know too much but don't try to 'bluff' your client. Find out the answers.

Your client should feel welcomed, respected, valued and individual.

All clients will remember a bad experience for far longer than a good one. If your diary is full and you can't fit a client in, always, always take a name and contact number for them and run a cancellation list; you never know when you will suddenly find yourself with a large space to fill if somebody cancels at short notice. This way your book stays full and the client you ring back to accommodate is impressed."

Jacqui Bostock

The role of the receptionist

Clients attending a beauty therapy salon like to feel relaxed and able to enjoy quality time in a pleasant environment. The receptionist can start the process the moment the client enters the salon by using their **interpersonal skills** effectively, as follows:

- Make eye contact with the client.
- Smile and have a friendly manner.
- Be calm and gently spoken.
- Give the client individual attention and show respect.
- Show genuine interest in the client.
- Be sensitive to the needs of clients and therapists.
- Take care not to do or say anything that could offend, particularly if it involves race, gender or religion.
- Ensure client confidentiality at all times.

Salon reception duties involve:

- keeping the reception area clean and tidy
- welcoming and receiving people entering the salon
- making appointments
- handling enquiries
- dealing with client payments
- selling products
- ensuring that product displays are well stocked.

Everyone working in a busy salon will have to carry out reception duties from time to time, so it is important that all members of staff are aware of the procedures for dealing with clients and the manner in which they should be treated.

> **Key term**
>
> **Interpersonal skills** – sometimes known as 'people skills', interpersonal skills are those used by people to interact with each other; this includes communication and behaviour.

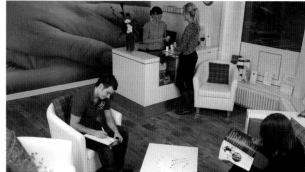

△ The reception area gives the client their first impression of the salon

 Remember . . .

The reception area is at the heart of the salon. The therapist relies on the receptionist to ensure appointments are made accurately and clients are treated with courtesy.

Outcome 1: Maintain the reception area

The reception area

This is the first part of the salon that the client comes into contact with. It must give a good impression by providing an area that reflects the high standards of hygiene and cleanliness, personal attention, comfort and relaxation that are associated with the beauty therapy salon.

The reception area must be kept clean, tidy and comfortable, by ensuring that:

- carpets are vacuumed regularly
- retail displays are dusted and neatly arranged to attract the client's attention
- there is a good supply of information leaflets
- used coffee cups etc., are removed
- flowers or plants are fresh and cared for
- magazines are kept up to date and stacked tidily.

Remember . . .
The reception area should be checked throughout the day to ensure it is clean and tidy.

The reception desk

The reception desk must be well equipped. Reception resources include:

- A telephone and answering machine: an answering machine is useful for the therapist who works alone and is unable to answer the telephone during treatments. It also allows clients to contact the salon out of hours to request appointments, make enquiries or cancel appointments. All messages should be dealt with promptly and those requiring a return call must be dealt with immediately.
- Computer: a computer has become the most widely used and efficient means of storing and transferring information. Most large salons have a computer which can be used for making appointments, taking payments and maintaining accurate client records. When attached to the phone line, and with the appropriate software it is a means of communicating information. Email allows publicity of promotional events, appointment reminders, sending orders to suppliers and provides instant responses, providing all parties are linked to the internet.

A good supply of stationery is essential, including ballpoint pens, pencils, spare till rolls, notepads, date stamp and salon name stamp. Other important items include:

- appointment book (if a computer is not used to book appointments)
- appointment cards
- receipt pad (for when a cash register which automatically issues a receipt is not used)
- message pad
- record cards
- calculator (which is useful when using a manual till, for calculating Value Added Tax (VAT) or when totalling a number of retail items).

Cash registers

Computerised cash registers

Computerised systems that incorporate records of stock levels and clients, for example, may be used in large salons. The computer is usually attached to an automatic till that records the transaction, stores the money and produces the client receipt. Some salons may also have a facility on the till to take debit and credit payment cards.

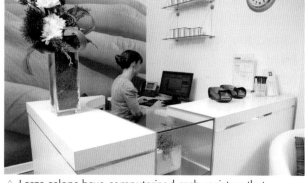

△ Large salons have computerised cash registers that incorporate records of stock levels and client details

Electric cash register

An automatic electric till is used by most salons. This records the transaction on a till roll as well as producing a receipt for the client. Cashing up is automatic on the press of a key and subtotals can be made at any point in the day by pressing specific keys.

Manual till

A manual till, which is a lockable drawer, may be all that is required in a small salon. Any transactions must be recorded by hand. It is more likely that errors will occur with this system and their credit card equipment. Due to the different types of tills, payment methods and salon policy, you will need to be trained in all aspects of payment procedures for your salon.

Cash float

A cash float in the cash register is necessary to ensure that there is sufficient change when dealing with cash transactions. The receptionist must make sure that there is change available throughout the day. This means thinking ahead and changing notes as necessary. Change may be kept in the business safe or arrangements may have to be made for change with a bank. It can be very annoying for the client to be kept waiting while the receptionist hunts for the correct change.

The cash float may also be used as petty cash. **Petty cash** is used for small incidental items such as fresh milk, postage stamps or cleaning materials. It is essential that receipts for petty cash purchases are retained for the salon accounts.

> **Key term**
>
> **Petty cash** – a small amount of money put aside to pay for incidental items such as milk for client's tea and coffee.

Facsimile (fax)

This is a very useful and quick means of transferring black-and-white documents such as invoices. The document is transmitted via the telephone line from one fax machine to another.

Credit card terminal

Credit card equipment is required if a salon chooses to accept credit cards. For a small salon that only deals in small transactions, it may not be worth the fee that the credit card company requires. If the business is authorised to accept credit cards, vouchers and a transaction printer will be necessary. (See also computerised cash registers above.)

Filing cabinet

For the storage of client record cards.

Waste bin

To keep the reception area free from waste paper and other items.

Retailing

An important part of the receptionist's role is **retailing**. This should support the therapist when selling to the client during the treatment and increase the salon's profit margins through retailing to 'walk-in' clients. The receptionist is often responsible for monitoring the sales of retail products from the shelves and producing reports for the salon owner or manager. It is important to maintain the levels of stock on retail shelves displayed within the reception in order to maximise retailing opportunities and maintain an attractive reception display. With efficient working systems between the receptionist and the person responsible for stock ordering, the right levels of stock are available to retail.

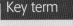

> Key term
>
> **Retailing** – activities relating to the selling of products to a client.

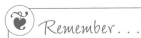

Remember . . .

Knowledge of the products and cosmetics available for retail is essential for the receptionist to effectively and confidently retail products to a customer.

The receptionist has a golden opportunity to promote products to the client by ensuring that:

- the product display units are eye catching, well stocked and dusted daily
- packaging is undamaged
- product leaflets are available in rest areas for the client to read
- display and advertising posters are up to date and in good condition.

It may be necessary for the receptionist to process stock orders. This will involve receiving goods and checking delivery notes for discrepancies and damaged goods. It is important to check for any leaking products through damage to the containers and ensure that packaging is intact and undamaged. Any such damage must be reported to the company immediately.

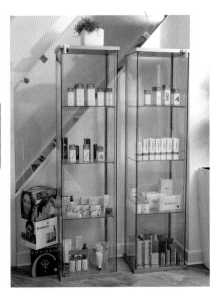

△ Product display units should be eye catching and well stocked

Legislation relating to salon treatments and goods sold in the salon

The receptionist must be aware of the law as it relates to the services the salon offers and the cosmetics and products available for retail. The Acts are:

The Sale of Goods Act 1979

This was the first of the laws that required **goods** to be accurately described without misleading the customer. The law takes into account:

- the suitability of the goods for a particular purpose
- the quality of the goods
- the description provided.

> **Key term**
>
> **Goods** – services or products.

The Supply of Goods and Services Act 1982

This went further than the 1979 Act to include **standards of service**, which should be:

- of reasonable quality
- described accurately
- fit for the intended purpose.

The Act also required that the service provided to a customer should be:

- carried out with reasonable skill and care
- within a reasonable time
- or a reasonable cost.

> **Key term**
>
> **Standards of service** – the treatment provided by the therapist is professional and meets the requirements of the industry.

The Sale and Supply of Goods Act 1994

This amends the previous Acts by introducing guidelines on defining the quality of goods.

Trade Descriptions Act 1968

This Act states that manufacturers, retailers or service industry providers must not mislead customers by making false claims about the products or services that they sell.

Client hospitality

The receptionist must make the client feel welcome by speaking to them as soon as they enter the salon, then helping them with their coat and offering them a seat. Magazines should be available with an offer of coffee or other beverages. A drinks machine can be a very useful asset in a reception area, allowing clients to help themselves. This can save both the receptionist and the therapist time. Information on treatments should be readily available for the client to browse through.

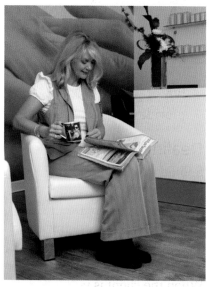

△ Always make the client feel comfortable

Outcome 2: Attend to clients and enquiries

A receptionist needs to show professional and non-discriminatory behaviour towards all clients and visitors to the salon and should always act within the limits of their authority.

Handling enquiries and giving information

Good **communication skills** are an essential part of the beauty therapist's job and the role of the receptionist.

Communication skills are used to give and receive information. They include:

- speaking clearly
- listening carefully
- reading carefully and writing clearly
- effective use of body language
- good personal presentation.

A potential client will usually require details of treatments and products available in the salon. The receptionist should be able to explain the benefits of a treatment, how long it will take and the cost. You can offer the client the salon's treatment price lists and/or product leaflets. Information should be as accurate and as helpful as possible. It should be offered in a caring and discreet manner. If you do not know the answer to a question, ask another member of staff.

Providing help and support in the salon

It is sometimes necessary to provide support for the therapists when they are very busy and falling behind with their appointments. You may be required to:

- liaise with the therapist and client, keeping them both informed of any delay
- tidy or prepare work areas
- provide coffee and magazines for the client.

Dealing with delays

Should there be any delay, the client must be informed as soon as possible and given an estimate of how long the delay will be.

If there is any change to the appointment, the client should be politely informed and offered alternatives.

Saying goodbye to the client.

When the client is ready to leave, the receptionist must ensure that she has been offered another appointment and deal with any retail requirements. The client should be helped with their coat and thanked as they leave the salon.

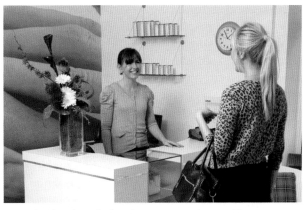

△ Make the client feel welcome. Greet them with eye contact and a smile

> **Key term**
>
> **Communication skills** – used to give and receive information.

> ☆ **Hints and tips**
>
> Being friendly does not require you to be the client's friend. It is important to maintain a 'professional distance' from a client and it is a balance of caring and listening without becoming involved. Do not discuss your personal details, give out your personal mobile number or discuss personal circumstances such as your relationship with your boyfriend.

Answering the telephone

It is important to answer the telephone promptly, on the second or third ring. The salon will usually have a standard response when answering the telephone. The name of the salon, your name and an offer of help should be included. You should answer with a friendly, clear and enthusiastic manner. A dull voice will give an impression of boredom and disinterest. Do not use slang and sloppy speech.

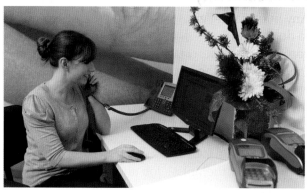

Listen carefully to what the client has to say and respond in a positive way, either by making an appointment, answering a question, taking a message or offering to call back if necessary. Repeat back to the caller the main points of the conversation, such as their full name or initials (remember there are lots of Smiths), telephone number and the details of the appointment you have made for them. Always do something positive rather than say 'No' or that you don't know. Use the client's name as you speak to them. Not only is this polite, but it will help you to remember their name in the future. Always end by thanking the client for calling.

△ Respond in a friendly, clear and enthusiastic manner when making appointments on the telephone

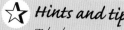 **Hints and tips**
Telephone manner is very important and requires practice to feel confident.

Taking messages

It may not be possible for a client to speak to a particular member of staff, whether on the telephone or face-to-face. A receptionist must be able to take accurate information from the client and judge the urgency of the call. A message that is clearly an emergency must be dealt with immediately. All messages must be acted on as soon as possible. Some messages may be confidential and will therefore require direct contact with the individual therapist concerned.

A system should be in place so that no message is overlooked. You might consider using a notice board in the staff room or behind the reception for messages. It should be displayed so that messages can be seen clearly. Message pads of bright coloured paper can be placed on the reception desk. Carbonised paper is useful as it ensures that there are two or more copies as a record of all messages received in the salon.

☆ **Hints and tips**
Confirming appointments: Repeat the date, time and treatment to the client and wait for their response.

Client records

Client records need to be available for the therapists. They should be updated by the therapist and filed after use.

Many large organisations use computer software to coordinate client appointments, client records and stock records. The receptionist in this case will be responsible for entering accurate data into the computer for each client, including:

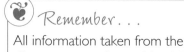 Remember . . .
All information taken from the client must remain confidential. (See the Data Proteection Act.)

- client appointments
- client's record card, including up-to-date personal data, accurate information regarding contraindications and medical history, and treatments carried out
- products used or purchased, providing the salon manager with information for stock control.

Confidentiality

Any information given by the client, perhaps for the record card or to do with the type of treatment they request, must be treated as confidential. It should not be discussed, other than in a professional capacity, with other members of staff. Some treatments, such as epilation (permanent hair removal), require detailed information on the client's health and medication. This information must be treated with sensitivity. Some clients requiring treatment for permanent hair removal may not wish other clients, who may be acquaintances, to know about it.

Some clients, wishing to be friendly, may involve you in gossip. Try to change the subject by choosing a more general topic. Never answer questions about other clients. Always respond by saying that you do not have the information or that it would be inappropriate to answer the question. The best way to avoid difficult or unprofessional conversation is to remain businesslike and deal only with the reception duties.

 Remember . . .

Some questions from a client enquiring about treatment may be of a sensitive nature and must therefore be handled carefully. If necessary, refer the question to the most appropriate member of staff.

Types of confidential information

These include the following:

- client record cards
    - name, address, telephone number
    - medical information
    - treatment information
- client's financial transactions
    - how much they spend
    - how payment is made
- information relating to the business
    - salon financial matters
    - treatment routines
    - product formulations
- staff records.

Such information must be available only to the business and its therapists. It should be kept in a locked filing cabinet or on a secure computer.

The Data Protection Act

The purpose of the Act is to protect people from having information about themselves freely available to others. The 1998 Act extends the 1984 Act to bring legislation in line with Europe and provide a much broader scope to include electronic data.

If the salon handles personal information about their clients there are a number of legal obligations to protect this information.

The Act includes both manual and electronic data, i.e. personal information held about the client on treatment consultation cards or details held on a computer regarding contact information, attendance at the salon, treatments and amount paid for treatments.

Only relevant personal data should be collected. This could bring into question the huge amount of information contained in some client treatment record cards. Any organisation that keeps information on record about people (staff or clients) must comply with the Act.

The legal requirements include:

- Any personal information about the client must only be recorded and retained on seeking explicit permission from the client.
- The client has a right to access any information held in client treatment record cards or data held on a computer.
- Only collect and retain information that is required for carrying out safe and efficient treatment, i.e. contraindications for the specific treatment.
- Releasing any personal details to third parties without specific consent is not permitted.
- Ensuring that all information is relevant, accurate and up to date.
- Information is only retained for as long as it is needed.
- Provide access to the person's own record if requested.
- Keep data secure through careful storage of paper systems and through up-to-date security measures on a computer such as data encryption.
- Provide staff with training on data systems and security and how they are affected by the Data Protection Act.

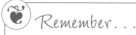 *Remember...*

Any organisation that retains personal information should register with the Data Protection Registrar.

Activity

Look at the client record system in your salon and evaluate whether it meets the requirements of the Data Protection Act.

Use the questions below as possible areas for discussion:

- Is there a code of practice for dealing with personal information?
- Where are records stored?
- Who has access to them?
- Do the clients sign to show they give permission for their personal details to be kept?
- Are the clients aware of their rights under the Act?

Dealing with problems and the dissatisfied client

The receptionist has to handle a range of problems that can affect the smooth running of the salon. Examples include:

- a client who is late for their appointment
- a client who demands treatment that is not booked and therefore no time has been allowed
- a client who is dissatisfied with their treatment
- a therapist who is delayed taking their clients for treatment.

Each of these situations needs to be handled sensitively. Listen to the client carefully, without making judgements or excuses. In the case of a client who is late or where a treatment has been incorrectly booked, it will be necessary to speak to the therapist concerned to see if they have time to fit the client in to their appointments schedule. Do not attempt to make decisions without consulting the therapist.

If a client has a complaint about a treatment, discuss the problem with the therapist concerned or a senior member of staff straight away. Reassure the client that the matter will be dealt with. Do not try to make amends yourself by offering free treatment, for example. This would be beyond the limits of your authority. The manager will follow the salon policy on complaints and decide what action should be taken.

Your job is to keep the client calm, ensuring that they are dealt with promptly. The complaint should be logged by recording the date, time, name of client, details of the problem, how it was handled and by whom.

Outcome 3: Make appointments for salon services

Booking appointments

Perhaps the most complex and important job for the receptionist is booking appointments. These can be made by the client in person or by telephone. Mistakes can cause frustration and delay to both therapists and clients and may lead to loss of takings. There is nothing more annoying for a client than to find that the appointment they booked has not been written down or that the information on their appointment card is incorrect. Equally, the therapist will not be pleased about the disruption this may cause to other clients during the day.

Each salon will have its own system of booking appointments. A special printed book or loose-leaf sheets in a file may be used, or a computerised system that uses specialist software. The appointment book is an important business record, which must be retained for auditing purposes.

The receptionist must:

- be polite and deal with clients promptly
- ensure that there is a good supply of pencils, pens, appointment cards, an eraser, ruler and message pad
- prepare appointment pages for several weeks in advance

Activity

Look around your reception area and make a list of:

- the things that you think attract clients to the salon
- any improvements that the salon could make to encourage clients to return.

- be aware of therapists' times in the salon, taking account of part-time staff, holidays and so on

- book all appointments in pencil so that they can be adjusted easily and neatly

- understand abbreviations and the timing of different treatments

- have a salon price list available

- be aware of individual clients and their special requirements

- know how to book courses of treatments and schedule follow-up appointments

- work closely with the therapists, seeking their advice on how appointments and clients should be scheduled. Remember that therapists will know the individual needs of their clients and how long they require to carry out treatments.

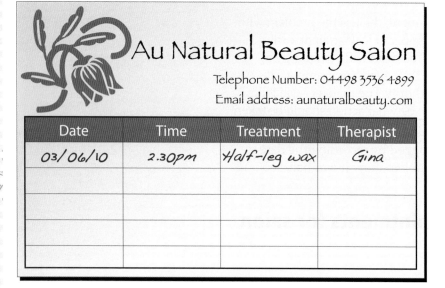

Au Natural Beauty Salon

Telephone Number: 04498 3536 4899

Email address: aunaturalbeauty.com

Date	Time	Treatment	Therapist
03/06/10	2.30pm	Half-leg wax	Gina

◁ Example of an appointment card

 Remember...

Allow extra time for new clients who require facial treatments, to give time for a full consultation. Specialist treatments such as masks may require longer and should be charged accordingly.

 Remember...

The receptionist should know about:

- each treatment on the price list

- the time needed to carry out treatments

- the cost of treatments

- which retail products can be sold to clients after their treatment.

Abbreviation	Meaning
DNA	did not attend
C	cancellation
Tick	client arrived

Treatment	Abbreviation	Approximate timing
Half-leg wax using warm wax	1/2/Leg cool	30 mins
Underarm wax using hot wax	U/a hot	15 mins
Manicure with paraffin wax treatment	Man/pw	1 hour
Cleanse with evening make-up	C/eve m/up	1 hour
Eyelashes brow and tint	LBT	30 mins
Full body massage	B/M	1 hour
Eyebrow shape	EBS	15 mins
Manicure	Man	45 mins
Full leg wax, bikini, under arm	FLW/bik/u/a	75 mins
Facial	Facial	60 mins
Ear-piercing	E/P	15 mins
Pedicure	Ped	50 mins

◁ Abbreviations and timings used in booking appointments

Missed appointments

Unfortunately it is quite common for people to make an appointment, and then not to turn up. The salon should have a clear policy on missed appointments.

The policy may state:

- 24 hours notice of cancellation is required.
- There is a small charge for missed appointments.
- A deposit is required for long appointments.

The policy must be made clear to the client by placing a notice on the reception desk or including a statement on the appointment card.

The policy may be difficult to enforce but it gives a clear message to the client that they should cancel appointments they do not wish to keep as early as possible.

Activity

Use the log below to record the range of clients and activities. This will provide evidence for your portfolio.

Log of visitors to reception				
Dates on reception				
	With appointments – name	Without appointments – name	Requiring salon services	Having business with the salon
New clients and visitors	1.			
	2.			
	3.			
	4.			
	5.			
	6.			
	7.			
	8.			
Existing clients and visitors	1.			
	2.			
	3.			
	4.			
	5.			
	6.			
	7.			
	8.			
Assessor/supervisor signature				
Students signature				

△ Reception visitors log

A telephone log may go towards assessment evidence for your portfolio.

Name of person requesting price lists	Name of person requiring information regarding services	Name of client booking a treatment	Communication with individuals on the premises
Complaints regarding services and products	Business calls from suppliers of goods and services	Person seeking employment, course details	Internal calls
Please note down the date and the person's name			
Assessor/Supervisor Signature			
Student Signature			

△ Reception telephone log

Outcome 4: Handle payments from clients

Calculating and taking payments

The duties carried out by the receptionist will ultimately affect the whole business. The care required when recording information, whether it is client details on a record card, treatment information in the appointment book or accuracy in handling money, is crucial to the business. For example, the reception desk must be fully equipped to ensure time is not wasted searching for a pen for a client to write a cheque.

The salon should have a policy and procedures for dealing with customers at the payment point.

The receptionist must be able to:

- establish the client's preferred method of payment
- provide accurate information to the client on charges by providing an itemised bill
- be accurate when totalling bills and giving change
- issue receipts
- check that retail purchases are in line with the client's requirements
- handle a range of payment methods such as cash, personal cheques, credit cards, debit cards, cash equivalents (e.g. gift vouchers)
- record the transaction.

Payments in cash

The basic procedure will be as follows:

- You will receive information from the therapist on the treatment the client has received. An itemised docket or bill is required. This may also include retail items.
- Total the bill and inform the client of the cost.
- Key in the amount(s) into the cash register
- Ask the client how they would like to pay.
- When payment is in cash, accept the money and look carefully at the notes, you have been given. Look for a water mark and metallic strip. There are special facilities for detecting forged notes. It is a good idea to place the note(s) on the till while you calculate the change.
- Count out the change into the client's hand and ask them to confirm that it is correct.
- Place the note(s) from the top of the till in the till drawer in the appropriate section and close it.
- Give the client a receipt and thank them.

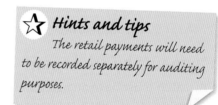

★ *Hints and tips*
The retail payments will need to be recorded separately for auditing purposes.

Payments by cheque

The procedure is as follows:

- Before accepting a cheque, make sure the client has a cheque guarantee card. This card guarantees payment up to a certain amount, usually £100 or £250.
- Check the card details are valid (i.e. expiry date, signature).
- Write the card number on the back of the cheque.
- Make sure that the signature on the card matches the one on the cheque.

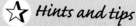

> ☆ *Hints and tips*
>
> *Using cheques as a method of payment is being phased out by banks. The chip and pin payment using debit and credit card are regarded as a more secure method, decreasing the chance of fraud.*

1. Cheque

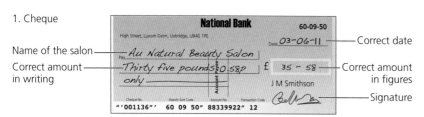

Name of the salon

Correct amount in writing

Correct date

Correct amount in figures

Signature

2. Debit card and cheque guarantee card

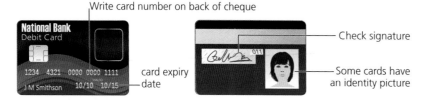

Write card number on back of cheque

card expiry date

Check signature

Some cards have an identity picture

◁ Check cheques and cheque guarantee cards carefully

When receiving payment by cheque follow the details shown in the illustration. Do not rush: take time to check all the details carefully.

Look closely at the signature on the cheque and make sure it matches the signature on the client's cheque card.

When you are satisfied, accept the cheque and give the client a receipt.

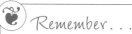

> 💗 Remember . . .
>
> A cheque that is made out incorrectly may result in the bank delaying payment or refusing to pay the money into the salon account.

Payments by credit card

The salon must have an agreement with companies such as Visa or Mastercard if they want to accept credit cards. The credit card company makes a charge, usually a percentage of each transaction.

An electronic terminal is supplied which provides receipts for both the client and the salon.

If a client wishes to pay by credit card, this is the procedure to follow:

- Look closely at the card and check the hologram and bank name.
- Check the expiry date on the card. If it is out of date, do not accept it. Request some other form of payment.
- Follow the instructions detailed below for debit and credit cards.

A computerised terminal may be used for credit cards and debit cards. The procedure to follow is described below.

Payments using debit cards/credit cards

An electronic payment system such as Maestro, Switch or Cirrus is used by many people instead of cash or cheque. The system uses debit cards, which are issued by the bank. (These cards may also act as cheque guarantee cards.)

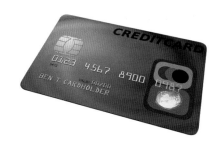

△ Look closely at credit and debit cards, checking the hologram, name and expiry date

You may be familiar with this system from supermarkets and other shops where payment points or checkouts have this facility. If the salon has a debit/credit card terminal the procedure is as follows:

- The terminal is linked to a main computer, which recognises the customer's card as it is swiped.
- The details of the transaction are keyed into the terminal and the client is requested to enter a PIN (Personal Identity Number).
- a printout authorising payment direct from the customer's account is produced.

If a card is declined during processing the client should be asked to offer another means of payment. This must be handled discreetly and without causing embarrassment.

Always follow the salon's policy.

Payment by cash equivalents

Cash equivalents are gift or discount vouchers. Gift vouchers are prepaid vouchers that are treated in the same way as cash. Most vouchers are dated to be used within a certain time, usually six months or a year from the date of purchase. The vouchers should indicate the value clearly and will usually be sold as £1, £5 or £10 'notes'. Each voucher should show the name of the salon, a signature and a number that corresponds with an entry in a book recording the date it was sold. This will guard against the possibility of fraud.

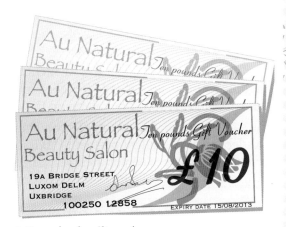

△ Example of a gift voucher

Discounts and special offers

Discount vouchers are a way of promoting salon services and may be part of an advertising campaign in the local paper, for example '10% off when you spend £40 or more on presentation of this voucher' or 'A free manicure with every full facial on presentation of this voucher before Saturday 15th June'. These discount vouchers are a form of payment and must be collected for the salon records.

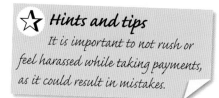

☆ *Hints and tips*
It is important to not rush or feel harassed while taking payments, as it could result in mistakes.

Dealing with payment discrepancies

In a busy environment such as the beauty therapy salon, mistakes can be made. These may not be noticed until the end of the day.

Discrepancies that result in invalid payments include:

- unsigned cheques
- incorrect date on cheques
- suspected fraudulent use of a payment card
- foreign currency (usually only small amounts in coins)
- out-of-date gift vouchers
- incorrect calculation of bills
- giving the wrong change
- pressing the wrong keys when entering amounts into the cash register.

These should be dealt with as soon as possible by contacting the client, if appropriate. If an error such as accepting a cheque without a cheque guarantee card has occurred, the cheque may bounce. This happens if there are insufficient funds in the client's account and may lead to loss of the payment by the salon. The cheque can be presented to the bank again, but if there is no money in the client's account the salon must stand the loss.

Fortunately, illegal transactions are not common, but the receptionist must be aware of the possibility of a client using forged notes, or a stolen credit card or cheque book.

If you have any doubt about the payment being made by a client, a senior member of staff should be called immediately. This must be done discreetly and without alarming the client.

The salon will usually have a policy on handling situations such as bad debts and fraudulent payments. Your job will be to take advice from the manager or senior therapist. Check what situations you have authority to deal with as they arise.

How to keep cash and other payments safe and secure

To keep payments safe and secure:

- Money should not be left on the premises overnight.
- The till drawer should be left open overnight to show that it is empty.
- An electric till should be installed. This ensures that takings are locked away, that there are receipts and a record of transactions on the till roll.
- The salon owner will decide who has access to the till security code or keys and who is responsible for cashing up at the end of the day. Any discrepancies should be dealt with immediately.

Activity

As part of your duties as a receptionist, you will be required to 'cash up' at the end of the day, keeping a copy of the dockets or takings sheet.

Write a brief explanation of how your particular system of recording works. Remember there are many different methods of keeping financial records.

Get your supervisor or assessor to check the accuracy of your records and ask them to sign to show that all financial transactions that you were responsible for were correct for the day.

Test yourself

Test yourself on reception duties by answering the following questions. For multiple choice questions, there may be more than one correct option.

1. When accepting a debit/credit card as payment, always check:
   a) the name of the bank that issued the card
   b) the account number
   c) the signature
   d) the hologram.

2. Good communication is an essential part of the receptionist's job. Give three examples of communication skills the therapist should use to deal with a client at the reception desk.

3. When handling enquiries on the telephone, you must:
   a) smile
   b) speak clearly
   c) make eye contact
   d) talk about the weather.

4. Which Act of Parliament governs the way a salon handles a client's personal information?

5. Give three important details that must be recorded in the appointment book when making an appointment for a client.

6. If a client makes a complaint to the receptionist, it should be handled by:
   a) listening attentively and not making judgements
   b) becoming angry
   c) ignoring the client
   d) offering a free cleanser.

7. From whom would you seek advice regarding an enquiry that is not your responsibility?

8. What payment discrepancy could be applied to cash payments?

9. What information do you need in order to deal with requests for an appointment?

10. How do you show that you are listening closely to what people are saying to you?

Are you ready for assessment?

It is necessary to make an action plan at the beginning of your course to enable you to watch your progress in both your learning and assessment and to review what you have achieved.

The following checklist will help you to be fully prepared.

1. **Practical observation**

    Your assessor will look at how you:

    - maintain the reception area
    - attend to clients and enquiries
    - make appointments for salon services
    - handle payments from clients.

2. **Knowledge and understanding**

    What you must know:

    - Salon and legal requirements.
    - Communication.
    - Salon service, products and pricing.
    - Calculating and taking payments.
    - Making appointments.

    To ensure that you have the necessary knowledge and understanding of reception duties your assessor will:

    - ask you questions before, during and after carrying out reception duties
    - ensure that you have completed project work and written tests relating to the unit
    - check that you have recorded in a log/diary your experiences while on reception
    - ensure that you have collected evidence for your portfolio, for example copies of messages taken
    - check that you have covered the range in your candidate logbook.

Sources of evidence

- Reception diary recording visitors to the salon, transactions dealt with, enquiries dealt with, etc.
- Copies of messages taken.
- Photographs of the reception area.
- Recording of telephone conversation.
- Video.
- Copy taken from appointment book.
- Cash sheet.

 Remember . . .
Always keep your logbook handy.

 Remember . . .
The reception area and the receptionist will give the first impression to the client.

 Remember . . .
Your assessor will observe your performance on at least three occasions and must cover all four outcomes of this unit.

 Remember . . .
Collecting evidence from simulation activities may be used e.g. dealing with an angry client role play.

Chapter 3
Unit G20: Make sure your own actions reduce risks to health and safety

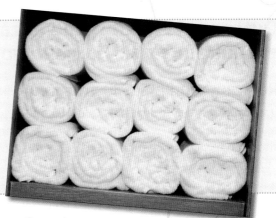

Learning objectives

This chapter covers the knowledge and procedures surrounding Unit G20 'Make sure your own actions reduce risks to health and safety'.

There are two learning outcomes for Unit G20 and they are:

1 Identify the hazards and evaluate the risks in your workplace.
2 Reduce the risks to health and safety in your workplace.

In order to be competent in health and safety you will need to show consistent practice and knowledge in both of these outcomes when applied to the practical skills and services within this qualification.

Unit G20 'Make sure your own actions reduce risks to health and safety' is a mandatory unit in Level 2 Beauty Therapy General and Make-Up routes and Level 2 Nail Services. It is worth four credits.

Introduction

The workplace can hold many dangers and it is everyone's responsibility to ensure that the salon is a safe and hygienic environment. The beauty therapist has additional responsibilities when working with clients. There is a **legal requirement** to ensure that the general public are not at risk when visiting the salon and receiving treatment.

Meet the professional

"As a therapist working in a busy salon you have a responsibility to clients and colleagues to provide a safe working environment. If you see a wet patch on the floor, don't wait, clean it up immediately. If equipment is not working properly report it. Don't leave it for someone else to do. It should be second nature to clean, sterilise and prepare a working area. Commit yourself to being a hygienic therapist. Dirty, unhygienic salons are the perfect way of losing clients. In the past I have walked into salons and straight back out again!

If you are unsure about something ask a supervisor. The only stupid question is the one you don't ask.

Never let your insurance expire, even for a day.

Remember your own health too. Always maintain good posture when performing any treatment, from massage to pedicures. Never put yourself at risk. Make sure there are always two therapists in the salon."

Jacqui Bostock

Outcome 1: Identify the hazards and evaluate the risks in your workplace

Relevant workplace instructions

It is important for individuals to understand clearly their role and responsibilities for health and safety within the workplace. Salons should have set procedures or rules for the safe day-to-day running of the salon.

It is the responsibility of the employer to safeguard the health, safety and welfare of everyone in the workplace by ensuring equipment is provided and maintained, strict hygiene procedures are followed and that safe working practices are identified in policies and procedures. The employer is ultimately responsible for enforcing safe working practices. They should do this by ensuring that:

1. Health and safety legislation is adhered to and information updated.
2. **Risk assessments** for all working procedures are carried out; hazards identified and reduced.
3. Staff are trained and competent in the use of health and safety equipment and procedures.
4. Staff are informed of changes within health and safety procedures.
5. Reporting systems are in place for the reporting of accidents and incidents within the workplace.
6. A healthy working environment is maintained by the provision of clean, tidy, well-lit and ventilated work areas.

Generally, an employee has responsibility to do the following.

1. Follow health and safety procedures and policies as instructed by the employer.
2. Be active in the implementation of such procedures.
3. Use health and safety equipment if it is provided.
4. Report any variance from health and safety policy or procedure.
5. Report accident and incident using the reporting system provided.
6. Report broken or dangerous equipment.
7. Report new hazards or those activities that have become more hazardous.

It is important to identify which workplace instructions are relevant to you.

Levels of responsibility

A supervisor has responsibility for others in the workplace. They must:

- monitor and report on aspects of health and safety practice such as accidents
- train junior members of staff in salon procedures to maintain health and safety, for example sterilising methods, preparation of the treatment room
- take on the responsibilities of the manager in their absence.

> **Key term**
>
> **Risk assessment** – a process that assesses the hazards and risks involved in a workplace activity such as a beauty therapy service. Procedures called controlled measures are then put in place to reduce the risks and therefore make the service safer.

The therapist is required to carry out a range of treatments competently and safely. They must:

- take responsibility for care, maintenance and safe storage of equipment and products
- work hygienically and safely by following salon practice on preparing for treatments and clearing away after clients
- report any hazards to the designated health and safety representative (usually the owner or manager)
- ensure the treatments they carry out on their clients meet health and safety requirements, i.e. contraindications are checked before the start of the treatment, manufacturer's instructions are followed
- ensure personal presentation and conduct meets salon policy.

The golden rule of health and safety

It is the responsibility of all employees to work and behave in a safe manner with due consideration for everyone, i.e. fellow workers, clients and visitors to the salon.

Harmful working practices

Health and safety practice is based on assessing the risks and hazards in the salon and putting controls in place to reduce them.

For example; a trailing flex from a piece of electrical equipment is a **hazard**. The **risk** is that someone may trip over it. If it is trailing across a busy walkway the risk of someone tripping is high but if it were moved so that it ran along very close to a wall the risk would be lowered. Moving the flex would be the **control**.

There are many hazards within a workplace such as a beauty salon, spa, nail bar or clinic. Other possible hazards in the salon include:

- faulty electrical equipment
- spillages on the floor
- overheating depilatory wax
- toxic or flammable products
- poor lighting
- carpet or flooring that is poorly fitted
- poor ventilation
- lifting heavy objects
- using chemicals.

Everyone has a responsibility to work safely and to avoid anything that could create a health and safety risk.

Evaluating the risk – risk assessment

Under the **Management of Health and Safety at Work Regulations 1999**, the employer should carry out risk assessments of the activities in the workplace and make arrangements to implement necessary controls.

Health and safety

Ensure that you understand your responsibilities for health and safety in the salon and carry out your work practices in line with salon rules and regulations and the Industry Code of Practice (HABIA).

Key term

A **hazard** is anything with the potential to cause harm.

A **risk** is the likelihood of the hazard harming someone.

Control is reducing or eliminating the risk.

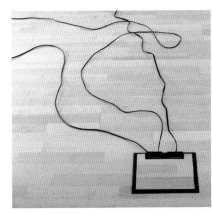

△ Trailing flex from electrical equipment is a hazard in the salon

The regulations state that employers with five or more employees need to record the findings of the risk assessments and write a health and safety policy for the salon. This identifies how health and safety is managed in the business, including the necessary controls to reduce the risks identified.

It is also required that a risk assessment be performed to regulate employees' exposure to substances that may cause ill health or injury under the **Control of Substances Hazardous to Health Regulations 1988 (COSHH)**.

The high-risk aspects of working as a beauty therapist

Certain aspects of performing treatments as a beauty therapist have a higher potential for risk than others. For example, performing a facial treatment with a piece of electrical equipment is a higher risk than performing one without equipment.

Activity

What other health and safety hazards are there in the salon? The beauty therapy salon carries risks relating to the use of chemicals and electrical equipment as well as those of falling, fire, infection, scalds, burns and cuts. Look around the salon you are working in and make a list of the hazards that could put you or your clients at risk of injury.

☆ *Hints and tips*
As far as the law is concerned, 'ignorance is not bliss'. Saying 'I didn't know' will not protect you, as it is your duty to find out.

Activity

Look at the table below. Try to place each of the beauty therapy services listed below in the correct column: high risk, medium risk, or low risk. An example has been done for you.

High risk	Medium risk	Low risk
Electrical facials		Manual facials

Beauty services: manicure, paraffin wax manicure, pedicure, heated bootee pedicure, eyebrow shaping, eyelash tinting, leg waxing, day make-up, application of strip false lashes, nail art, nail extensions, ear piercing, floatation treatments.

There are other hazards within the workplace that do not relate directly to performing treatments, but to the workplace environment. These hazards could relate to your immediate work area (for example a broken window) or to your wider working environment (for example a dark stairwell or unclean toilets).

High risk	Medium risk	Low risk
Dark stairwell	Broken window	

Dealing with hazards

Part of your responsibility as a therapist is to be aware of hazards in all aspects of your job and the workplace. If the hazard is a low risk and it is within your responsibility to reduce the risk, then you should do so. At other times it may be necessary for you to report the hazard and place a warning sign to protect the safety of others who may come across the hazard.

The employer should provide a reporting system for employees to report health and safety issues. Accidents in the workplace are often the result of unsafe working conditions or poor working practices. Staff may carry out treatments incorrectly or take unnecessary risks through lack of knowledge or training.

Any accident that occurs in the salon must be recorded in an accident book. If the accident is serious or if there are incidents of disease in the salon, a report form must be completed and sent to the Health and Safety Executive (HSE). The senior member of staff responsible for health and safety in the salon must be kept informed and take responsibility for the correct procedures being carried out.

Reporting accidents

Serious accidents or those that reoccur frequently are reported to the HSE in accordance with the **Reporting of Injuries, Diseases and Dangerous Occurrences Regulations 1985 (RIDDOR)**. These regulations ensure that any incident occurring in the workplace and leading to an injury or a condition resulting from a work activity is recorded and in the case of serious injury resulting in an absence from work or death, reported to the HSE within 10 working days. If any harm comes to a client or an employee through an unsafe action or procedure on your part or through neglecting to take action, the employer and yourself are deemed responsible and a prosecution may be made against both parties.

Activity

Look at the table on the left. Try to place each of the workplace hazards listed below in the correct column: high risk, medium risk, or low risk. An example has been done for you.

Workplace environment hazards: a wet floor, a plate glass shop front, a step down into a storage area, a fire door that sticks, carpet flooring, peeling paintwork, broken light fitting, curtains, visible water pipes, a cluttered corridor, a busy reception area, high shelving in a storage area.

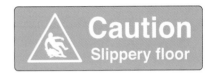

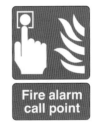

△ Examples of warning signs

A vast amount of health and safety legislation applies when working in a salon, although it is not specific to just the beauty industry. To place the legislation into a beauty therapy context the hair and beauty industry authority or HABIA have written approved '**Codes of Practice**' that offer practical examples of good practice. They give advice on how to comply with the law by, for example, providing a guide to what is 'reasonably practicable'. For example, if regulations use words like 'suitable and sufficient', an approved Code of Practice can illustrate what this requires in particular circumstances.

Au Natural Beauty Salon

INCIDENT REPORT FORM

This form must be completed following an incident or illness by the person making the report. It should be completed immediately following the incident and handed to the salon manager who will forward to the Health and Safety Officer as appropriate

Date _____   Time incident took place _____

Location of incident _____

Name of injured person _____

Address _____

Email address _____   Tel. No _____

Description of accident/illness:

Account of injury/illness (tick the relevant boxes):

First aid given ☐   Ambulance called ☐   Taken to hospital ☐

Relative called ☐   Treatment continued ☐

Signature of injured/ill person _____

Signature of person(s) attending the incident _____

Any preventative action or safety recommendations _____

Signature of Salon Manager _____

◁ An incident report form

Activity

Ask to see the accident book in your salon. Note the types of accidents recorded and discuss with a colleague how they might have been avoided. Can you spot any trends (for example falls or injuries due to a specific treatment)?

The accident book

Keeping a record of all accidents, no matter how small, is essential. The entry in the accident book should be completed as soon as possible by a member of staff who saw the accident and can give an accurate account of what happened.

Details noted in the accident book should include:

- the personal details of all those involved
- date and time of the accident
- details of the place where the accident occurred
- a brief description of what happened and the resulting injury/illness
- a description of the first aid given
- whether the emergency services were called or the person(s) taken to hospital. If so, it is likely that the accident would be regarded as serious and an incident report form would also be required.

The law relating to beauty therapy practice

An outline of some of the important pieces of health and safety legislation

It is important that everyone in the salon is aware of the law as it relates to them. The employer should provide training and ensure leaflets and a poster on health and safety is displayed at all times in the salon. The following legislations and regulations are relevant to working in the beauty therapy industry and each will look at the application to the therapist, the salon and the client and incorporate the industry's Code of Practice (HABIA).

Health and Safety at Work Act 1974

This is the main Act of Parliament governing the duties and responsibilities of employers and employees while at work. The Health and Safety at Work Act (HASAW) is an 'enabling' Act that covers a whole range of legislation relating to health and safety. All individuals have responsibility for health and safety while at work. The findings of the Health and Safety Executive and the demands of European legislation have led to a number of new laws.

Regulatory Reform (Fire Safety) Order 2005

This fire safety legislation has significantly changed fire safety in practice. It places the responsibility for fire safety on the 'responsible person'; this may be the employer, landlord or others with any control over the building. It states that the responsible person must do the following.

Provide a suitable and sufficient level of fire precautions. These should include:

- appropriate measures to reduce the risk of fire
- appropriate measures that will limit the spread of fire
- appropriate measures of detection and giving warning in case of fire
- appropriate measures to ensure that means of escape can be effectively used at all time
- appropriate portable *fire extinguishers* for the risk identified in means of fire fighting

★ *Hints and tips*
Codes of Practice are recognised by the Health and Safety Executive and therefore have special legal status. A person can be prosecuted for having not followed an agreed industry code of practice even though it is not part of any law. For example, if you perform an eyelash tint on a client without first performing a skin test and the client gets an allergic reaction, they can prosecute the salon and the individual therapist.

Activity

Access a copy of the HABIA Codes of Practice by downloading the document from their website www.habia.gov.uk

★ *Hints and tips*
The HSE website is a valuable source of information.

- appropriate signs and notices to enable persons to escape safely
- ensuring persons understand the action to be taken in the event of fire on the premises, including:
  - Instruction and *training* of staff
  - Measures to lessen the effects of fire.

  If you employ five or more people, you must carry out and record the findings of fire risk assessment to comply with the new fire legislation.

The risk of fire in the beauty salon

Electrical equipment constitutes a significant hazard in the beauty salon. The amount of electrical equipment used in the salon increases the risk of:

- electrical fire
- shock and burns
- fire and explosion when in contact with flammable liquids or aerosols.

Overloading electrical circuits or not following electrical safety procedures (for example ignoring worn cables) are the most common causes of electrical fires. Switching off all equipment at the mains immediately after use will help to prevent this type of fire.

Chemicals that are flammable (such as nail polish remover and surgical spirit) are a fire hazard and must be handled and stored in accordance with COSHH regulations.

Depilatory wax and paraffin wax, if overheated, will give off fumes and may ignite. Thermostatically controlled heaters must be used and maintained regularly. Never leave heated wax unattended and do not carry heated wax from cubicle to cubicle.

Fires may be started by carelessness and poor working practices (for example, drying towels over electrical or gas heaters, leaving unused appliances switched on, discarded cigarettes). A no-smoking policy should be in force in the salon to reduce the risk of fire.

Emergency evacuation procedure

1. Each business premises should have an evacuation procedure that takes account of the emergency exit routes and fire escapes from the building.
2. Make sure you know where fire-fighting equipment is kept and how to use it.
3. You must take responsibility to inform your clients, who may be receiving treatment in different parts of the salon. Direct them to the nearest safe exit.
4. Switch off electrical equipment close by you at the mains.
5. Ensure that everyone has left the premises and is congregated well away from the building.
6. If the fire is small and can be safely tackled with a fire extinguisher, this can be carried out. However, you should not take any risks and the premises must be vacated quickly, closing as many doors as possible.

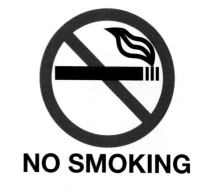

NO SMOKING

△ A no-smoking policy should be in force in the salon

 Health and safety

Check the emergency evacuation procedure for your salon and identify your role in an emergency.

7. At the earliest possible time, the emergency services should be contacted by dialling 999 (see below). Give the exact address and details of the emergency.

8. Not all emergencies are caused by fires. Bomb scares require you to evacuate premises as quickly as possible, to get well away from the building and to follow police instructions.

9. Toxic fumes or gas leaks may also require clients and employees to be evacuated from the building.

10. The salon should have regular emergency evacuation practice to familiarise staff with the procedure.

Fire-fighting equipment

Fire extinguishers

Different fire extinguishers are made to deal with different types of fire. Since 1997, all fire extinguishers in the UK must be coloured red, except for a small band or patch of colour using the standard colour code to distinguish the type of extinguisher and the type of fire on which it can be used.

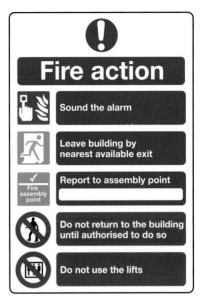

△ All salons should have an emergency evacuation procedure

KNOW YOUR FIRE EXTINGUISHER COLOUR CODE

WATER	DRY POWDER	FOAM	CO₂ CARBON DIOXIDE	VAPOURISING LIQUIDS
Unsafe all voltages. Wood, paper, textiles, etc.	Safe all voltages Flammable liquids	Unsafe all voltages Flammable liquids	Safe all voltages Flammable liquids	Safe all voltages Flammable liquids

△ Each type of fire should be dealt with using a different fire extinguisher

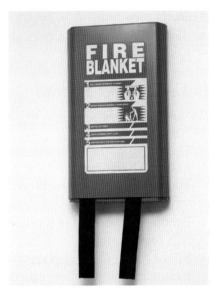

△ Fire blanket

Fire blanket

This is a fire-resistant material used for smothering a fire, for example burning wax or oil, or for wrapping around a person if their clothes are on fire.

Emergency procedures in the event of an accident

The procedure when calling the emergency services is as follows:

1. Dial 999 (check whether your phone line requires an additional number – usually 9 – to get an outside line).

2. Speak clearly, stating what the emergency is and where you are.

3. Listen carefully to any instructions you are given.

4. Return to a safe place or to the client.

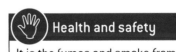

Health and safety

It is the fumes and smoke from fires that can kill. The building must be evacuated immediately.

Health and Safety (First Aid) Regulations 1981

These regulations cover requirements for the provision of first aid. It is advisable for someone in the salon to be trained in first aid but it is not required by law for a small business. Your local St John Ambulance (St Andrews Ambulance in Scotland) or Red Cross will be able to give you details of courses.

The first-aid box

It is however, a requirement by law to have a first-aid box. The employer will have the responsibility for the provision and maintenance of the first aid box and ensuring that it is adequately stocked. The first-aid box should contain:

- assorted plasters, individually wrapped
- medical wipes individually wrapped
- triangular bandages
- sterile eye pads
- different sizes of sterile dressings
- safety pins
- disposable plastic or rubber gloves
- cotton wool.

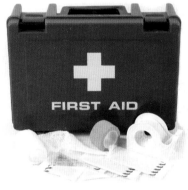

△ First-aid box

First aid for minor accidents

It may be necessary for you as the therapist to deal with minor accidents.

- Dizziness: sit the person down near an open window for fresh air. Loosen clothing around the neck. Placing the head between the knees will help to bring blood to the head but care must be taken with elderly people.
- Fainting: as above, but if possible lie the person down with their legs raised.
- Minor cuts: put on disposable gloves and apply pressure with a clean dressing. Follow procedure for handling contaminated materials on page 64.
- Epilepsy: a person suffering from an epileptic fit may injure themselves by falling or hitting furniture during an attack. Do not try to restrain them but ensure that their airways are clear and furniture and equipment is moved away. When the attack is over, cover the person with a blanket and allow them to rest.
- Minor burns or scalds: hold the area under cold running water for at least ten minutes.
- Nose bleed: bend the head slightly forward and squeeze the bridge of the nose until bleeding has stopped.
- Electric shock: do not touch the person but disconnect the appliance at the mains immediately. Lie the person down and check their breathing.
- Cosmetics in the eyes: apply cotton wool soaked in water. Allow the water to run through the eyes but do not allow the person to rub their eyes.

 Health and safety

Painkillers should not be issued by a first-aider and therefore should not be part of the first-aid kit. Only a medical practitioner should issue painkillers. Antiseptics should not be part of the first-aid kit because, if they have been used previously and the top not secured, they may contain germs.

Activity

Ask to see the accident book in your salon. Note the types of accident recorded. Is there a particular trend in the types of accidents? (For example falls or allergies due to a particular treatment.)

The Health and Safety Information for Employees Regulations 1989

These regulations require the employer to disseminate health and safety information and changes to all employees, which may include displaying a poster telling employees what they need to know about health and safety.

Cosmetic Products (Safety) Regulations 2008

As part of Consumer Protection legislation, this law requires cosmetics to comply with correct labelling to have safe formulation and be fit for the purpose intended.

Insurance

While every effort must be made to prevent injury and disease, unforeseen circumstances may lead to accidents in the workplace.

The Employers Liability (Compulsory Insurance) Act 1969

The law requires the employer to provide insurance cover against claims for injury or illness by an employee as a result of his or her normal working practice. The certificate of insurance must be displayed in the workplace.

Public Liability Insurance

The employer is not required by law to take out insurance to cover claims from the public, but is well advised to do so. It is becoming increasingly common for clients to sue businesses for damage to personal property or injury as a result of an accident in the salon.

Professional Indemnity Insurance

Professional indemnity insurance is part of the service offered by becoming a member of a professional organisation. Your annual subscription entitles you to liability cover against claims by clients for personal injury. Some treatments carry more risk than others, for example electro-epilation and ear-piercing. It is advisable to have appropriate professional indemnity insurance. It should be noted, however, that this insurance is only valid if industry Codes of Practice are followed.

Inspection and registration

All businesses must comply with the law on health and safety. To ensure this, the environmental health department of the local authority will appoint an Environmental Health Officer (EHO) to visit and inspect the premises.

This inspector has the authority to demand that any hazards identified during the inspection are dealt with by the employer within a given period of time. This is called an 'improvement notice'. Should the employer not comply with the notice by removing the danger within a given period of time, closure of the business can result, with the local authority issuing a 'prohibition notice'.

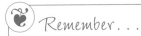

Remember...

In the event of an accident or incident a client can prosecute both the salon and the therapist.

Outcome 2: Reduce the risks to health and safety in your workplace

Everyone in the salon, whether they are staff, clients or visitors has a responsibility to act in accordance with safe practice as outlined by the law.

The beauty salon carries risks relating to:

- the building (such as falling on stairs or fire evacuation)
- the equipment used for treatment
- the products and chemicals used in treating the client.

Safe working practices are important in reducing the risks involved with hazardous activities. In general you should do the following:

- Never ignore any risk. Try to put things right, or report it immediately to a senior member of staff if it is beyond your capabilities.
- Always read manufacturers' instructions.
- Do not attempt to do treatments that you are not fully trained to do.
- Keep accurate records of client treatments including contra-indications, contra-actions and any incident associated with the client's time in the salon.
- Always follow strict hygiene procedures.
- Consider the risks involved in using products which may cause an allergic reaction or dermatitis.
- Be aware of the risk of repetitive strain injury when carrying out certain treatments.
- Always ask if you do not know how to do something that may put you at risk, particularly when dealing with electrical equipment, heated substances such as wax, or products whose ingredients and effects you do not understand.

Staff training in health and safety is the responsibility of the salon owner or manager and should include:

- induction of new staff
- safe systems of work
- fire prevention
- risks and hazards found in the salon
- fire evacuation procedures
- emergency procedure in the event of an accident
- first aid.

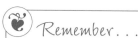

Remember...

Ignorance is no defence when it comes to the law. To say 'I didn't know' will not protect you.

Promoting a safe working environment

When working in the hair and beauty sector employers have legal responsibilities to provide a healthy and safe environment for all people working or visiting the salon under section 2 of the Health and Safety at Work Act 1974. The requirements for this environment are laid down in the Workplace (Health, Safety and Welfare) Regulations 1992. They place a duty on employers to make sure that the workplace is safe and suitable for the tasks being carried out and that it does not present risks to employees and others.

The regulations cover all aspects of the working environment, including:

- maintenance of the workplace and equipment
- ventilation, temperature, lighting
- cleanliness and disposal of waste materials
- room dimensions for working space and seating
- condition of floor and walk ways
- windows, skylights and ventilators and the ability to clean windows safely
- sanitary conveniences, washing facilities, drinking water
- accommodation for clothing, facilities for changing
- facilities for rest and to eat meals.

Heating

The minimum temperature in the workplace should be 16°C (60°F). However, the temperature in the salon should be around 20–23°C (68–75°F) as clients will be removing clothing. It is essential that the client is warm to encourage relaxation. An exercise room would need to be maintained at a lower temperature, around 17°C (63°F).

Thermostatically controlled heating will ensure that the salon remains at a constant temperature. Make sure that you know how to control the heating.

Ventilation

Adequate ventilation is equally important. Air conditioning is the most efficient method of ensuring clean air. Special consideration should be made for specific treatments such as nail extensions, which require extractor fans in the direct work area to remove strong smells and dust particles. Open windows will help remove strong smells from cosmetic preparations, fumes from chemicals and stale air, which is caused by a build-up of carbon dioxide and pungent smells.

Exercise rooms and wet areas must have very efficient air circulation and good extraction systems: air conditioning is ideal. Poor ventilation can result in headaches, dizziness, nausea, fainting and fatigue.

Lighting

All areas of the salon should be well lit, particularly stairways and fire escapes. Treatment areas where cosmetics are used should have natural daylight to ensure that make-up colours are not distorted. Matching make-up with skin tones or the client's clothing is an important aspect of applying cosmetics. 'Daylight' lamps can substitute for poor natural light where necessary.

Lights should be checked regularly, replacing flickering fluorescent tubes or changing the angle of lights that cause unnecessary glare.

Dimmer switches in treatment rooms will enable the therapist to regulate the amount of light according to the treatment being carried out, for example during facial massage lights should be dimmed.

Washing and toilet facilities

The law makes it very clear that an adequate supply of clean hot and cold water should be available in the workplace, with separate washing facilities away from areas where food may be prepared or consumed.

The number of toilets required is governed by the number of employees. A toilet must be available for clients. It is essential that toilets are spotlessly clean and checked regularly to ensure that there is a good supply of toilet tissue, disposable hand towels and soap and the waste bin is emptied regularly.

Salon cleaning

It is very important for the salon image, and to prevent the spread of infection, that the premises are kept very clean. Floors and windows should be cleaned once a week. This may be done by a cleaner employed out of business hours. Other daily cleaning jobs must form part of the salon routine, with all staff taking responsibility for completing jobs. This is usually done on a rota basis.

The Local Government (Miscellaneous Provisions) Act provides the local authority with powers to inspect the premises for hygiene and cleaning practices, in particular disposal of waste, cleanliness of floors, work surfaces and sterilising procedures.

Salon duties

The duties of a therapist go beyond providing services to clients; they also include the following:

General cleaning

Floors may be cleaned out of business hours. However, it is important that any spillages are wiped up immediately. Wet floors should have a clear sign to stop people walking over them until the surface is dry and safe to walk on. Carpets should be vacuumed as required and any worn or frayed areas secured to avoid tripping.

Laundry

There must be sufficient clean towels, sheets and headbands to supply the salon. Laundry needs to be sorted and put into machines for washing regularly throughout the day. Washed towels need to be dried, folded neatly and stacked on shelves for easy access by the therapists. There should be sufficient washing powder and fabric softener available at all times. In order for the laundry to run efficiently, the machines must be in full working order.

The salon may choose to send towels out to a commercial laundry although this practice will prove to be expensive. It will be necessary to count soiled towels to go out and clean towels when they return. Paperwork will need to be kept up to date to check the accuracy of invoices before payment.

Activity

It is essential that hygiene and safety tasks are carried out daily. Using the information in this chapter, devise a salon rota to ensure that all daily tasks are completed. Use your rota to allocate tasks to the staff (students) in the salon and check at the end of the day that the jobs have been completed to your satisfaction.

You will need to discuss the rota with the manager and the staff. Outline how the jobs should be carried out and how you intend to check at the end of the day. Remember to give feedback on how well the duties have been carried out.

Evidence for assessment: the rota is valuable evidence for your portfolio. Remember to get your teacher or assessor to date and sign the rota, to observe you allocating jobs and monitoring that they have been carried out.

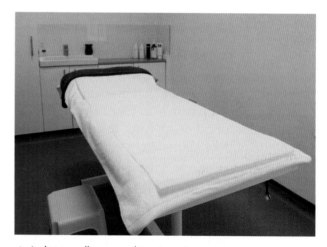

△ A clean, well-prepared treatment room

Waste disposal

Each work area must have a small waste bin with a lid and a foot pedal to avoid using hands to open. Used cotton wool and tissues must be placed in the bin, not left lying on the trolley, couch or floor. This bin should be emptied after each client into a large receptacle for disposal at the end of every day.

Specialist or contaminated waste such as disposable epilation probes are placed in a special yellow plastic container called a **sharps box**. This container must be handled with care and removed for incineration at appropriate intervals. Contaminated waste, i.e. with blood or serum on it, should be placed in a bin liner tied securely for incineration.

Broken glass must be disposed of carefully by wrapping in newspaper before placing in the bin.

> **Key term**
>
> A **sharps box** is a special yellow container for disposal of specialist or contaminated waste.

Basins and wet areas

Blocked basins must be dealt with immediately to avoid unpleasant smells. The S-bend under the basin has a screw cap that can be opened to remove blockages. Basins and shower cubicles must be wiped down after use with disinfectant. A ceramic cleaning fluid should be used at the end of the day to remove oil and lime scale. These can accumulate, leaving unsightly stains that can harbour germs. Disinfectant should be poured down the drains at the end of every day. Saunas and steam baths require regular, thorough cleaning using disinfectant. The warmth and moisture provide the perfect breeding ground for germs.

Trolleys and work surfaces

Surfaces that are dusty and have creams, oils or wax spilt on them look unsightly, unprofessional and will harbour infection. Spillages must be wiped up immediately and all work surfaces kept clean throughout the day.

Detergent will remove oils and creams. Products like depilatory wax should be left to cool before being picked off the surface. Wipe over with surgical spirit.

Hand mirrors are often neglected and left smeared with fingerprints. Handing a dirty mirror to a client is not acceptable.

Equipment

Electrical equipment must be wiped over before and after use with a damp cloth to remove dust and any products that may have accumulated during treatment.

At the end of the day a final check must be made to ensure that all electrical appliances and salon equipment is switched off and disconnected.

 Remember . . .

Note any electrical faults, switch off the machine, place a clear 'out of order' sign on the machine and report the defect to the salon manager immediately.

Client refreshment facilities

Clients are often offered drinks or snacks in the salon. Hygiene procedures must be very strict when preparing food and drinks. If hot and cold drinks are supplied to the clients, they must be prepared in an area that is suitable, away from treatments and chemicals. The client should consume refreshments in a suitable room or rest area, away from chemicals. Disposable containers must be used if there are not adequate facilities for preparing drinks and washing up.

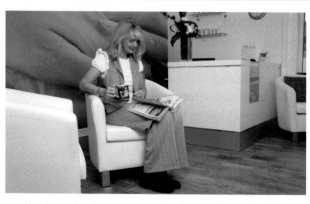

△ The client should consume refreshments in a suitable room or rest area away from chemicals

Salon hygiene

Everyone must be aware of the importance of carrying out strict hygiene procedures to protect themselves, other therapists and clients from infection. Guidelines laid down in the beauty therapy Codes of Practice outline hygiene procedures. These are particularly important when the treatment involves skin piercing (see Chapter 15). Sterilisation and disinfection is an essential part of salon duties for the therapist. Methods of sterilisation and disinfection can be found in Chapter 1.

The therapist must be able to recognise skin disease and disorders associated with the area of the body being treated (see the relevant chaper for more details) and carry out the meticulous hygiene procedures that are outlined in this chapter.

Infection

Infection is caused by micro-organisms that invade the body and cause inflammation. These include:

- bacteria
- viruses
- fungi.

Procedures to prevent infection are:

- Wipe down equipment with disinfectant and/or warm soapy water after use.
- Clean and sterilise small tools.
- Always use clean towels, linen and disposable products.
- Check personal appearance.
- Ensure good personal hygiene by showering daily, using deodorant as appropriate.
- Always wash hands before and after treating a client.
- Cover any cuts or open wounds on the hands with a waterproof adhesive dressing.
- Check client for contraindications before starting treatment.
- Keep product jars and containers clean and free from drips.
- Dispose of waste in a closed bin (recycle where possible).
- Place soiled laundry in a basket for laundering.

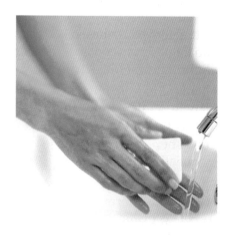

△ Wash hands before and after treatment or as often as necessary during the treatment

Environmentally friendly working practices

Under the Environmental Protection Act 1990 and The Controlled Waste Regulations 1992 it is important for a beauty therapy business to consider the environment.

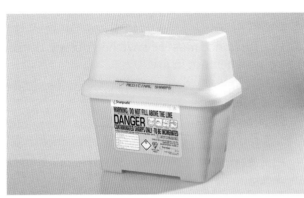

- Buy products in larger, economy sizes and dispense as required to avoid waste.
- Dispose of chemicals correctly (contact the environmental health department at your local council for advice) Do not pour chemicals down the sink.
- Recycle packaging appropriately.
- Switch off electrical equipment when not in use.
- Switch electric lights off in rooms not in use.
- Use long-life light bulbs to reduce use of energy.
- Control the heating in the salon by using the thermostat, taking account of external weather conditions.
- Cut down on disposable products unless for strict hygiene requirements.

△ Dispose of waste correctly

Health and safety regulations

To reduce the risk of some common hazards in the workplace, a number of regulations should be in place. The following are examples of those regulations that apply to working in the beauty industry.

Provision and Use of Work Equipment Regulations 1998

These regulations require that equipment provided for use at work, including machinery, is sourced from a reputable supplier and complies with safety guidelines as appropriate. For example, the presence of the 'British Kitemark' on a piece of equipment shows that it conforms to the appropriate 'British Standard' and is safe and reliable.

The Electricity at Work Regulations 1989

Beauty therapists use a range of electrical equipment, which must be tested by a qualified electrician at least once every five years but more frequently if the equipment is in constant use. A sticker will usually be placed on each item giving the date it was tested. A record of equipment inspection and servicing must be made available on request.

When using any electrical equipment you should make the following checks:

- Equipment should not be used near basins or where liquids are likely to be spilt on the appliance.
- Cables, flexes, connections, sockets and plugs must be intact, with no exposed wiring.

 Health and safety

Do not touch sockets, connections, plugs or wires with damp or wet hands. If you come across faulty or damaged electrical equipment, take it out of use immediately by placing a clearly written 'out of order' sign on it. Report the fault to the manager.

- There must be sufficient sockets at every workstation and the use of adapters should be avoided.
- The appliance should be on a level and stable trolley.
- The appliance must be switched off and disconnected from the mains when not in use.
- Cables and flexes must not be allowed to trail across the floor as they could cause someone to trip.
- Electrical equipment should be stored carefully by winding flexes and cables smoothly round the appliance.
- At the end of the working day someone must be responsible for checking that all appliances are switched off and disconnected.

The Personal Protective Equipment at Work Regulations (PPE) 1992

The regulations state that employers must provide suitable and sufficient protective clothing and materials.

- Salon dress, aprons, disposable gloves and masks are examples of the PPE that should be adequate to protect therapists.
- Protective clothing and materials should be available to protect the client.

Salons have set professional work wear for all staff. The salon uniform should present a smart, clean image as well as being a means of protecting the therapist from chemicals that may be absorbed into the skin. The uniform may also protect from possible cross infection. The uniform should be changed daily and should only be worn in the salon, to avoid picking up odours or grime from outdoors.

It is essential that clean towels and linen are available to each client. Disposable paper such as couch roll and tissues need to be readily available.

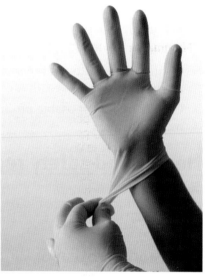

△ Therapists should wear latex gloves to protect themselves from risk of infection

Control of Substances Hazardous to Health Regulations 1988 (COSHH)

The employer is required to regulate employees' exposure to substances that may cause ill health or injury. The potential risks to all those working in the salon are assessed. This process is called risk assessment and is normally carried out by the salon manager.

Hazard warning symbols appear on packaging and notices around the workplace.

The following grid gives you examples of chemicals currently used in the salon, with recommendations for storage and handling.

	Specification	Health hazard	Use/ handling	Storage	Disposal	Caution/ action
Aerosols	Hairsprays Nail dry sprays Surface cleaners	Flammable	Do not smoke. Keep away from eyes. Use in well-ventilated areas.	Cool, dry place. Avoid sunlight. Avoid excessive heat	Do not pierce or burn container (explosive).	In case of fire, evacuate areas known to contain aerosols.
Caustic	Cuticle remover	Substances that can burn the skin.	Keep away from eyes. Do not use on sensitive skin.	Cool dry place.	Wear gloves. Mop up spills with damp cloth (rinse well)	Eye/skin contact – use eye bath or wash area with plenty of water. Ingestion – drink plenty of water.
Flammable	Acetone Astringent Eau de cologne Equipment cleaner Flowers of sulphur Nail polish remover Nail polish thinners Rose water Solvents Surgical spirit Witch hazel	Flammable vapours	Do not smoke. Label clearly. Good ventilation.	Distinguish inflammables from flammables Store in cool place. Keep sealed. (Look at labels.)	Seek advice from EHO if disposing of large quantities.	Wash skin or eyes immediately. Remove to fresh air if inhaled.
Sensitising	Acrylic nail powder Chemical peels Equipment cleaner Gluteraldehyde solution Lash tint Nail glue Nail off remover Nail primer Resin gel	May cause allergic reaction.	Wear disposable gloves.	Cool, dry place.	Use normal disposal methods or contact EHO if large amounts.	Eye/skin contact – wash off immediately. Inhalation – move to fresh air. Ingestion – seek medical advice
Skin bleach	All bleach products Hydrogen peroxide	May cause skin irritation.	Wear gloves. Avoid inhalation.	Cool, dry place.	Do not incinerate. Dilute to mop up spillages. Wash powders down the drain.	Eye/skin contact – wash off immediately. Inhalation – move to fresh air then seek medical advice.
Fine powders	Acrylic nail powder Bleaches Bronzing powders Calamine powder Face powder Flowers of sulphur Fuller's earth Kaolin Magnesium carbonate	Inhalation can cause irritation.	Avoid inhalation by wearing a mask.	Cool dry place. Closed container.	Treat as domestic waste. Flowers of sulphur is a fire hazard.	Eye/skin contact – wash off immediately.

△ Storage, handling and disposal guidelines for chemicals in the salon

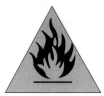
Highly Flammable

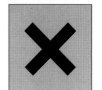
Harmful

Explosive

Toxic

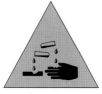
Corrosive

Oxidising

△ You should be familiar with hazard warning symbols

The Manual Handling Operations Regulations 1992

These regulations require everyone in the workplace to minimise risks from lifting and handling large or heavy objects. The beauty therapist must take particular care when moving equipment or boxes containing stock in the salon.

Equipment should be fixed on a suitable trolley and free-standing equipment should be on castors for ease of movement around the salon. Trolleys must be checked regularly to ensure that they are stable and that the castors run freely. However, equipment should not be moved unnecessarily, in particular equipment containing hot liquids such as wax.

Manual tasks risk factors

Poor posture when lifting heavy items can cause injury.

Working postures for the beauty therapist can cause aches and pains and in the long term result in serious injury.

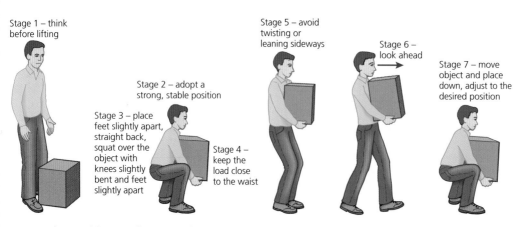

Stage 1 – think before lifting

Stage 2 – adopt a strong, stable position

Stage 3 – place feet slightly apart, straight back, squat over the object with knees slightly bent and feet slightly apart

Stage 4 – keep the load close to the waist

Stage 5 – avoid twisting or leaning sideways

Stage 6 – look ahead

Stage 7 – move object and place down, adjust to the desired position

△ Learn how to lift correctly, so you do not strain your back

Examples of posture problems associated with treating clients:

- back bent or twisted, shoulders raised in an unnatural position when carrying out massage
- repeated movements or awkward posture over a long period of time when leg waxing
- back bent when doing manicure/nail art
- poor standing posture when applying make-up.

Awkward posture requires greater muscular effort and leads to fatigue, particularly when the position is held for a long time.

The employer should ensure that the equipment can be raised or lowered to meet the needs of all the therapists working in the salon. Hydraulic or manual lift couches and stools should be available.

The Local Government (Miscellaneous Provisions) Act 1982 (Local Authority Licensing)

The beauty therapist carries out some treatments (such as ear-piercing, micro-pigmentation, waxing, eyebrow shaping and electrical epilation) that require particular attention to hygiene. This is due to the increased risk of cross-infection from blood or body fluids coming into contact with the therapist, equipment or other clients.

Guidelines are available from the local authority and under the local by-laws inspection of the premises to check hygiene procedures will be necessary. When the Environmental Health Officer (EHO) is satisfied that the premises are of the required standard, the business will become registered and receive a certificate. An officer will pay particular attention to:

- cleaning and sterilising of implements
- safe working practices with materials such as disposable needles
- salon cleaning to a high standard
- therapists' personal hygiene and working practices.

Licensing by the local authority covers a range of activities including ear-piercing, electrical epilation, hairdressing/barbering and other professions such as acupuncture and tattooing.

Local authorities are not expected to assess the treatment techniques used by the therapist; however, they have to ensure adequate levels of training and competence exist.

Age restrictions can be enforced under the by-laws. It is recommended that clients under 16 have a parent or guardian present and that a consent form is signed prior to treatment. A declaration and proof of age can also be insisted on under the by-law. This is a further indication of the importance of thorough and careful consultation, with fully completed records.

Health and safety

Staff should be trained in correct lifting techniques and good posture when carrying out treatments.

Activity

Working in a small group and using the internet find your local authority local by-laws relating to the beauty therapy salon. You may find that different local authorities have different information and slightly different regulations. This is because by-laws are based on local needs and the interpretation of government guidelines may vary to meet these needs.

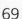

> ### Want to know more?
>
> The Health and Safety Executive provide information and leaflets to help the employer and staff of a business to implement health and safety legislation and particularly the risks and hazards found in the work place. More information is available online at www.hse.gov.uk.
>
> Your local council Environmental Health Department is also a useful source of information that relates to local issues. It is also your licensing authority. Beauty therapy premises must be licensed to carry out the range of beauty treatments. The beauty therapist must also be registered with the Council. For further information look at your local council's website.
>
> **Training**
>
> You should take every opportunity to attend training courses on health and safety practice and these may include:
> ☞ in-house staff training courses
> ☞ equipment suppliers' demonstrations and training
> ☞ product manufacturers' training courses.

Test yourself

Test yourself on health and safety by answering the following questions:

1. The act that covers local by-laws for hygiene procedures in the salon is the:
   a) Workplace (Health, Safety and Welfare) Regulations
   b) Personal Protective Equipment at Work Regulations
   c) Local Government (Miscellaneous Provision) Act
   d) Control of Substances Hazardous to Health Act.

2. The Electricity at Work Regulations require the therapist to:
   a) switch on an electrical heater at the start of the day
   b) ensure that all electrical equipment in the salon is in safe working order
   c) wear rubber gloves
   d) know the symbols on fire extinguishers.

3. When making a visual check on electrical equipment before switching a machine on, you must look at:
   a) the red indicator light that tells you the machine has mains power
   b) the manufacturer's instructions
   c) all the dials and switches
   d) the cables and flexes for loose wires or exposed wires.

4. Give two ways of avoiding straining your back when picking up a heavy object.

5. Give two reasons why salon dress/overall should be worn when working in the salon.

6. List four possible hazards found in the beauty salon.

7. Give three examples of environmentally friendly work practices.

8. What does the abbreviation COSHH stand for?

9. Define the terms:
   a) risk
   b) hazard

10. List four types of fire extinguisher and what each is used for.

Are you ready for assessment?

The following checklist will help you to be fully prepared for your assessment

1. **Practical observation**

   Identify the hazards and evaluate the risks in your workplace
   Reduce the risks to health and safety in your workplace

   Your assessor will look at how you:

   - identify salon practices which could harm you or others
   - identify those responsible for health and safety in your salon
   - correctly report health and safety hazards
   - demonstrate health and safety good practice throughout the service
   - carry out all treatments with regard to the salon's health and safety instructions and supplier's or manufacturer's instructions
   - ensure your personal appearance and behaviour meets salon rules and health and safety requirements
   - follow good practice which takes account of the environment.

2. **Knowledge and understanding**

   What you must know:

   - What hazards and risks are.
   - Health and safety legislation and workplace policies.
   - Risks to health and safety in your own work role and what precautions you must take.
   - Your responsibilities for controlling and reporting health and safety risks.
   - The importance of suppliers' and manufacturers' instructions in safe working practice.
   - The importance of personal presentation and professional behaviour in maintaining health and safety in the salon.

   To ensure that you have the necessary knowledge and understanding of health and safety procedures your assessor will:

   - ask you questions before, during and after carrying out the treatment
   - ensure that you have completed project work and written exercises relating to the unit
   - check that you have recorded in a log/diary procedures you have carried out showing that you are aware of risks and hazards in the salon
   - observe you at least twice demonstrating safe working practice
   - check that you have covered the range in your candidate logbook
   - require you to take a test.

 Remember...
Always keep your logbook handy.

 Remember...
It is important that you understand the terms hazard, risk and control.

 Remember...
Simulation is not a valid means of assessment for manicure service.

 Remember...
Health and safety is an important part of the salon's working day. Good practice is essential.

Sources of evidence

- Take part in an evacuation procedure (fire practice)
- Health and Safety training in the salon and training course
- Risk assessment you have completed and recorded
- Reporting a hazard in the salon using the correct procedure
- Discussion on possible risks and how to prevent them

Part 2: With the client

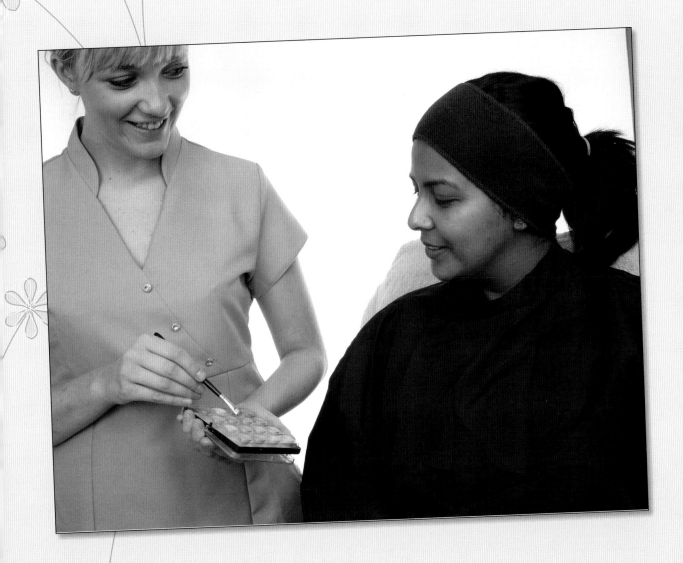

Chapter 4
Unit B4: Provide facial skin care treatment

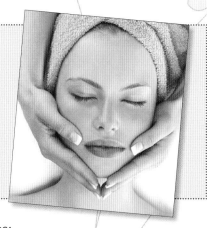

Learning objectives

This chapter covers Unit B4 'Provide facial skin care treatment'. It is about facial skin care for a variety of skin types, skin tones and age groups.

There are four learning outcomes for Unit B4 and they are:

1 Maintain safe and effective methods of working when improving and maintaining facial condition.

2 Consult, plan and prepare for facial with clients.

3 Improve and maintain skin condition.

4 Provide aftercare advice.

You will need to be competent in all of these outcomes to be competent in manual facial therapy, qualify for insurance and perform the treatments on members of the public.

Evidence requirements

Your assessor will need to observe you perform this treatment successfully on at least three occasions on different clients. You must:

1 Demonstrate the use of consultation techniques:
- questioning
- visual
- manual
- reference to client records.

2 Take one of these necessary actions:
- encourage the client to seek medical advice
- explain why the treatment cannot be carried out
- modify the treatment.

3. Treat skin types:
- oily
- dry
- combination.

4. Treat two of these skin conditions:
- mature skin
- sensitive skin
- dehydrated skin.

5. Use these types of facial product:
- eye make-up remover
- cleansers
- toners
- exfoliators
- moisturisers
- specialised skin products.

6. Use these massage mediums:
- oil
- cream.

7. Use these massage techniques:
- effleurage
- petrissage
- tapotement.

8. Use these mask treatments:
- setting
- non-setting.

9. Provide this type of advice:
- suitable aftercare products and their use
- avoidance of activities which may cause contra-actions
- recommended time intervals in between facial treatments
- home-care routines.

Introduction

Facial therapy is a very rewarding aspect of being a beauty therapist. To make a fundamental difference to the appearance and condition of a client's skin and the consequential increase in their self confidence gets to the heart of the 'therapy' in beauty therapy.

Unit B4 'Provide facial skin care treatment' is a mandatory unit in the Level 2 Beauty Therapy qualification in both the General and Make-up routes and is worth eight credits.

Meet the professional

"Start analysing your client's skin the minute they walk through the door! Look and listen: are the client's expectations from the treatment realistic? There are many treatments available and a 'quick fix' treatment might not be suitable.

A skin care treatment will probably be your client's only chance of an hour's relaxation, so make it a perfect, personal, prescription treatment. Make the treatment stand out and something they won't forget and they will want to come back to your salon again!"

Jacqui Bostock

Outcome 1: Maintain safe and effective methods of working when improving and maintaining facial skin condition

Much of the general information you need to be competent in this outcome is dealt with in Chapter 1 'Professional skills' and Chapter 3 'G20 Make sure your own actions reduce risks to health and safety'.

Legal requirements

The following table gives a summary of the relevant health and safety legislation that applies to facial skin care treatment.

▽ Relevant legislation as it applies to facial skin care treatment

The treatment room	Health & Safety at Work Act 1974	General safety of staff and visitors to the salon including clients
	The Workplace (Health, Safety & Welfare) Regulations 1992	Governs the working environment including ventilation, temperature and lighting, etc.
	Regulatory Reform (Fire Safety) Order 2005	The safe evacuation of the building in an emergency such as a fire
Equipment	Provision and Use of Work Equipment Regulations 1998	Governs the acquisition of safe and reliable equipment
Facial skin care products	Control of Substances Hazardous to Health 1988	Governs the exposure of persons to substances likely to cause harm including flammability and the effect on the tissues
	Cosmetic Products (Safety) Regulations (2008)	Requires cosmetics to comply with correct labelling, to have safe formulation and be fit for the purpose intended
Disposal of waste	The Controlled Waste Regulations 1992	Governs the correct disposal of contaminated waste, i.e. that contaminated with blood or other bodily fluids

There are other legal requirements for treating clients, such as your responsibilities surrounding treating minors, avoiding discrimination and complying with data protection law. You will find details in Chapter 1.

Facial skin care service times

The recommended maximum service time for a facial is 60 minutes. However, specialist facials may require longer, following manufacturer's instructions. You should check your column in the appointment book before starting work and refer to salon records of previous visits, where appropriate, for details of service times.

If the client is new, you should have all the necessary paperwork ready for completion. You should also check the range of products available to ensure you can offer options to suit the individual's need and your recommendations following initial consultation.

Preparation

Safe and hygienic practices within a salon environment are crucial to prevent cross-infection. Tools, materials and equipment must be sterilised before and after each client. Linen should also be changed after each client. The recognition of contraindications is of vital importance to prevent cross-infection.

It is essential to create a calm and relaxing environment for the client. The salon furnishings and equipment should be appropriate and fit for the purpose. The client may be apprehensive, particularly if it is their first visit. It is important to avoid delays and you should have everything prepared and ready for the client's arrival. This will also increase salon efficiency if you work within the time parameters for each treatment.

Personal appearance

The client is coming to you for a range of treatments and services that will help to maintain or improve a particular condition or meet a specific need. You are therefore perceived to be a professional, an exponent of your craft. It is important that your image projects your expertise. Your appearance will indicate to others how much care and pride you take in your role. In the beauty business an appropriate image is paramount. You may be very confident and knowledgeable in the services and products offered, but if your appearance is not appropriate it sends the wrong message to the client. (See also Chapter 1, which deals with personal appearance in more detail.)

Client record cards

The systems for recording findings will differ from one salon to another. It is usual for salons to design their own system of record cards based on their 'house style'. Salons also use treatment plans. A treatment plan is a record of the proposed schedule of treatment and the therapist's recommendations. Plans may be one double-sided form or two separate ones.

Remember a treatment plan should include:

- client's full name
- client's usual skin care routine
- result of skin analysis
- contraindications
- recommended treatments and products – including costs and duration
- outcomes of treatment
- contra-actions
- aftercare advice given
- client's signature
- record of client feedback.

A record card should include:

- client's full name
- client's address and telephone number(s) (and e-mail address)
- date of birth
- medical history.

Remember . . .

Your appearance should project the pride you take in your role as a skin care therapist. Clients look to you to provide a professional treatment for their skin and it is important that you maintain their confidence in your abilities by being presented appropriately. You only have one chance to make a first impression!

Remember . . .

It is important to record your findings neatly; other therapists may need to refer to the records.

Outcome 2: Consult, plan and prepare for facials with clients

Contraindications

Accurate inspection of the skin is vital in assessing the client's needs and for the identification of contraindications. The tables below show the contraindications that are specific to facial treatments. They are separated into those requiring medical referral and those that restrict treatment within the localised area.

Contraindications that require medical referral are largely infectious skin disorders and diseases.

Health and safety

It is essential that you have a clear understanding of the structure and function of the skin, bones and muscles of the head, face and neck, and composition and function of blood and lymph. See Chapter 19 for full details.

▽ Contraindications requiring medical referral

Disease or disorder	Cause	Appearance
Impetigo	Caused by the invasion of streptococcal or staphylococcal bacteria	Fluid-filled blisters that rupture and form a yellow crust. Highly contagious. Commonly found around the nose and mouth in children
Furuncle and carbuncle	Caused by staphylococcal bacteria	Commonly known as boils. Appears red, swollen and painful with a pus-filled head. Commonly found on the neck but can appear anywhere on the body. A group of furuncles together are known as carbuncles
Conjunctivitis	Commonly caused by a bacterial infection but can be a complication from a viral respiratory infection such as colds or flu	Highly infectious condition affecting the membranes of the eye, which appears red and puffy, feels irritated and 'gritty' and may weep. The eye lids may stick together after a night's sleep

Disease or disorder	Cause	Appearance
Stye	Caused by staphylococcal bacteria invasion through poor hygiene or using contaminated cosmetics	A red and painful swelling in or on the eyelid with pus formation and weeping
Folliculitis	Invasion of the hair follicles of staphylococcal bacteria	Appears as a red rash with the formation of pustules that may be itchy. Common in the beards of men through poor hygiene when shaving
Herpes simplex	Caused by the herpes simplex virus type 1 (HSV-1)	Commonly found on the lips, mouth and nose. Begins as a burning or itching sensation followed by the formation of fluid-filled blisters, which weep to form a yellow crust or scab. Commonly known as cold sore(s)
Herpes zoster	Caused by the varicella zoster virus (the same virus that causes chickenpox)	Pain or tingling on one side of the body, followed by the formation of fluid-filled blisters, which weep and form crusts. Common on the body but may affect the face, mouth, eyes and ears
Warts	Caused by the human papilloma virus. Warts on the feet are called verrucae	Appear as firm nodules of keratinised skin. Common on the hands and feet but can be found on the face

Ringworm or tines	Caused by a fungus that lives off the dead keratinised cells of the skin, hair and nails. Tinea corporis is tinea of the body; Tinea capitis that of the scalp and Tinea pedis is also known as 'athlete's foot'	Appears as red, itchy scaly patches that can appear anywhere on the body. The skin heals in the centre of the patch first, so as the condition spreads outwards, 'rings' are formed
Pediculosis	Caused by the infestation of parasitic lice	The lice are often difficult to see but their egg cases (known as 'nits') can be seen attached to the hair shaft close to the scalp. Commonly found above and behind the ears and often accompanied by intense irritation
Scabies	Infestation by a mite called acarus scabiei commonly known as 'itch mite'	The mites burrow into the skin to lay their eggs leaving a red 'track' which is extremely irritating.

Other contraindications that require medical referral are:

- systemic medical conditions such as epilepsy, diabetes, heart and vascular conditions
- severe skin conditions such as severe psoriasis, eczema or acne.

Contraindications that restrict treatment include:

- recent scar tissue
- eczema
- allergies
- cuts
- abrasions
- bruising
- vitiligo
- styes.

The key to improving the condition of the client's skin is the correct analysis.

Remember . . .

It is very important that you **do not** inform the client of your diagnosis of the contraindication, as you are not qualified to do so and may alarm or embarrass them. Instead, you should ask the client to seek medical advice from their GP.

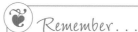
Equipment checklist

To carry out a skin analysis you will need:

✔ good lighting or additional illumination
✔ a magnifying lamp.

Identifying current skin care routine

You must be prepared to look at the skin with care and talk to the client about their current skin care regime. You should ask all clients to tell you about their perceptions of their skin. It is important to find out what skin type the client believes they have. This information will provide you with clues to any anomalies you may notice during your inspection. It will also help you to make your own decision. Some conditions can be exacerbated by clients who have inaccurately identified their skin type and used unsuitable products, upsetting the skin's sensitive acid mantle.

Men and women

Beauty treatments are now popular with both female and male clients. There is a wide variation in both skin characteristics and skin types. It is important to understand and recognise these differences when analysing skin and planning treatments.

Male skin

In recent times, the popularity of male grooming products has encouraged men to seek salon-based therapy treatment for a range of skin conditions.

As with female skin, male skin has many different characteristics and types. The hormonal differences (particularly testosterone) gives male skin a thicker epidermis, which creates a tougher, more resistant and less sensitive skin than that of females. The male hormones also cause the skin to be oilier and more acidic. The aging process of male skin is less dramatic than for female skin, with male skin retaining a higher degree of elasticity. However, the daily shaving regime can leave the skin prone to infection and sensitive from skin rashes, in-growing hairs and excessive dryness caused through continual use of soap-based shaving foams and gels, which strip the skin's natural acid mantle. Often, this will have been further exacerbated by poor skin care and neglect of basic treatments such as regular moisturising.

The male grooming industry is now very popular and while most products are based around shaving needs, there are now also aftercare products that are designed to calm, moisturise and soothe sensitised skin. The development of bespoke male therapy salons or clinics is also increasing the popularity of male skin care.

Skin colour

All skin types function in basically the same way, irrespective of gender, type or colour. The colour of skin is determined by pigmentation caused by the amount of melanin present. Melanin is constantly produced to maintain the skin's natural colour. There are, however, important differences in the skin characteristics of people from different ethnic groups.

Remember . . .

Don't rely on the client's diagnosis of their skin. Come to your own conclusions.

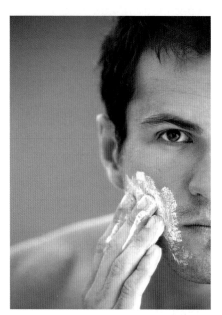

△ The daily shaving regime can leave male skin prone to infection and sensitivity

Remember . . .

Men tend to have firmer neck muscles, partly because shaving requires tightening the platysma and sternocleidomastoid muscle.

'White' skin

This type of skin has very little defence against ultraviolet light and burns easily. The group has problems with spots and blemishes, particularly through puberty, but may also have a tendency towards sensitivity and dryness during the twenties and thirties. The delicate nature of the skin means that premature signs of ageing occur in the early thirties. The pale tones of the skin are usually accompanied by fair, red or mid-brown hair.

'Yellow-toned' skin

This group has a tendency to skin displaying a mild oiliness, a consequence of which is a delay in the skin's ageing process. There is also more sudoriferous activity. The signs of ageing will generally start during the late thirties and early forties. This skin is prone to hyper-pigmentation and, therefore, any blemishes on this type of skin should be treated with care. Relatively minor skin damage (sometimes even expressing of comedones) can lead to hyper-pigmentation. Hair colour is usually mid- or dark-brown to black.

'Black' skins

This describes a range of dark skins that may vary in tone from light to dark with a wide variety of undertones. There is generally more sebaceous and sudoriferous activity in this group. The skin does not display signs of the ageing process until the forties are reached. The first sign can be greying of the hair. It is easy to mistake the sheen on dark skins as excessive oiliness. The sebaceous glands are larger, however, the darker the skin and more reflection of light occurs. This reflected light can be mistakenly diagnosed as too much oil. Another common mistake, particularly on dark Asian skins, is the identification of comedones on the centre 'T' panel. Close and careful examination will actually show the presence of dark facial hair around the nose and forehead, not comedones. It should be noted that black skins easily form keloid scars (an over-thickening of the skin) when damaged and caution should be exercised. Dermatosis papulosa nigra is a condition found on the cheeks and across the nose on the skin of both males and females of African origin. Black raised spots of varying sizes can be seen.

A lack of pigmentation, usually in irregular patches, is known as **vitiligo**. Dark irregular patches of pigmentation are known as **chloasma**. Corrective make-up techniques can be used to disguise both conditions.

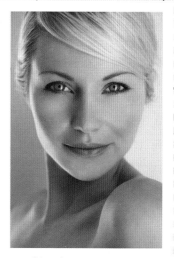

△ White skin

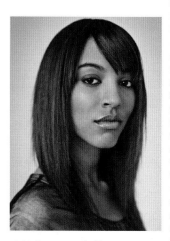

△ Yellow-toned skin

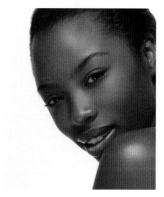

△ Black skin

General differences

1. Skin cancer is rare in darker skins as the pigmentation filters ultraviolet radiation.
2. The epidermis on dark skins is thicker.
3. Acne is rare in darker skins, despite having more sebaceous glands.
4. Paler skins are more prone to product-related allergies.
5. Dark-skinned people have a greater heat tolerance due to the increased number of sudoriferous glands.
6. Paler-skinned people have a greater tolerance to extremes of cold.
7. Black skin desquamates (naturally sheds surface cells) more easily than white skins.

Skin types

There are three main skin types:

1. oily
2. dry
3. combination.

Oily skin

Oily skin is usually coarse in texture and appears shiny, particularly around the nose, chin and forehead. Comedones and open pores will be present. The coarse texture is due to pores, which have been stretched by a previous blockage.

The skin will appear coarse and grainy. It will be moist and the epidermis will appear thick. It will be sallow (have a yellowish hue).

The cause of oily skin is an over-secretion of sebum, caused by hormonal imbalance, for example through the effects of puberty. Male skin has a greater tendency to be oily than female skin.

Dry skin

Dry skin appears taut. Fine lines may be evident and there may be flaky patches. There is a tendency for dilated capillaries: these are the permanent dilation of tiny capillary blood vessels. Blood has leaked from the capillaries leaving a spidery appearance across the cheekbones and around the nose (sometimes referred to as couperose tissue).

The skin will be fine in texture, sensitive and finely lined but will have a coarse surface. It is unlikely that the skin will have any comedones or open pores.

The causes of dry skin are:

- not enough sebum, with low fluid content in the upper layers of the skin
- excessive use of soaps and degreasing agents such as astringents
- exposure to sunlight without due care and attention
- extremes of temperature
- central heating, which will also have a drying effect.

Combination skin

The face has a central panel commonly referred to as the 'T' zone, which includes the forehead, nose and chin. In this skin type these areas will appear oily and congested, while the rest of the skin may be dry. This is one of the commonest skin types.

Mature skin

'Mature skin' describes skin that has started the ageing process. It lacks natural oil (sebum) and moisture. Character lines and wrinkles begin to form around the muscles of facial expression. There is some loss of underlying muscle tone and the subcutaneous (fatty) layer is shrinking.

Young skin

Skin treatments are becoming increasingly popular with a younger clientele. Young skin can present a variety of characteristics. Typically, it is firm to the touch, even in texture and colour with few blemishes. However, some young clients may have seborrhoeic conditions caused by the onset of puberty. This is readily identified by oily skin with enlarged pores and comedones.

Skin conditions

You will also need to recognise and differentiate between skin types and skin conditions. The following are skin conditions that you should be able to identify:

- sensitivity
- comedones
- milia
- dehydrated
- broken capillaries
- pustules
- papules
- open pores
- hyper-pigmentation
- dermatosis
- papulosa nigra
- pseudo-folliculitus
- keloids
- in-growing hair
- seborrhoea.

Sensitive

Sensitive skin is thin; it can become blotchy and is quickly irritated. It may be recognised by its high colour and warmth. There may be fine, dilated capillaries around the cheeks and nose.

Comedones

Comedones are also referred to as 'blackheads'.
Comedones are formed when sebum is trapped
within a pore; keratinised cells at the top of the pore
multiply and block off the exit from the sebaceous
gland. The surface of the blocked pore becomes black
due to oxidation (a chemical reaction when exposed
to air). When there is a build-up of sebum it may
cause the gland to erupt, which will allow sebum into
the lower levels of the skin. When this occurs, it leads
into the formation of a papule. If it becomes infected
it will become a pustule.

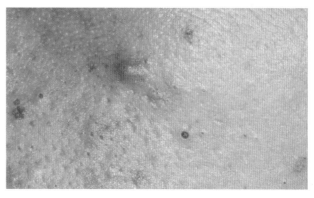

△ Comedones

Milia

Milia are small dots of sebum trapped within a blind duct. They are
common on dry skin types, particularly around the eye and cheek
area. They appear as white pearly nodules and are a clear indication
of a tendency towards dryness in that localised area. If the milia are
not established it may be possible to disperse with gentle massage. If,
however, there is a hardened mass then it will be necessary to remove
the milia using a sterile lance on pre-warmed skin. The tops of the milia
are split using the sterile lance and the sebum is lifted out. The skin is
then left to heal. Milia should never be expressed in the way that other
spots and blemishes may be. It would cause the client a great deal of
discomfort and may lead to permanent damage of the skin.

Dehydrated

Dehydrated skin lacks moisture and appears dull. It may become
itchy and tight. It may also have a smooth sheen but must not be
confused with oily skin. Any skin type can become dehydrated and it
should be considered a temporary condition.

Seborrhoea

Seborrhoeic conditions are caused by overactive sebaceous glands,
creating too much sebum on a skin that is already naturally oily. It is
a common condition in young people and is particularly associated
with the onset of puberty. It may also be the start of acne if it is
left untreated. The sebaceous secretions are increased and the skin
becomes grainy, with enlarged pores and comedones. The pores can
become blocked with the sebaceous secretions. As the hormones
settle down the condition subsides.

Couperose

Couperose refers to dilated capillaries found on the cheeks and around the nose. The walls of the capillaries lose their elasticity and remain permanently dilated, giving the skin a pronounced redness. Dilated capillaries appear on fine, sensitive, dry skin, or can be the result of years of exposure to extremes in temperature, i.e. cold winds and extreme heat. Spicy foods, alcohol and very hot drinks can also be contributing factors.

The 'danger triangle'

The danger triangle covers an area from the centre of the eyebrows at its tip, spreading outwards to the lower lip at its base. The client should be advised not to express spots around this area. Important blood vessels lie directly under the area and if the skin is damaged, they may be prone to bacterial infection. This may cause a condition known as **deep cavernous thrombosis**.

Ageing and the skin

The general signs of skin ageing usually appear around the age of 40 and increase with the onset of menopause. However, skin ages at different rates depending upon several factors. These include ethnic group, hereditary or health-related factors and the treatment the skin has received. Incorrect cleansing, harsh treatment, overexposure to ultraviolet light, smoking, poor nutrition, stress and extremes of temperature all play a part in the ageing process. Despite the best possible skin care regime, the underlying muscle structure tends to lose its tone and inevitably, a softening of the features occurs. In men, this softening occurs later than in women.

The softening of the skin and decrease in muscle tone creates character lines, particularly around the muscles of expression. There is a loss of elasticity in the skin and the expression lines become permanent. This effect is caused by the breakdown of collagen and elastin fibres within the dermis. It is the bundles of collagen that make the young skin supple and smooth.

The formation of wrinkles occurs along the lines of facial expression. (This is why wrinkles are often referred to as 'character lines'.) The regular contraction of the muscle forms the lines and, while the skin can stretch easily, it cannot contract in the same way as muscles do. Because of this, the skin loses its elasticity and the lines deepen.

A combination of these factors indicates skin ageing. The appearance of the skin reflects the underlying changes that are taking place.

The physical and physiological signs of ageing

The following features are signs of ageing skin:

1. Circulation slows down, so that waste is not removed as efficiently.
2. The elasticity of the skin decreases and character lines are formed.
3. There is an accelerated growth of fine lanugo (baby hair), particularly on the cheek and upper lip.
4. There is a decrease of skin permeability, leading to gradual dehydration.
5. There is an increase in hyper-pigmentation, for example chloasma.
6. The skin becomes noticeably thinner, especially around the eyes.
7. The capillary network can be more easily ruptured due to the inelasticity of the skin.
8. There is a decrease in sebum production.
9. There is a decrease in the activity of the sudoriferous glands.
10. The basal cell metabolic rate slows down.
11. There are open pores present.

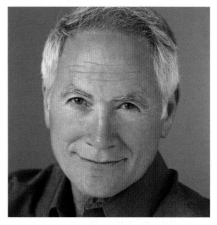

△ Ageing male skin

Analysing skin

It is essential that time is given for a full consultation and skin analysis. (You will find full details of how to carry out a client consultation and how to prepare a treatment plan in Chapter 1.)

Take care not to make a superficial diagnosis, but to ask appropriate questions, to look at the skin closely (preferably using a magnifying lamp) and to touch the skin to judge texture, temperature and muscle tone.

A common error is to fail to talk to the client about their skin care routine and their own perceptions of their skin. Correct analysis is like an investigation, which will require good detective work to find the clues and piece them together. It is important to gather as much information as possible. The client may be using inappropriate products, which are stripping the skin's protective acid mantle. This leaves the skin feeling taut, shiny and prone to infection and bacterial invasion. Clients may feel that their skin is oily because of the effect of using these products and will mistakenly use a product for oily skin, which will be too harsh and will exacerbate the problem.

The group who are most likely to fall into this trap are those going through puberty. Companies still specifically target this vulnerable group with products so harsh they can upset the delicate skin balance at an early age. Incorrect selection of products can also sensitise areas. If the product is too strong it can induce vascular response, which can result in the underlying capillaries stretching or dilating. In some cases the capillaries may rupture.

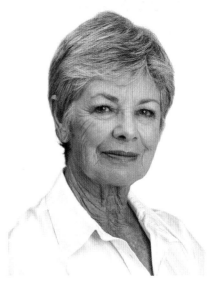

△ Ageing female skin

 Remember . . .

The longer the client uses inappropriate products, the more the body attempts to restore the acid mantle through increased secretions. This may lead to even more shine.

Remember . . .

The therapist must take care when analysing darker skins, as imperfections readily visible on a lighter skin may not be immediately noticeable.

Look out for clients who use sunbeds or those who have recently been exposed to sunlight. They will display signs of dehydrated skin, but this is likely to be a temporary state. A note should be made on the record card and subsequent changes recorded. The range of false or self-tanning products, while harmless, can prevent an effective diagnosis. It is possible, even weeks after application when the skin colour has normalised, to have open pores still stained with the product. The clear, liquid-type products are more likely to do this than the cream formulations. It may require a series of exfoliating treatments to remove the problem. Clients should be advised of the correct application of such products.

It is important not to rush the skin analysis and you should allow at least five minutes in the treatment schedule for a thorough analysis.

> **Remember . . .**
> You must treat the **current** condition of the skin. It is vitally important that you conduct a thorough analysis each time the client visits and note all changes.

Outcome 3: Improve and maintain skin condition

Products

You must be familiar with the range of available products in order to make the correct selection for each individual client. You need to know which products are required for each treatment.

Cleansers

A good cleansing medium should:

- remove make-up, dirt and grime effectively
- be suitable for the client's needs
- be easily applied and easily removed.

There are several types of cleansing preparation available: creams, milks, lotions and soapless cleansers and bars.

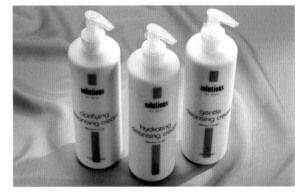
△ Cleansers

Creams

These are ideal for mature skin conditions and for dry skin types. They are designed to dissolve the pigmented waxes that are found in make-up products. They are usually water-in-oil emulsions and therefore do not soak into the skin. They have a cooling effect on the skin and are easily removed.

Milks

These are available in various consistencies. Milks are liquid and are mostly made from an oil-in-water emulsion. They are not very effective in removing a heavy make-up and are mainly used for superficial cleansing.

Lotions

Cleansing lotions are particularly useful on congested or oily skin. They leave very little residual oil on the skin after removal. However, they can be very strong so it is important that you know the product and that the skin has been accurately analysed.

Soapless cleansers (facial wash) and cleansing bars

These products are becoming the popular choice. They have changed the concept of cleansing, particularly in relation to the male market. Many clients will inform you that they prefer to use soap and water because they do not feel that their skin has been properly cleansed otherwise. This range of products now allows clients to use gentler complexion soap with water. Cleansing bars are made from soft soap but have a carefully balanced pH, which does not leave the skin feeling tight and shiny. They leave the skin at the correct pH balance and are particularly effective on seborrhoeic and acned skins. Soapless cleansers are made from laurel sulphates and soap bars contain potassium palmitate.

Toners

Toner is used at the conclusion of the cleansing treatment and prepares the skin for make-up application. It removes any product remaining on the skin after cleansing or the removal of a face mask. Toners dissolve surface oil and have an antibacterial effect. They may also have a refreshing effect, depending upon the type selected. Toner refines the pore size as it evaporates, leaving the skin prepared for an application of moisturiser.

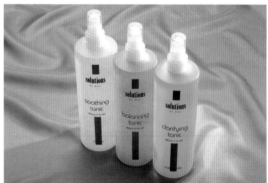

△ Toners

Toners are made from infusions of herbs and flowers, such as witch hazel, orange flower water, rose water, with small amounts of glycerine in distilled water. Other ingredients could include zinc sulphate and potassium sulphate. Toners also contain varying amounts of alcohol, which determines their strength. As with cleansing products, there is a wide range to choose from.

Skin tonics

Skin tonics include astringent solutions, which can be very strong. The amount of alcohol present and the active ingredient, for example witch hazel, will determine which tonic you select for a particular client's skin. If more than 20 per cent alcohol is present, use should be restricted to oily skin types. An astringent removes the surface oil and can disturb the skin's pH balance. It would therefore be contraindicated on blemished or sensitive conditions, as it could be an irritant. Witch hazel has astringent properties and should also be used with caution.

Skin fresheners and bracers

These have a much gentler effect. The action is a refreshing but mild one and these products are suitable for dehydrated, dry, delicate and mature skin conditions. They contain only small amounts of alcohol and do not remove oil as efficiently as their stronger counterparts. Dilutions of orange flower water or rose water are examples.

Eye make-up remover

These specially designed products need to have certain characteristics. They must not be heavy in texture, highly perfumed or excessively creamy, but must be effective in removing densely pigmented waterproof products. They are based on a mineral oil such as liquid paraffin or soft waxes such as paraffin wax.

Exfoliants

Exfoliants aid desquamation (the skin's natural shedding of surface cells). They smooth the surface of the skin, prepare the skin for further treatment and stimulate the blood and lymphatic flow, thereby aiding the elimination and absorption of waste products. All skin types benefit from using exfoliating products.

They fall into two categories: pore grains or facial scrubs, and peeling creams.

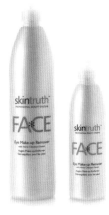

△ Eye make-up remover

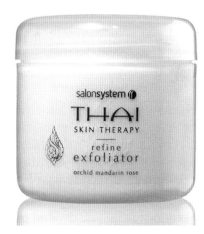

△ Exfoliants

Pore grains or facial scrubs

These are made up of detergent and small grains of almond shell, oatmeal and pumice or ground fruit kernels. They have a detergent cleansing action and when gently massaged over the skin remove surface adhesions, leaving the skin soft and smooth. Frequent use should be restricted to those with an oily skin. Those wishing to refine and tone can use them, but not often.

Peeling creams

These are based on clay and other natural biological ingredients. They are applied to the skin and allowed to dry. They can then be lifted off the skin or gently rolled using friction to slough off dead cells. These are effective on all skin types, particularly those conditions that require gentle treatment.

Massage mediums

Massage can be carried out using a variety of mediums. Most, however, will be based on either a cream or an oil formulation, which may have added ingredients to suit the individual needs of the client's skin. Mediums contain mineral oils, beeswax or paraffin wax and a large percentage of distilled water.

Moisturisers

Moisturisers comprise an oil and water emulsion. They can be presented in either a cream or liquid form.

They readily evaporate from the skin, leaving a fine film of **emollient**. An emollient is a substance that softens the skin by increasing its water content and keeps it soft by slowing moisture loss. The gentle evaporation produces a cooling sensation, which temporarily refines the pores and leaves the skin feeling soft and supple. The moisturiser leaves an aqueous film on the skin, which is ready for make-up to be applied.

Moisturisers also supplement the skin's water content by attracting water from the atmosphere by the means of a **humectant** (water-attracting) product. Glycerol, sorbitol and glycol are examples of humectant materials.

All skin types require the use of a moisturiser. Moisturisers prolong the appearance of make-up: they prepare the skin for the application of foundation by smoothing the surface. They also protect the skin from the pigments in the make-up. Moisturiser should always be worn even if make-up is not; it will protect the skin from the elements and pollutants in the atmosphere.

The choice of moisturiser will depend on skin type.

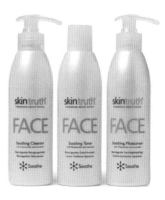

△ Cleanser, toner and moisturiser

Remember . . .

Always check the content of products, particularly toners, to assess their suitability. Manufacturers are legally required to list product ingredients.

Specialist skin products

Eye creams, gels and lotions

These specialist products are used to temporarily minimise the appearance of 'crow's feet' and character lines; they may also have a temporary tightening effect. The creams are formulated in the same way as moisturisers. They contain cocoa butter and vegetable oils. Petroleum jelly and a high wax content are avoided as they can cause puffiness around the delicate eye area. Eye gels often contain astringents, such as witch hazel. They have a cooling and firming effect on the delicate tissue surrounding the eyes. Lotions are similar to gels. They are usually applied onto a dampened pad of cotton wool and placed over the eyes. They produce a soothing, refreshing effect on the eyes.

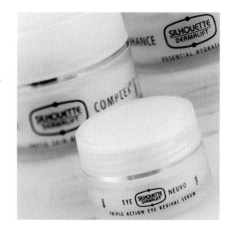

△ Eye cream

Acne products

There are certain products that are now recognised as irritants to acne. These are products that contain petroleum jelly, lanolin and some vegetable oils. There are specifically designed lotions, which are spirit-based in a chemical formulation to prevent infections. The use of soapless cleansers facial wash and cleansing bars, as described earlier in this chapter, are particularly effective on acned skins.

Neck creams

Neck creams are rich moisturising creams that may contain other active ingredients, such as collagen. The action of these rich formulations is primarily to soften, tighten and tone the skin.

Lip balms

These are a range of specifically designed products for softening and protecting the lips. They form a protective film and prevent moisture loss. They are formulated from varying mixtures of oils and waxes and may contain colour pigments.

Night creams

Night creams are emollients and are generally heavier and thicker than other skin creams. They are usually formulated from a range of products including animal fats, vegetable oils, cocoa butter, olive and almond oils and beeswax. The action of a night cream is to soften and hydrate the skin. Most products contain a humectant.

Preparation for treatment

Reception

The appearance of the salon and the manner in which the client is greeted are of vital importance. It is essential that there is a professional atmosphere at all times, in which the client feels comfortable and uninhibited. If the atmosphere at the reception is professional, it will instil confidence in the client.

Trolley

The trolley should be clean and tidy and contain all the products needed to carry out the required service or treatment. You will also require a magnifying light.

You should also have ready and prepared:

- the client's record card or treatment plan
- a protective headband
- towels
- a hand mirror.

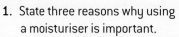

Activity

1. State three reasons why using a moisturiser is important.
2. List two qualities of an eye gel, cream or lotion.

Facials are performed on the client in a reclining or semi-reclining position. The treatment chair or couch should be capable of adapting to meet the requirements of the treatment. The height of the couch is important both for client comfort and for the beauty therapist. Back problems are common among therapists and therefore it is important to prevent such problems by correct positioning. The beauty therapist normally works from behind the client and may be seated or standing to carry out the treatment. There should be pillows and covering available for the client during treatment to provide warmth and to promote relaxation. If you are working in a cubicle, it should have screening, which will ensure complete privacy from the rest of the salon.

You should have a steamer and brush cleanse unit available.

Preparing the client

The client should be given very clear instructions about what to do. Hair and clothing should be protected. You should ask the client to remove all necklaces and earrings and to put them somewhere safe. You should ask the client to remove their outer clothing and offer them a robe or towel to protect their modesty. The client will expect privacy. When the client is settled on the chair or couch, ask them to remove or slip down any underwear straps that will inhibit the facial treatment.

The client's head should be slightly elevated and their hair should be protected using a headband or other suitable covering. Finally, wash your hands. You are now ready to commence treatment.

The facial

The facial is carried out in stages:

- superficial cleansing
- deep cleansing
- extraction (if required)
- facial massage
- application of face mask
- removal of mask and prepare client to leave

Cleansing

Cleansing usually comprises two stages. The first stage is to remove surface oil and make-up. The second stage is to deep-cleanse the skin. The analysis of the skin type will be carried out after the superficial cleanse. You may be expected to conduct cleansing in a

> ### Equipment checklist
>
> You should have the following items on your trolley:
>
> ✔ cotton wool – dry and dampened – to remove cleansing products and for applying products such as toners
> ✔ tissues to blot the skin and to remove cleansing products
> ✔ a selection of bowls for holding dry cotton wool and dampened cotton wool
> ✔ spatulas to remove creams and products from containers, and to mix face mask formulation
> ✔ a selection of skincare products. Always remember to replace lids, use spatulas to remove products or in the case of liquid products pour into the palm of your hand
> ✔ face mask brush to apply formulation (do not remove from steriliser until ready to be used)
> ✔ facial sponges to remove product, to remove face mask formulation
> ✔ a covered waste receptacle.

Health and safety

Always ensure that your client sees you wash your hands. This will instil confidence and demonstrate good hygienic practice.

Activity

Compare facial record cards with a fellow student. Design a record card for your own use. (See also Chapter 1.)

routine that has been adopted as the house style in your salon or training institute. However, the routine will be based on common principles and practices.

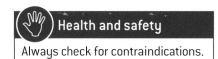

Health and safety

Always check for contraindications.

Procedure for a superficial cleanse

This is always carried out, whether the client is wearing make-up or not.

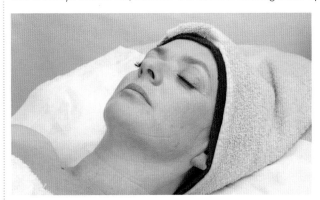

1   Ask the client to close their eyes and select a suitable cleansing product.

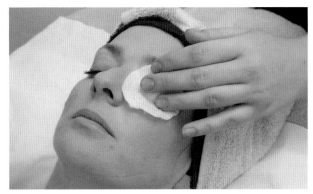

2.   Apply the selected product using small gentle circular movements. Avoid exerting too much pressure over the eye. Apply to upper lid, lashes and under the eye.

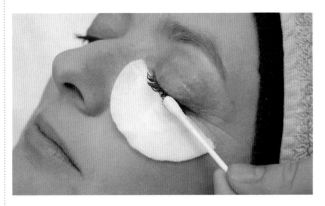

3.   If the client is wearing mascara, place a dampened pad of cotton wool under the lashes and apply eye make-up remover with either fingers or cotton bud until the mascara has dissolved.

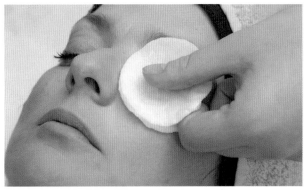

4.   Remove the loosened make-up and cleanser using dampened cotton-wool pads. Ensure you support the skin as you work.

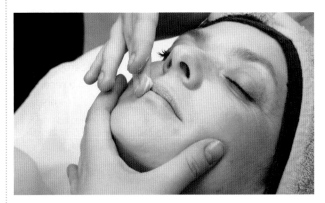

5.   Select a suitable product for the lip area. Apply using gentle circular movements.

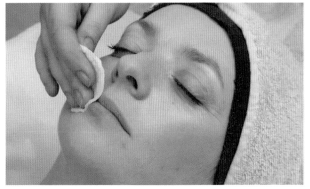

6.   Remove the loosened lip cosmetic and cleanser with dampened cotton wool. Blot the lips using a tissue.

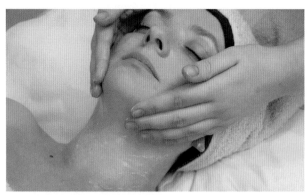

7. Select a suitable product for the face and neck. Apply the selected product using light, upward movements on the cheeks, forehead and neck.

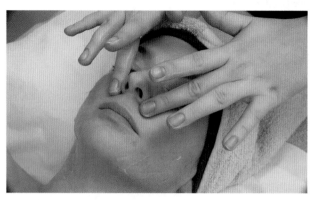

8. Work the product into the folds around the nose and chin.

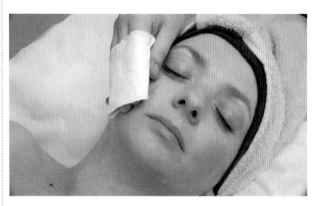

9. Remove the cleansing product by initially blotting with soft facial tissues. Tissues are used for their absorbency when using greasy or oil-based products. Dampened cotton wool may be used to remove water-soluble debris from the skin. The skin is clean when the cotton wool shows no soiling.

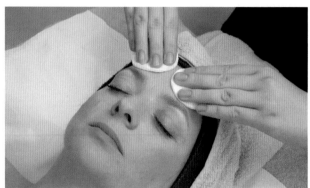

10. Apply mild toner, using dampened cotton-wool pads.

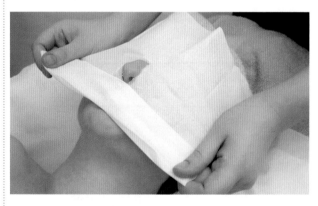

11. Blot the skin using a facial tissue. Place a hole in the centre for the nose and blot. Then fold the tissue down onto the neck and blot again.

Remember . . .
Always cleanse the lip and eye areas first. This will prevent the spreading of densely pigmented make-up over the face and neck.

You should allow at least five minutes in the treatment schedule for superficial cleansing.

Deep cleanse

You should carry out an analysis of the skin before commencing the deep cleanse. Analysis should be carried out at each visit and you should not simply accept an earlier diagnosis.

The aim of the deep cleanse is to:

- soften and loosen comedones and other skin blockages
- increase circulation
- remove any remaining make-up preparation
- increase desquamation.

It is important that you adapt movements and pressure according to the client's needs. Each movement should be repeated at least six times, unless otherwise stated.

Procedure for a deep cleanse

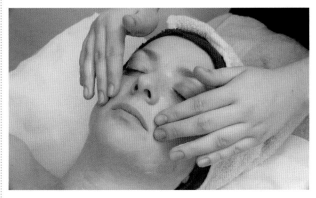

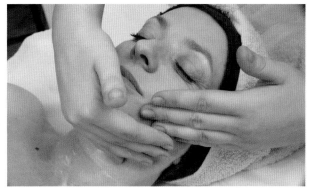

1. Select a suitable cleansing product. Place hands at the base of the neck. Work upwards over the platysma muscle to the jaw (mandible bone), using a light, flowing movement. Sweep across the mandible. Apply a light sweeping stroke down either side of the neck, following the sternocleidomastoid muscles.

2. Using a light sweeping movement work along the mandible from one side to the other.

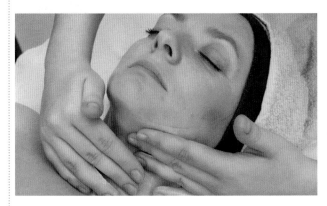

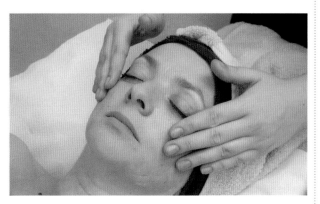

3. Starting at the chin, use small circular movements, moving slowly up to the sides of the nose. Glide along the cheeks (zygomatic muscle and zygomatic bone) without exerting pressure, and back to the chin

4. Slide hands along each cheekbone and up to the forehead.

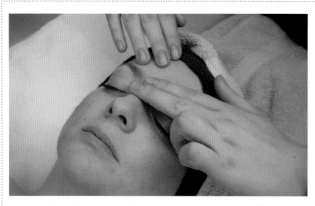

5. Gently slide the hands down over the nose and back along the cheeks.

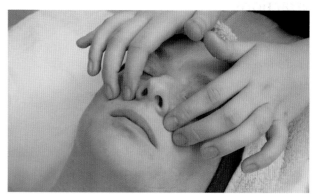

6. Using small circular movements work around the base of the nose.

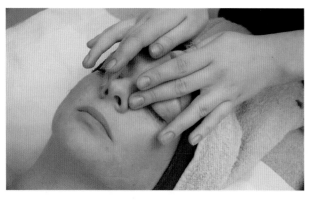

7. Slide the fingers down the top and sides of the nose, using alternating strokes.

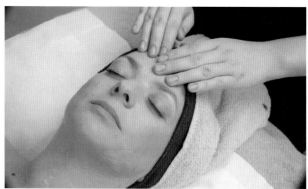

8. Using large circular movements, work across the forehead, slide across the cheekbones and back up to the forehead.

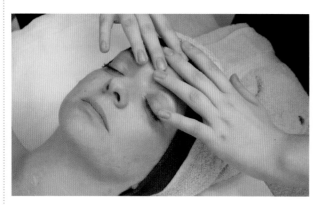

9. Using the pads of the fingers, perform a scissor or zigzag movement across the forehead, working from one side to the other.

Always conclude a facial routine by applying slight pressure at the temples, which indicates the end of the routine.

Remove the cleansing product by blotting the surface with tissues then using dampened cotton-wool pads. It is vitally important to ensure all trace of cleanser is removed. You should check around the hairline, under the jaw and in the folds of the skin. You may then apply toner.

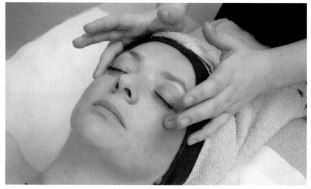

10. Stroke around each eye using the ring finger and gently perform a lifting movement, three times under each eyebrow.

You should allow at least 10 minutes for deep cleansing in the treatment schedule.

 Remember...

Always work the chosen cleansing medium between both hands to warm the product and to provide slip.

Extractions

After a deep cleanse, skin blockages should be extracted.

Comedones

Comedones will have been loosened following a deep cleanse. Extraction of skin blockages can take place at this point. The skin should be warmed, using hot dampened cotton-wool pads, a steamer or heated towels.

Steaming

The steamer should be filled in accordance with manufacturer's instructions. It is usual to fill the steamer using distilled water. This prevents the element furring up with limescale, which can cause the unit to spit boiling water.

The duration of treatment will vary between 3 and 20 minutes. Positioning of the unit will depend upon skin type:

- 25cm (10in) for oily skin
- 30cm (12in) for normal skin
- 40cm (15in) for dry skin.

If the client has dilated capillaries or very sensitive skin you should avoid stimulating the circulation. In these cases, steaming would not be indicated.

Most steamers have an ozone facility within the unit. The use of ozone is particularly beneficial to those who have a blemished skin. It is drying and has an antibacterial effect. There are restrictions governing the use of ozone, however, and it is important that you check with your local health authority before offering the facility. The ozone option is not required for warming the skin.

Heated towels

A towel can be soaked in hot water, wrung out and wrapped around the face, leaving a space for the nostrils to enable the client to breathe.

When steaming has been completed, the skin should be blotted. Extractions should be carried out using fingers covered with tissue or a comedone extractor. If the fingers are used, a rolling, pressing motion should be used until the comedone is expressed. If a comedone remover is used then gentle, even pressure should be applied over the blockage. You should work with caution to prevent exerting too much pressure, which may cause bruising.

Milia

Milia should also be removed following steaming. However, they should never be expressed by exerting pressure. They are usually formed into a hard pearly lump when they have become established. Following steaming, the milia is gently exposed using a sterile lance. The lump can be lifted out. Great care must be taken to prevent infection.

Health and safety

You must make all the precautionary safety checks before using a steaming unit:
- Ensure that the unit is not overfilled.
- Make sure that it is on a safe, solid base.
- Place the unit at the correct distance for the skin type.
- There should be no trailing wires or flexes.
- Check that the vapour is evenly emitted before directing towards the client.

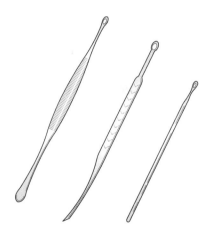

△ Types of comedone extractor

Activity

1. State the differences between a superficial cleanse and a deep cleanse.
2. What precautions should be taken when carrying out extractions?

Facial massage

The benefits of massage

1. Cell division in the epidermis is optimised, resulting in an improvement in the appearance of the skin.

2. As the epidermis is being replaced frequently, the skin feels soft and smooth.

3. Skin colour is improved due to the increase in local blood circulation.

4. The collagen and elastin fibres maintain their elasticity, improving skin tone.

5. Skin texture is improved by the increased health of the epidermis and dermis.

6. Puffiness around the eyes is reduced due to the removal of excess tissue fluid.

7. Fine lines are reduced by the increased activity of the epidermis.

8. Dark circles around the eyes are reduced by the increase in blood circulation and waste removal.

9. Removal of waste products from muscle tissue prevents fatigue and gives a subsequent improvement in muscle tone.

10. Continued good lymph drainage combats the signs of ageing, resulting in the client looking young for longer.

11. Acned or spotty skins are improved as there is a reduction in the risk of infection, so fewer spots result.

12. Skin healing is improved so scarring is less likely and there may be an improvement in scars already present.

13. If spots or other infections occur, the healing process will be quicker.

14. Skin appendages benefit, in other words, hair and nails grow stronger and more quickly

All good facial treatments should be aimed at improving the skin tone and texture, firming the underlying muscles and tissue structure. A good facial massage will cleanse, tone and refine the skin, strengthen the muscles and relax the client. The stimulation of the circulation will increase cell regeneration and maintain the correct oil and fluid balance of the skin. By understanding the classification of massage movements and their effects, the therapist can tailor a massage to suit the need of the individual client.

The facial massage is based around three types of movements – **effleurage**, **petrissage** and **tapotement**.

Each of these movements has a specific purpose. You may be expected to learn a routine that has been designed as the salon or training institute's house style. Whatever routine is adopted, it will be based on these three massage movements.

Effleurage

Massage always starts with effleurage. This is a series of light, continuous stroking movements that are designed to relax the client and are used to link up other movements and manipulations within the routine.

Effects of effleurage:

- increases blood circulation
- increases lymphatic drainage
- aids desquamation
- promotes relaxation.

Petrissage

Petrissage is a series of compression movements that include kneading, knuckling, lifting, rolling and pinching. The movements are intermittent and deeper than those employed in effleurage. They are used over soft tissue.

Effects of petrissage:

- increases blood circulation
- improves lymphatic drainage
- improves muscle tone
- increases mitosis (the process by which cells reproduce)
- aids desquamation.

Tapotement

Tapotement movements are applied in a light, quick, stimulating manner. They include movements such as slapping and tapping. They should be applied in a continuous rhythmic series of strokes.

Effects of tapotement:

- stimulates the nerve endings
- increases blood circulation
- improves lymphatic drainage
- tones the skin.

The repetition of movements will depend upon the needs of the individual client. The routine should take between 15 and 20 minutes of the recommended 60 minutes' duration for a facial. The selection of a suitable massage medium will depend upon client need, but will usually be a cream or oil-based product.

Procedure for a facial massage

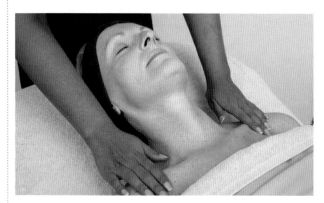

1. Place fingers on the pectoral muscle at the base of the sternum. Slide across and around the shoulder (deltoid muscle). Turn the hands and slide back along the trapezius muscle to the neck.

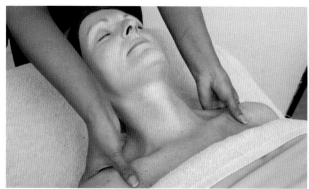

2. Slide the fingers to the deltoid and use circular thumb-kneading along the trapezius to the top of the spine. Slide back and repeat.

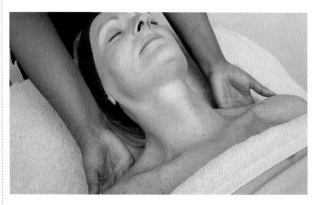

3. Place the fingers on trapezius, at deltoid, and proceed with deep circular finger kneading.

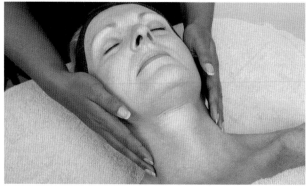

4. Place the fingers at the back of the neck and vibrate up the back of the neck.

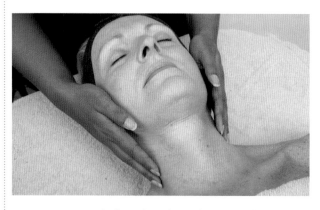

5. Carry out circular kneading along platysma and sternocleidomastoid.

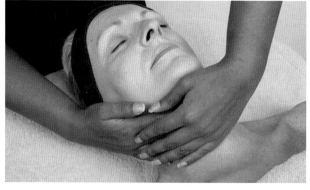

6. Cup hands one above the other, place on the sternum, slide up the left side of the neck, across the jawline and down the right side.

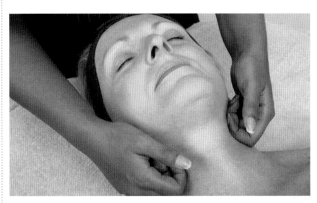

7. Bend the fingers and, using the knuckles, knuckle up and down the neck area.

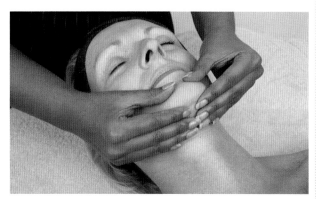

8. Place the thumbs on the centre of the chin. With first fingers placed under the jaw, slide the thumbs firmly down the platysma.

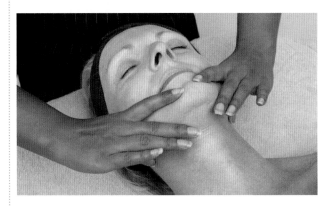

9. Bring the first fingers onto the chin, slide along the jawline to the ear, change and slide down to the chin.

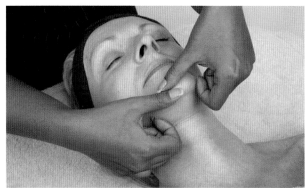

10. Place the thumbs one above the other on the chin and proceed with circular kneading along the jawline to the ear and back. Reverse the circling and knead to the other ear.

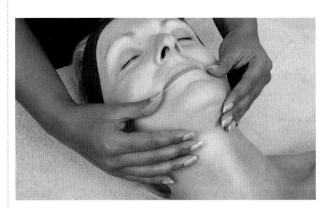

11. Place the thumbs at the corners of the mouth and lift the mouth with a flicking upward movement.

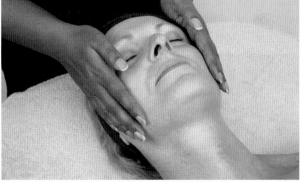

12. Clasp the fingers under the chin, turn hands, unclasp and slide the hands up the face towards the forehead.

13. Place the hands on the forehead at the temples and stroke upwards from the eyebrow to the hairline from left to right.

14. Using the ring finger, draw a figure of eight around the eyes.

15. Repeat movement 12.

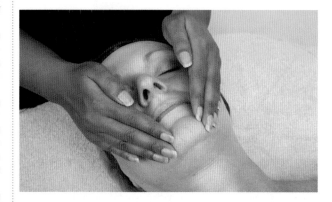

16. Carry out circular kneading from the chin.

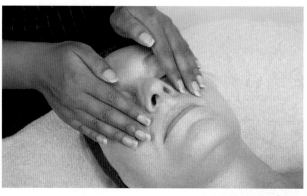

17. Carry out circular kneading from the nose.

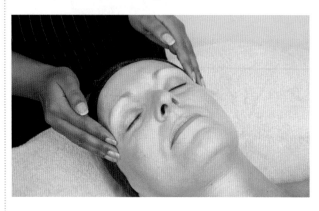

18. Carry out circular kneading from the temples.

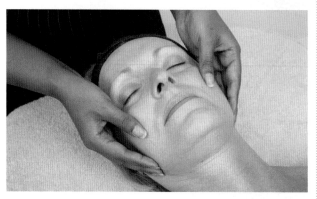

19. With thumbs on the cheeks, carry out deep circular kneading to the cheek area.

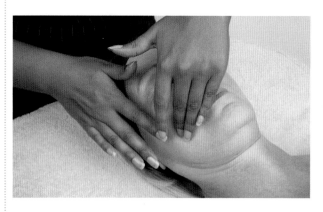

20. From left to right, tap along the jawline.

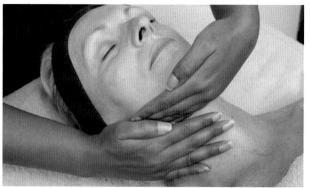

21. Cup the hands and lift the masseter muscle on each side of the face and release.

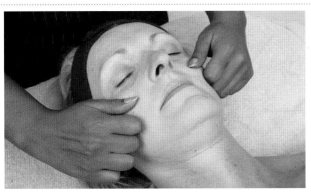

22. Using thumb and forefinger, proceed with a deep rolling pinching movement to the cheek area.

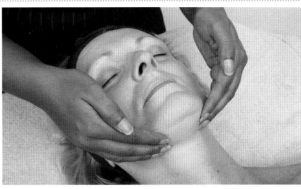

23. Place the pads of the fingers on the mandible and proceed to work towards the ear, using a lifting movement.

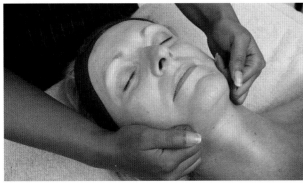

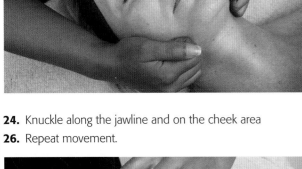

24. Knuckle along the jawline and on the cheek area

26. Repeat movement.

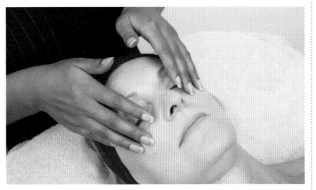

25. Using the palm of the hand, slap along the jawline from ear to ear, lifting the muscles.

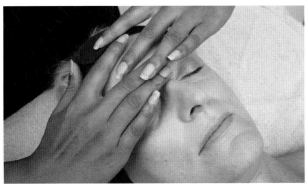

27. Scissor movement to forehead.

29. Repeat movement 13.

30. Repeat movement 1.

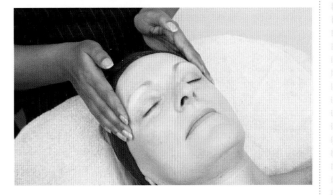

28. Using pads of the fingers, tap gently around the eye area.

31. Slide the hands across to the temples and apply slight pressure to signify the end of the routine.

Face masks

Face masks complement the beneficial effects of the cleansing routine. They have deep-cleansing qualities and may contain active ingredients to hydrate and soothe the skin.

Face masks are based upon different formulations, which vary according to the ingredients used and the action required. A sound knowledge of the actions and effects of the basic ingredients will allow you to formulate preparations to suit the need of the individual. The timings for face masks within the 60-minute treatment schedule will vary depending on the type selected. A face mask doesn't usually take more than 20 minutes.

The mask is generally applied at the end of the facial treatment. However, some facial routines may specify the application of the mask at a specific point, designed to achieve maximum benefit.

There are several types of mask. They can be formulated to suit all skin types. They are:

- **setting masks**. These masks dry on the skin. They include clay-based masks and peel-off masks (used on oily skin to remove excess oil and deep cleanse)
- **non-setting masks**. These masks do not set but are cooling and soothing on the skin. They include biological and clay-based masks, to which oil is added
- **specialised masks**. These are masks that include paraffin wax, oil masks, gel masks, thermal masks and cream masks (used on specific conditions such as very dry skin).

Different face masks have different beneficial effects on the skin. They may:

- soothe and calm
- soften
- improve desquamation
- moisturise
- deep cleanse
- have a slight bleaching effect
- remove excess oil
- stimulate circulation.

General contraindications to face masks are as follows:

- infections like herpes simplex or impetigo
- recent scar tissue
- cuts and abrasions
- highly sensitive or sensitised skin, for example through sunburn.

The mask should be applied onto skin that has been thoroughly cleansed. In some cases, the mask may be applied over the massage medium when carrying out specialised treatments. However, the skin will normally be completely free of all traces of product. Skin analysis and inspection was discussed earlier in this chapter. It is very important that you examine the skin thoroughly to enable you to make an informed decision about the most suitable formulation for the client.

Activity

1. What adaptations could you make to the facial massage routine for a client with dry or sensitive skin?

2. How much time should you allow for the facial massage?

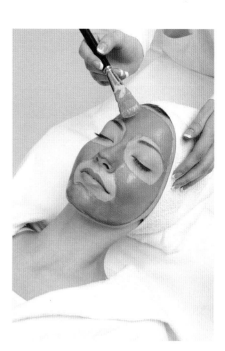

△ Applying a face mask

The mask should be mixed with a spatula, not a brush. This will ensure an even distribution of ingredients. If a brush is used to mix, the neck of the brush becomes clogged with the formula. Masks can be applied with a brush or spatula, depending on type. They should be applied evenly, especially clay-based masks mixed to a setting formula. If they are unevenly applied they can evaporate too quickly, giving a burning, itching sensation on the skin.

Soothing, refreshing eye pads made from witch hazel or water can be applied.

> **Remember...**
>
> You should ask the client whether or not they like eye pads, as some may feel claustrophobic and prefer to have their eyes open.

Setting masks

Clay-based masks

Clay masks are made from a variety of clay and powdered mineral ingredients. The basic ingredients are:

- **Calamine** – this is a pale pink powder. It is ideal for sensitive skin conditions. It soothes inflamed skin, calms high colour and has a very gentle effect. It is usually mixed with orange flower water or rose water.
- **Magnesium carbonate** – this is a bright white powder. It has slightly astringent properties and is particularly effective on skins with isolated blemishes. It is commonly used in conjunction with other powders because of its effects.
- **Kaolin** – this is a dull white powder, stronger in effect than magnesium carbonate. It has a drawing effect, which is deep cleansing. It increases blood circulation and removal of waste products.
- **Fuller's earth** – this is a greyish-green powder. It is the strongest of all the powders and is usually mixed with witch hazel. Fuller's earth should only ever be used on oily or seborrhoeic conditions. It induces a fast vascular response and is very stimulating. It aids desquamation and has a deep cleansing action.

> **Remember...**
>
> Oil can be warmed prior to mixing. This is particularly good for clients with a mature, dehydrated skin.

A combination of these ingredients is mixed with an active liquid ingredient to form a paste. These liquids are as important as the powders and, therefore, should be prescribed with care. They include:

- **Witch hazel** – an astringent, which has a stimulating and drying effect. Used on oily skins.
- **Rose water** – a mild tonic effect. Used on dry skins.
- **Distilled water** – used on normal skin.
- **Orange flower water** – similar to rose water, but slightly stimulating.

Vegetable oils have a softening and moisturising effect. They are particularly good for mature skins and dehydrated conditions. A few drops can be added to the clay mask.

The face mask paste is mixed to a smooth, even consistency and applied to the face and neck using a sterilised brush. Care should be taken to avoid the hairline, septum, mouth and eyes. As the mask dries the moisture in the formulation evaporates and has a tightening effect on the skin. Impurities are brought to the surface of the skin and the clay powder absorbs excess oil and removes surface adhesions.

Once the mask has dried, it should be removed using warm water and sponges. Once all trace of the mask has been removed, the skin should be wiped over with dampened cotton wool.

Peel-off masks

Peel-off masks have become increasingly popular. They are not as strong as clay-based masks. Peel-off masks fall into two categories: those based upon waxes (paraffin wax), gums, latex and plastic resins, and those that are gel-based. They may be water-based or, for quicker drying, may contain alcohol. They are applied in their liquid state and left to dry on the skin.

This group of masks is easier to apply than clay masks and are gentler on the skin. The wax- and latex-based products form a seal on the skin, which induces heat and prevents moisture escaping from the skin enabling the moisturising product to be more readily absorbed. The effect on the skin is cleansing and, through the creation of heat, promotes an **erythema** (slight redness). They are suitable for all clients except those who are very sensitive or who have a couperose skin.

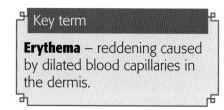

Gel-based masks are cooling and slightly astringent. Peel-off masks are designed to be lifted off the skin when dry, taking softened surface adhesions off the skin.

Non-setting masks

Biological masks

Non-setting masks are usually cooling and refreshing on the skin. They have different effects depending on the type of preparation used. Biological masks are based on wholly natural ingredients such as herbs, vegetables, fruits, flowers and plant extracts. They are applied in a light film over the skin. This does not harden but becomes firm and drier depending on the binding agent, for example honey.

Natural ingredients can be sliced, chopped up and pulped and placed directly onto the skin or onto a gauze to aid removal. The ingredients may be mixed with honey, cream, egg white or yoghurt. This will lessen the astringent effect of some ingredients.

Most soft fruits have an acidic reaction on the skin and should be used with care. The enzymatic action of some fruits can soften and remove dead skin cells, but may also sensitise.

Herbs and vegetables can stimulate, balance and tone the skin. Plants can stimulate the circulation. Egg yolk whipped with honey has a moisturising effect. Whipped egg white or yoghurt has a drawing, tightening effect on the skin.

Specialised masks

These can be both setting and non-setting. They include:

- **Specialised cream masks** – these are usually part of a professional range that provides retailing opportunities for the therapist.

- **Paraffin wax** – an occlusive mask, particularly effective on mature skin types. Specialised products may be applied to the skin prior to application to enhance the effect.
- **Prescription masks** – usually gel based. These are a series of active products from which tailor-made masks can be created to suit the needs of the individual.
- **Thermal masks** – these masks either generate heat or require an external heat source.

Heat-generating masks are formed from a paste that is applied over a specialised cream or ampoule. The paste sets and generates heat as it hardens. The mask is lifted away in a solid form on cooling.

Heat-reliant masks are preparations that include the use of warmed oil to mix and bind formulations. A gauze is placed over the application and an infrared lamp may be used to further increase the warmth.

Outcome 4: Provide aftercare advice

This chapter has discussed treatments designed to improve the condition of the facial skin. To ensure optimum effectiveness of the treatment, the client should be advised on how to treat the skin between visits for professional facials, thus maintaining the condition.

This advice should cover three aspects:

1. General care of skin at home.
2. Treatment of skin following professional treatment.
3. Other factors.

General care of skin

The client may have been carrying out a particular skincare regime for years. Their routine may require adapting or changing completely. It is quite common to discover that a client's skin care routine is actually the cause of the skin problem. The therapist should ensure that clients are aware that their skin type will not always stay the same.

It is very important that the therapist is knowledgeable about the product range available in the salon. You should read all available information, as this will increase your confidence when advising your clients. Most salons stock a professional range. This means that it is a range that can only be purchased through approved salons. The client will see a better result if the products used in the facial treatment are complemented by professionally prescribed products to use at home. (You will find more about offering clients additional products in Chapter 17.)

Treatment of skin

Aftercare advice should also relate to special treatment of the skin following salon treatment. Clients should be advised that any erythema caused by treatment will quickly disperse and is temporary. They should also be told what activities and products to avoid. This will depend on the type of treatment. However, it is wise to recommend that the client avoids using sunbeds,

Activity

1. List the uses and effects of a Fuller's earth mask.
2. What is a thermal mask?
3. What is an occlusive mask?
4. What precautions should be taken when using biological masks?

Activity

1. Working with a colleague, design a face mask that contains natural ingredients.
2. List the formulation and the effect on the skin.

Remember...

If you are working in an assisting role you should ask the senior therapist if the finished effect needs any further treatment.

sunbathing, extremes of temperature or strong-scented products. Some facial treatments may carry on working for up to 24 hours and it is important for the client not to irritate the area, avoiding the application of make-up for several hours after treatment. Rough handling of the skin or using harsh, inappropriate products will only serve to undo the positive effects of the facial.

Other factors

A professional beauty therapy treatment will undoubtedly benefit and improve most skin conditions. It is important, though, that you consider other factors that may be the underlying cause of a skin problem or may influence the predicted outcome of the treatment.

Other factors that affect the condition of the skin include:

- stress
- smoking
- diet
- exercise
- sun exposure.

Stress

Stress is thought to be one of the main causes of premature ageing. It can affect the client's sleeping pattern, lead to depression, weight loss or gain and sallow, dull-looking skin. Relaxation activities such as massage could be suggested to help improve the condition.

Smoking

Smoking will also have an adverse effect on the skin. It can reduce the amount of oxygen reaching the skin, as the blood is polluted by the gases inhaled during smoking. This affects the oxygen reaching the cells and results in dryness and dilated capillaries. It will also cause the formation of premature lines around the lips. Of course, it has other very harmful effects on the rest of the body too!

Diet

Diet also contributes to healthy skin. There has been a culture of change in dietary habits over the last 20 years. There has been an increase in food allergies, fad dieting and eating disorders. Eating patterns have changed, with a greater reliance on snacks and processed foods. The effects of this change are evident in the increase in nutrition-related problems. A healthy body requires a balanced diet that contains a mixture of proteins, fats and carbohydrates. Fresh fruit and vegetables are daily essentials.

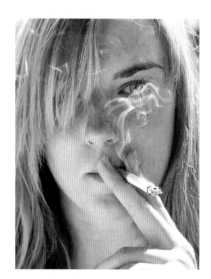

△ Smoking has an adverse effect on the skin and can cause the formation of premature lines around the lips.

Exercise

Exercise also affects the skin. If the client has a healthy, well-balanced diet and takes moderate regular exercise, they will look and feel better. They will have more energy and be less prone to tiredness and tension.

The therapist must understand the limitations of the professional salon treatment. It will help to improve the condition of the skin, but for how long and to what extent depends on other factors affecting the health of the client.

The condition of the skin is also affected by exposure to the sun.

Ultraviolet light and the skin

The effects of the sun and sunbeds on the skin are well documented. Articles appear each year in journals and magazines just before the summer holidays or the ski season, offering wise precautionary advice. It is important that, as a beauty therapist, you understand the long-term effects of exposure to sunlight.

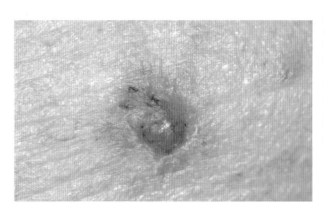

△ Ultraviolet rays are damaging to the skin and can cause skin cancer

Ultraviolet rays are damaging to the skin, although some types are more harmful than others. The amount of damage can be directly attributed to the length of time spent exposed to the rays. Damage can range from mild irritation to blistering, swelling and inflammation. Continued exposure to sunlight can cause permanent damage to the skin. The most severe and increasingly common danger is that of melanoma (skin cancer). Fair-skinned people are particularly prone to melanoma.

The colour of skin, as discussed earlier in this chapter, can be attributed to the amount of melanin present in the skin. The darker the skin, the higher the melanin content. Melanin protects the skin from the effects of sunlight. Therefore, darker skins are less prone to conditions such as melanoma and have more tolerance to ultraviolet exposure. It should be noted, however, that all skin types suffer from the effects of overexposure: excessive dryness and premature formation of wrinkles.

The skin becomes drier following exposure to ultraviolet light and eventually the collagen fibres, which give the skin its elasticity, break up. This is exactly the same process that occurs during ageing. It is the prolonged exposure that speeds up this process, resulting in premature ageing. The effects of ultraviolet exposure cannot be reversed.

Psoriasis and acne are the only conditions that can be improved through controlled exposure to sunlight. This works by causing the surface of the skin to peel slightly, unblocking the sebaceous glands and increasing desquamation (removal of skin cells).

Sunscreens

The client should always be advised to use a sunscreen. Products will indicate a sun protection factor (SPF) number on the packaging.

The SPF indicates the amount of protection provided by the product. Total sun block, for example, will range from SPF 60 to 95. Most skin foundations have an SPF of 15 to 20. The choice of sunscreen will depend on the skin type, the activity (sunbathing, swimming, skiing) and the area of the world in which the client will be exposed to the sun.

The following provides a guide on the level of SPF that is needed for each skin type:

- very fair, freckled skin which burns easily – use SPF 30+
- fair to medium skin – use SPF 20+
- skin that tans easily – use SPF 15+
- children must be always be protected using SPF 50+.

The area of the world where the skin will be exposed to the sun is another important factor to take into account. The sun is strongest in very hot climates (the tropics and places like Australia). The Mediterranean is very popular for beach holidays and the sun is also very strong there. Northern Europe and the UK are often regarded as safe areas for exposure to the sun. However, this is no longer the case due to changes in the Earth's ozone layer. The skin should always be protected from the sun, particularly around midday, and a minimum of SPF 15 should always be applied.

Fake tanning products

The known effects and dangers of the sun still fail to dissuade some clients. It may be prudent for the therapist to recommend fake tanning products. These used to be hard to apply, had an unpleasant smell and invariably dried in streaks on the skin. More recently, these products have become refined, effective and pleasantly scented. Application can be by massaging the product into exfoliated skin. A more popular method is spray tanning, which is the diffusion of the tanning agent through a high pressured fine spray.

Application

The skin should always be exfoliated and a light application of moisturiser applied. The skin should then be allowed to settle for a few minutes prior to applying the self-tanning product. Two or three light applications should be made, to avoid streaking. The client should be advised to reapply after a few hours, depending upon the depth of colour required. When applying to areas of the skin prone to dryness, such as knees and elbows, a small amount of moisturiser should be mixed with the self-tanning product.

It is important for the therapist to wash their hands thoroughly after application and the client should also be advised to do this if they are going to use the product at home.

Most fake tans contain dihydroxyacetone. This adheres to the keratin cells and stains them an orangey-brown. As the skin desquamates, the stained cells are shed, resulting in a gradual fading of the tan.

> 🌸 *Remember...*
>
> The therapist must always advise the client on sunscreen products and use the opportunity to sell suitable products to the client.

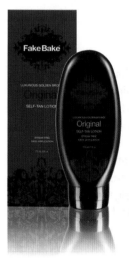

△ Self tan

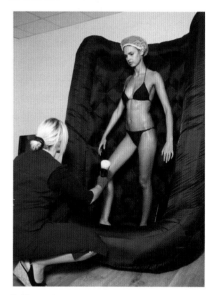

△ Spray tan

> ⭐ *Hints and tips*
>
> *The professional application of these products has become a very popular service offered by the beauty therapist and a good selling point for future treatment.*

Want to know more?

Invasive facial treatments

The past few years have seen a huge growth in the range of invasive anti-aging treatments. You should check with your client during the consultation and analysis stages whether they have undergone any of them, as this may affect the type of treatment you can offer and may necessitate modification of treatment routines.

The use of injectable products such as 'fillers' (for example Restylane® and Botulinum Type A (Botox®)) are becoming popular as they become more affordable.

After having fillers, clients should avoid facials or chemical peels until their skin has completely healed.

Botulinum toxin relaxes muscles. Micro-current facial treatments stimulate muscle, so should be avoided in areas where a botulinum treatment has been administered.

Micro-needling is where a roller with approximately 300 needles of 1–1.5mm in depth is used to penetrate the skin to stimulate growth of new collagen and other new skin cells.

Largely these treatments are not performed by traditional therapists but medical professionals only. They need specialist training and insurance.

Test yourself

Test yourself on providing facial skin care treatments by answering the following questions:

1 Give two possible causes of overactive sebaceous glands.

2 State two benefits of incorporating brush massage into the facial routine.

3 What are milia?

4 How should milia be removed?

5 What are the benefits in using a non-setting mask?

6. Give five physiological effects of facial massage.

Are you ready for assessment?

The following checklist will help you to be fully prepared for your assessment.

The range of clients/treatments you must cover:

- Equipment used in facial treatment.
- Various consultation techniques.
- Skin types.
- Skin conditions.
- Consider your actions if contraindications are present.
- Facial products.
- Massage mediums.
- Massage techniques.
- Mask treatments.
- Give treatment advice.

1. **Practical observation**

   Your assessor will look at how you:

   - prepare the treatment area, ensuring that you carry out safe and hygienic practice
   - prepare the treatment area with suitable facial equipment
   - consult with the client and prepare a record card
   - establish skin types – oily, dry or combination
   - establish skin conditions – mature, sensitive or dehydrated
   - use products and equipment to maintain skin condition
   - use massage techniques and a suitable medium for the client's skin type
   - apply mask treatments – setting and non-setting
   - carry out the facial in a commercially acceptable time
   - check with the client that the result is to the client's satisfaction
   - provide aftercare advice
   - demonstrate professional practice throughout the service
   - carry out all treatments with regard to health and safety.

2. **Knowledge and understanding**

   What you must know:

   - Organisational and legal requirements.
   - How to work safely and effectively when providing facial treatments.
   - How to consult, plan and prepare for treatment with clients.
   - Contraindications and contra-actions.
   - Anatomy and physiology.
   - Facial treatments.
   - Aftercare advice.

Remember . . .
Always keep your logbook handy.

Remember . . .
A clear understanding of skin types, thorough skin analysis and the choice of skin care products is the basis of good treatment.

Remember . . .
Your assessor will observe your performance on at least three occasions, each involving a different client.

To ensure that you have the necessary knowledge and understanding of facial services your assessor will:

- ask you questions before, during and after carrying out the treatment
- ensure that you have completed project work and written exercises relating to the unit
- check that you have recorded in a log/diary treatments you have carried out, with signed record cards showing that you have completed three facial treatments competently
- check that you have covered the range in your candidate logbook
- require you to take a test.

Remember . . .

Simulation is not a valid means of assessment for facial service.

Remember . . .

To enhance the experience ensure the client is comfortable throughout the treatment.

Sources of evidence

- Completed client record cards indicating the range of clients and skin types and conditions.
- Certificates of achievement from commercial courses (manufacturers hold courses for new products and treatments).
- Following your attendance at a course, ask your assessor to observe you showing your colleagues the skills you have learned.
- One-to-one tutorial with your assessor or salon supervisor to establish your progress and set targets. A copy of the tutorial report should be available for your portfolio.
- Client feedback.
- Project work.

Chapter 5

Unit B5: Enhance the appearance of eyebrows and eyelashes

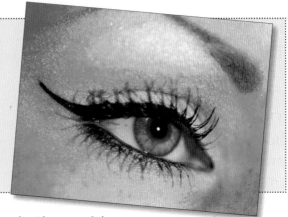

Learning objectives

This chapter covers Unit B5: eyebrow shaping, lash and brow tinting treatments and the application of artificial lashes.

> There are six learning outcomes for Unit B5 and they are:
> 1 Maintain safe and effective methods of working when enhancing the appearance of eyebrows and eyelashes.
> 2 Consult, plan and prepare for the treatment with clients.
> 3 Shape eyebrows.
> 4 Tint eyebrows and lashes.
> 5 Apply artificial eyelashes.
> 6 Provide aftercare advice.

You will need to be competent in lash and brow services, to qualify for insurance and to perform the treatment on members of the public.

Evidence requirements

Your assessor will need to observe you perform this treatment successfully on at least three occasions, involving different clients. They will also want to see you apply a partial set of artificial eyelashes and tinting eyebrows and eyelashes. You must:

1 Demonstrate the use of consultation techniques:
   - questioning
   - visual
   - manual
   - reference to client records.

2 Deal with one of these necessary actions:
   - encourage the client to seek medical advice
   - explain why the treatment cannot be carried out
   - modify the treatment.

3 Perform these eyebrow shaping services:
   - total reshape of the brow
   - maintenance of original brow shape.

4 Work with two of these colouring characteristics:
   - fair
   - red
   - dark
   - white.

5 Apply these artificial lashes:
   - strip lashes
   - individual flare lashes.

6 Use these products:
   - adhesives
   - solvents.

7 Provide relevant aftercare:
   - avoidance of activities which may cause contra-actions
   - recommended time intervals between treatments
   - suitable homecare products and their use.

Introduction

The eyes are an important facial feature and considered to be a woman's beauty asset. Emphasising and grooming the eye area enhances the face.

The eyes are one of the most sensitive areas of the body. The texture of the surrounding skin is very fine and there is very little subcutaneous fatty tissue to provide support. Therefore, the skin around the eyes can often look darker due to the fine texture. Also, the skin is stretched over a bony prominence in the skull, creating a sunken area between the bone and eyeball. No matter how beautiful the facial features are, if the client has dark circles under the eyes, tired eyes, unkempt eyebrows or straight eyelashes, the beauty of the other facial features will be diminished.

Treatments around the eye area are some of the most important of the salon services and they will have the most dramatic and immediate effect.

Unit B5 'Enhance the appearance of eyebrows and eyelashes' is a mandatory unit for both Level 2 NVQ Beauty Therapy General and Make-up routes and is worth five credits.

Hints and tips
Did you know that during a conversation with another person you would either look at their eyes or their mouth? Guess which one is the more popular.

Meet the professional

"An eyebrow shape is a very quick treatment but it still requires a full consultation. Even if it's a regular client, always check if they want anything different.

It's better to remove too little than too much. You can't stick it back on!

Listen very carefully to what your client wants regarding shape and final appearance. Just because you might want to try something different doesn't mean your client will want that. Make your suggestions to the client but remember that it is their decision.

You must always carry out a tint test, even if your client has had their lashes and brows tinted many times before. You need to make sure they are not going to react to the tint. Remember people can suddenly become sensitive to something they have had for years!

When tinting eyebrows, always consider the client's skin tone and natural/ dyed hair colour. The most effective method for building gradually to the desired colour is through the wipe-on, wipe-off technique. If your client is unsure how dark they want to go, you can build the colour up and show the client at each stage until the desired colour is achieved. They will appreciate the time you've taken and will trust you for a second visit."

Jacqui Bostock

Outcome 1: Maintain safe and effective methods of working when enhancing the appearance of eyebrows and eyelashes

As with all beauty therapy services it is important to fulfil service standards in regard to health and safety and sterilisation and to follow legal requirements. More on these aspects can be found in Chapters 1 'Professional skills' and 3 'Make sure your own actions reduce risks to health and safety'.

Legal requirements

The following table gives a summary of the relevant health and safety legislation that apply to lash and brow services.

▽ Relevant legislation as applies to lash and brow services

The treatment room	Health & Safety at Work Act 1974	General safety of staff and visitors to the salon including clients
	The Workplace (Health, Safety & Welfare) Regulations 1992	Governs the working environment including ventilation, temperature and lighting, etc.
	Regulatory Reform (Fire Safety) Order 2005	The safe evacuation of the building in an emergency such as a fire
Equipment	Provision and Use of Work Equipment Regulations 1998	Governs the acquisition of safe and reliable equipment
Lash and brow products	Control of Substances Hazardous to Health 1988	Governs the exposure of persons to substances likely to cause harm including flammability and the effect on the tissues
	Cosmetic Products (Safety) Regulations (2008)	Requires cosmetics to comply with correct labelling to have safe formulation and be fit for the purpose intended
Disposal of waste	The Controlled Waste Regulations 1992	Governs the correct disposal of contaminated waste i.e. that contaminated with blood or other bodily fluids

There are other legal requirements for treating clients, such as your responsibilities surrounding treating minors, avoiding discrimination and complying with data protection law. You will find details in Chapter 1.

Lash and brow service times

The table below provides the commercially accepted treatment times for lash and brow services.

▽ Lash and brow treatment times

Service description	Service time
Eyebrow shape	15 minutes
Eyebrow tint	10 minutes
Eyelash tint	20 minutes
Full set of artificial lashes	20 minutes
Partial set of artificial lashes	10 minutes

Preparation

The work area should be prepared with clean laundry after wiping down work surfaces with a suitable disinfectant. Equipment and tools such as tweezers should be sterilised and disposable items such as couch roll, cotton wool and mascara brushes should be used to avoid cross-infection.

The therapist's personal appearance should conform to industry expectations, details of which can be found in Chapter 1.

For certain lash and brow treatments a sensitivity or 'patch' test should be performed in order to protect the client from allergic reaction to products.

Patch testing for lash tinting and artificial lashes

Clients may insist that it is unnecessary as they have had their hair tinted or chemically treated before with no ill effect. You must ensure that the client appreciates the sensitivity of the area and that it is common for different areas of the body to be more sensitive than others. Skin sensitivity tests must also be carried out when applying artificial lashes.

Procedure for patch testing:

1. Cleanse an area of skin either behind the ear or in the fold of the elbow.
2. Apply a very small amount of the chemical to be used to the area. This may be mixed tint or adhesive depending upon the desired service
3. If testing for tint leave for five minutes and then wipe over area (if applicable). If testing for adhesive, wait until the adhesive has dried.
4. Advise the client to wash the area if an adverse (or positive) reaction occurs.

It is important that strong products for wiping/cleansing the area are avoided as the client may be reacting to them rather than the applied treatment product.

 Health and safety

It is vital that a patch test is carried out at least 24–48 hours prior to any treatment in the eye area that involves the use of chemical preparations. This should be made clear to the client when they make their appointment. Your salon will have an established procedure for this, which will ensure that all staff who book appointments are aware of the policy and can advise the client accordingly.

Clients should be advised what to expect from a positive reaction: there may be redness and irritation in the area. The client should be told to inform the salon if a positive reaction occurs and to apply a cooling, soothing product or cool water. If the reaction is severe or is prolonged, particularly if swelling develops, the client should be told to seek medical advice – either a pharmacist, their GP or in extreme cases go to the accident and emergency department of their local hospital.

A positive reaction to a patch test will mean that the client cannot have the treatment and this should be explained to the client in a supportive manner. A negative reaction will mean that the treatment can go ahead.

The date of the patch test and the outcome (positive or negative) should be recorded on the client's treatment plan or card.

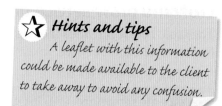

Hints and tips
A leaflet with this information could be made available to the client to take away to avoid any confusion.

Health and safety

It is important to patch test before every treatment as areas with a negative test result can become sensitised between treatments.

Personal protective equipment

One of the common work related conditions acquired by the frequent use of chemicals such as tint, hydrogen peroxide and adhesives is **contact dermatitis**. This condition occurs due to frequent exposure to chemicals where the natural protective oils are removed from the skin leaving the skin dry, red and irritated. It is common in the Hair and Beauty sector on the hands and fingers and the wearing of protective gloves is advised. Gloves should be powder-free, nitrile or vinyl gloves – not latex, which can exacerbate the condition.

Outcome 2: Consult, plan and prepare for the treatment with clients

Contraindications to lash and brow services

It is important to check for contraindications before eyelash and brows services.

The specific contraindications are:

- positive reaction to the patch test
- cuts and abrasions in the area
- bruised (black eye) eye area
- conjunctivitis
- watery eyes
- sties
- inflammation or swelling
- known allergy to cosmetics.

For more information on the correct professional consultation techniques to perform for lash and brow services please refer to Chapter 1.

Outcome 3: Shape eyebrows

Eyebrow shaping is one of the easiest ways of giving definition to the eye area. It is only necessary to remove a few hairs to create a groomed appearance.

Preparation of work area for eyebrow shaping

The couch and trolley should be prepared prior to the client's arrival. The trolley should contain the equipment listed below.

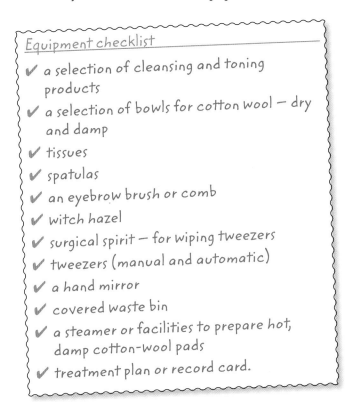

Equipment checklist

✔ a selection of cleansing and toning products
✔ a selection of bowls for cotton wool — dry and damp
✔ tissues
✔ spatulas
✔ an eyebrow brush or comb
✔ witch hazel
✔ surgical spirit — for wiping tweezers
✔ tweezers (manual and automatic)
✔ a hand mirror
✔ covered waste bin
✔ a steamer or facilities to prepare hot, damp cotton-wool pads
✔ treatment plan or record card.

 Health and safety

All tools and equipment must be sterilised in the appropriate way and should not be brought to the trolley until they are required for use.

Preparation of client

The client should be in a semi-reclining position and the hair and clothing should be protected.

The area to be treated should be cleansed and toned. It is important to tone to ensure all cleansing product is removed from the area.

It is important to discuss the desired effect with the client before starting to remove the hairs. Consideration should be given to the natural brow shape and the shape of the client's face. You should also take into account whether the client has had their brows shaped before. If this is the first time, it may be wise to shape them gradually over two treatments.

Once the desired outcome has been agreed, the brow area should be brushed against the growth to separate the hairs and then brushed into their natural shape.

 Health and safety

Always check for contraindications. Examples that prevent treatment are eye infections such as conjunctivitis and stye.

a) sweeping shape

b) angled shape

c) arched shape

◁ Eyebrow shapes

Methods of eyebrow shaping

Eyebrows can be shaped using a variety of methods. However, tweezers are the most popular method. Manual and automatic tweezers are available. Automatic tweezers are designed for speed and for removing a lot of hairs.

Manual tweezers are used for final shaping and tidying the brows.

> ☆ **Hints and tips**
> Selection of the type of tweezers should be left to the therapist. It is important that you feel confident with the selected tool.

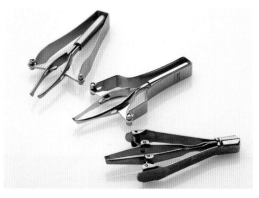

△ Automatic tweezers

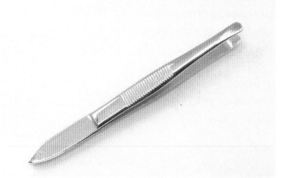

△ Manual tweezers

Procedure for shaping the brows

The brows should be warmed, using either a steamer or hot damp cotton-wool pads.

The brows should be measured using the following guidelines.

1. Hold the skin taut and remove hairs only in the direction of growth.

2. Wipe over constantly with warm, damp pads.

3. Brush the brows regularly to ascertain developing shape.

4. Do not work on one brow only; instead, remove a few hairs from each brow to maintain balance.

5. Hairs should only be removed from underneath the brow line.

6. Stray hairs at the temple area or above the brow should only be removed if they do not form part of the main brow growth.

7. Place removed hairs on a tissue. Do not leave on the skin.

> ✋ **Health and safety**
>
> Personal protective equipment in the form of powder-free, nitrile or vinyl gloves should be worn during eyebrow shaping services to protect from cross-infection by blood-borne viruses such as hepatitis.

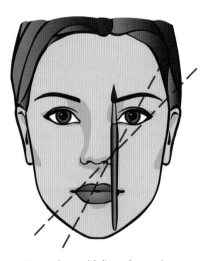

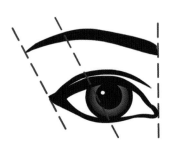

△ Measuring guidelines for eyebrows

8. When completed wipe over with a witch hazel or mild skin tonic pad to soothe the area
9. Show the client the finished result
10. Provide aftercare advice: avoid application of make-up until the erythema has gone and wipe over with soothing antiseptic cream.

Outcome 4: Tint eyebrows and eyelashes

Tinting the eyelashes or brows is one of the most natural and effective ways of enhancing and defining the eyes. It is particularly popular with clients for whom make-up is prohibited, for those who prefer a more natural look and those who are going on holiday or do not want to wear make-up. It can also be effective if the client has changed their hair colour or if they have grey or fair hair and wish to add definition to the eye area. Combining eyelash tinting with other eye services such as artificial lash application can give a natural appearance for special occasions or holidays.

You should allow 20 minutes for eyelash tinting in the treatment schedule and no more than 10 minutes for tinting the brow hairs. This will vary depending upon the client's natural colouring. Clients who have a lot of red in their hair colour may require a longer processing time to achieve a satisfactory result.

Preparation of the workstation

The workstation should be prepared prior to the client's arrival. The trolley should be prepared with the equipment in the following list.

Equipment checklist

You will need:
- ✔ a selection of bowls — for damp and dry cotton wool
- ✔ tissues
- ✔ a selection of cleansing and toning products
- ✔ petroleum jelly
- ✔ a small glass or non-metallic dish
- ✔ a selection of eyelash tints
- ✔ preformed tinting shields
- ✔ 10-volume (3 per cent) hydrogen peroxide
- ✔ orangewood sticks
- ✔ small brush
- ✔ spatulas
- ✔ eyebath and distilled water (for emergencies)
- ✔ a covered waste receptacle
- ✔ treatment plan or record card.

Activity

Collect images from magazines of models, both male and female.
- ❖ What do you notice about the shape of the eyebrow?
- ❖ Have the eyebrows been groomed?
- ❖ What is the effect?

Hints and tips
Ask the client to refrain from wearing mascara on the day of treatment. This will reduce the possibility of sensitising the area prior to treatment through cleansing the area.

Health and safety
All tools and equipment should be sterilised by the appropriate method. (See Chapter 1.)

Hints and tips
Ensure that the bottle of peroxide is kept tightly closed to maintain the strength of the peroxide.

Choosing the colour

Lash tint comes in a range of colours – black, brown, grey and blue. They can be mixed to provide a range of depth and tone of colour. As with all colour choice, the client may have a preference. However, certain considerations must be given to:

- the colour of the lashes
- the age of the client
- the hair and skin colour
- the client's usual make-up.

Applying black to a mature client with white hair would be harsh and would look artificial. However, black mixed with brown or grey would soften the colour. Younger clients can take black or black mixed with blue to give depth to the lashes.

Particular care must be taken when choosing colour for the eyebrows. Do not be tempted to use the same colour as the lashes. Brown is the most commonly used colour.

Preparation of the client

The client should be comfortably seated on the couch with their hair and clothing protected. The eyes should be cleansed and toned or a full cleanse carried out if the tinting is part of a facial.

Avoid cleansing the eyes with oily make-up remover as any oil or cream remaining on the lashes can prevent the tint from 'taking' properly.

The desired effect should be discussed. Always consider the different effects and depths of colour achieved by the various tints, depending upon the client's natural colouring. Pay careful regard to manufacturer's instructions, as they may vary.

The client should be informed that if at any time during the treatment they feel discomfort (a tingling or burning sensation), they should inform you immediately so that the tint can be removed.

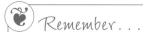

☆ *Hints and tips*
If in doubt as to the choice of colour, consider the colour of mascara your client normally wears.

Remember . . .
Begin by confirming that the client has had a satisfactory patch test. Establish and record the outcome of the test before proceeding with the treatment.

Health and safety

If the client does experience any contra-actions to treatment, the tint should be removed immediately and the eyes rinsed using an eyebath and distilled water, followed by a cold-water compress to soothe the eye.

Procedure for tinting the eyelashes

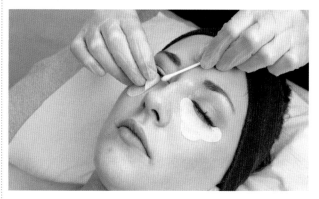

1. Place a dampened preformed tint shield under the lower lashes. It is advisable to coat the underside with petroleum jelly to help the shield to stay in place.

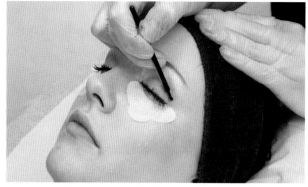

2. Using a clean, fine brush, apply petroleum jelly to the upper eyelid and underneath the lower lashes.

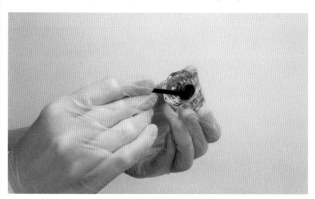

3. The tint should now be mixed. The formulation is usually 5–6mm of tint to 2–3 drops of 10-volume peroxide (the tint comes out of a tube rather like toothpaste – you will need to squeeze 2–4mm long). However, you should always refer to the manufacturer's instructions. Only a very small amount of tint is required. Do not waste products unnecessarily. Do not mix the tint until the client has been prepared. The tint will start working immediately and if it is not applied straight away the effect will be lessened. Always mix the tint formulation using an orangewood stick. Never use the applicator brush to mix as the tint will clog at the top of the brush head, causing a messy application.

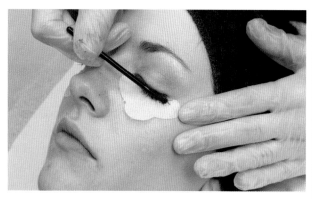

4. Apply the tint to the bottom lashes on both eyes using a small, sterilised, dry brush. Ask the client to close their eyes and apply to the upper lashes.

> ⭐ *Hints and tips*
> *Care must be taken when applying the petroleum jelly. This will act as a barrier between the tint and the skin. However, it will also act as a barrier to the tint if it comes into contact with the hair, preventing the tint working on the lashes.*

> ⭐ *Hints and tips*
> *Make sure that you take the tint application as close to the roots as possible. Use a clean finger to gently lift the underside of the eyebrow to expose the roots of the lashes. This is particularly important in both the application and the removal process.*

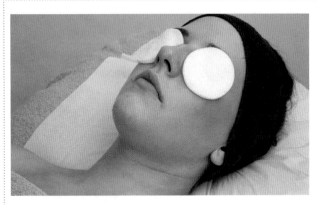

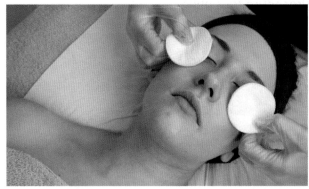

5. Place warm, dampened (not wet!) cotton wool pads over the tint to create warmth. This will assist in the development of the tint and will also help to prevent the client opening their eyes during the processing time.

6. The tint should be removed following the manufacturer's recommended processing time. This is normally around 10 minutes. The pad of cotton wool and the tint shield should be grasped and removed in a quick downward movement. This is carried out on both eyes. Ask the client to keep their eyes closed.

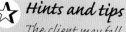

★ Hints and tips

The client may fall asleep during the process and could open the eyes if suddenly disturbed. It is therefore important to talk generally to the client, explaining each step in the procedure. It is also recommended that you inform the client not to open the eyes until instructed to.

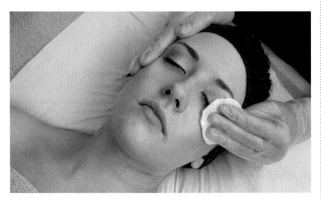

7. Dampened cotton-wool pads are then used to wipe the lashes. The area should be wiped until the cotton wool shows no evidence of any remaining tint.

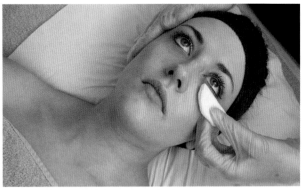

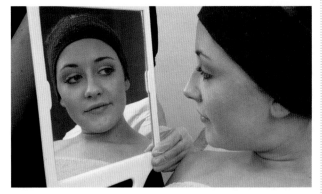

8. The client should now be asked to open their eyes. Using a folded, dampened cotton-wool pad, gently wipe the base of the lashes. Continue until the pad wipes clean.

9. Wipe over the eye area with tonic to remove the petroleum jelly and show the client the finished result.

Procedure for tinting the brows

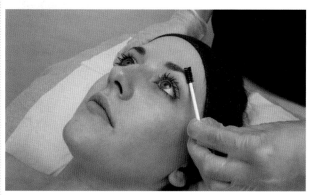

1. The brows should be brushed thoroughly to lift and separate them.

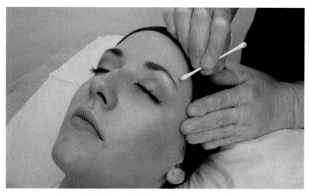

2. Petroleum jelly is applied to the surrounding area, taking care not to touch the hairs that are to be tinted.

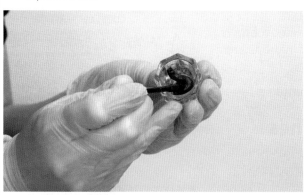

3. The colour should be chosen carefully and mixed as for lashes.

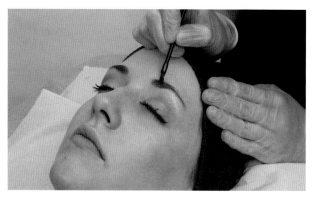

4. The tint is applied to the hairs of the brows, not the skin, to avoid harsh lines, applying against the growth of the brows.

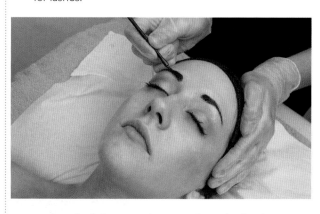

5. Apply to both brows and remove from the first brow immediately to assess the colour, which can 'take' very quickly. Then remove from the other brow immediately.

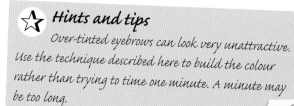

☆ *Hints and tips*

Over-tinted eyebrows can look very unattractive. Use the technique described here to build the colour rather than trying to time one minute. A minute may be too long.

☆ *Hints and tips*

The brows must not be shaped beforehand and on the same day as tinting. The area will become sensitised following the shaping procedure and the application of tint could cause irritation. The client could have the brows shaped after the tint or could book a shape for the next salon visit.

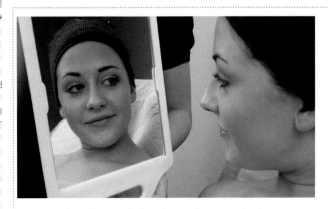

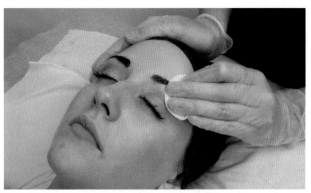

6. Discuss colour with the client using a hand mirror. Reapply if colour is not dark enough. It may take 3–4 applications to achieve the right depth of colour.

7. The area should then be wiped over with tonic pads to remove all traces of the petroleum jelly.

Clients may choose to have a range of treatments on their eyebrows and lashes. The recommended timings for typical combinations are:

- Eyebrow shape and lash tint: 35 minutes.
- Eyebrow tint, eyebrow shape and lash tint: 40–45 minutes.

Outcome 5: Apply artificial eyelashes

There are two methods of artificially enhancing the natural eyelash. The 'strip' method is temporary and the 'individual' method is semi-permanent. These are very popular salon treatments. Eyelash enhancements are particularly effective for those with short or straight lashes or those wanting a natural look while still defining the eyes. It is important for the beauty therapist to discuss with the client the options for lash enhancement. This should also include finding out whether the effect is for a particular event, for example a wedding or a holiday. This will assist you in advising the client on the most appropriate method.

Temporary (strip) lashes

The temporary or strip lash is made of natural hair or synthetic fibres woven onto a fine band or strip, which is pre-shaped and flexible to complement the curve of the eye. The strip lash is fixed using a latex-based adhesive, which is secured to the eyelid as close as possible to the natural lashes. This method is used extensively in fashion photography, on the catwalk and to enhance particular make-up looks. The client must be advised that they are temporary and should not be worn for more than one day. This makes them particularly popular for bridal make-up. The strip lashes are easily removed and the client can perform this without returning to the salon. To preserve the quality of the eyelash the client should be advised how to clean the lashes and how to store them for future use.

> ⭐ **Hints and tips**
>
> Excess grease on the lashes from oily eye make-up remover will act as a barrier to the chemical, therefore preventing a successful treatment.

Activity

1. List four safety precautions when carrying out lash and brow tinting.
2. List the treatment sequence you would follow if the client has booked for an eyebrow tint and shape.

Selecting the strip lashes

The lashes are available in a variety of colours and styles. They may be feathered, flared, very thick or fine. They can also be enhanced with crystals, jewels and other lightweight adornments. The client should be advised to purchase the strip lashes from the salon, as they would be trimmed specifically to fit her eye shape. The strip lash can then be tailored or shortened to ensure a suitable fit.

Preparation for treatment

Ensure you have the following items prepared and available on the workstation.

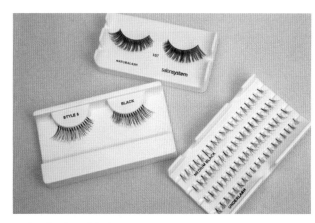

△ A selection of lash types

Remember...

Allow 10 minutes for the application of strip lashes and a further 10 minutes if they are to be applied as part of a make-up application. This will provide time to prepare the lashes as agreed with the client during the earlier consultation.

Remember...

Consider the client's age, the occasion and the desired effect. Strip lashes should complement the colour of the mascara application.

Equipment checklist

You will need:

✔ tissues
✔ cotton wool (dampened and dry)
✔ clean sterilised tweezers
✔ selected strip lashes
✔ adhesive (only use the recommended adhesive)
✔ mascara which complements the colour of the selected strip lashes
✔ sterilised scissors
✔ spatula
✔ clean orangewood stick
✔ clean, sterilised lash brush or clean, disposable mascara wand
✔ hand mirror
✔ eyebath and freshly prepared water for immediate eye irrigation in case of accident.

Procedure for applying temporary (strip) eyelashes

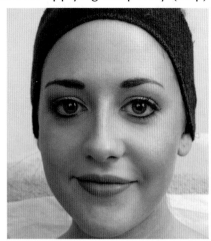

1. Complete the make-up application.

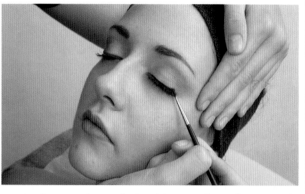

2. Eyeliner may be applied at this stage dependant upon the look required.

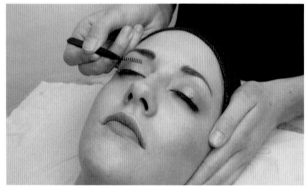

3. Ideally, apply the lashes from behind, with the client in a semi-reclined position.

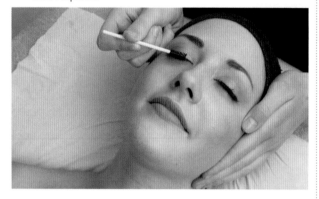

4. Brush the natural lashes.

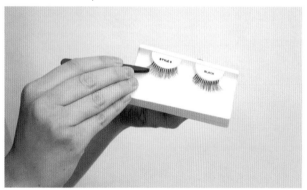

5. Using tweezers, firmly remove the strip lash from the packaging.

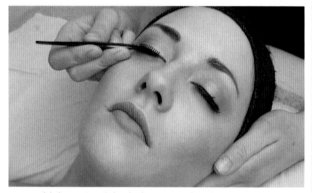

6. Hold the strip of the lash against the client's eyelid to determine fit.

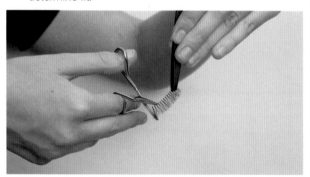

7. Trim to size using sterilised scissors.

 Remember . . .

If temporary lashes are to be applied as part of a make-up procedure they should be applied at the end of the make-up application.

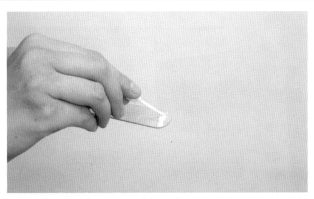

8. Apply a small amount of the adhesive to the spatula and replace the lid.

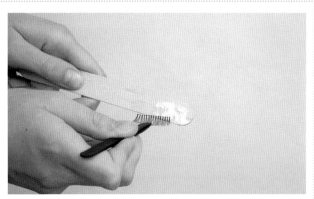

9. Using tweezers, hold the prepared lash and gently run the strip through the adhesive, ensuring the full length of the strip is covered.

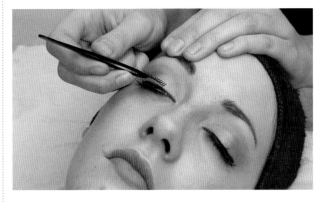

10. Gently lift the eyelid from under the eyebrow to ensure a good fit.

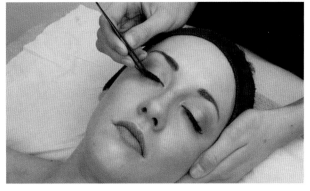

11. Place the lash onto the centre of eyelid, applying them as close to the line of the natural lashes as possible.

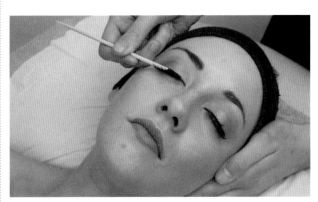

12. Using the clean orangewood stick, gently press the strip lash firmly into place along the length of the strip.

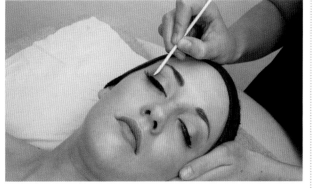

13. Check the adhesive is evenly distributed at both ends of the strip and using the orangewood stick apply additional adhesive if required.

14. Repeat the above procedure to the other eye.

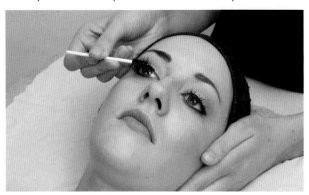

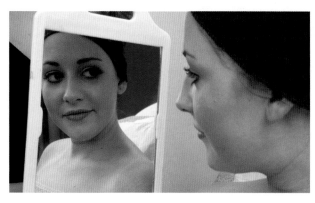

15. Once the adhesive has dried, usually the cream-coloured adhesive becomes clear. Using the mascara wand brush together the natural and false lashes.

16. Check the effect from the front of the client and show the client .

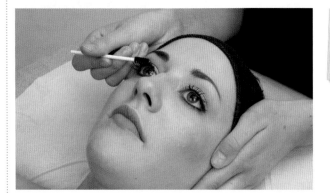

☆ *Hints and tips*

Be careful to only cover the fine strip with adhesive and not the lash hair.

17. Apply a coat of mascara if desired.

Removal and storage

The client should be advised to wear the temporary lashes for no more than one day and should be advised on the correct removal and storage of the strip lashes.

Removal:

1. Support the outer corner of the eye and gently pull away from the eyelid.

2. Using tweezers or firmly holding the strip lash, peel the adhesive from the lash strip.

3. Replace in the box, ensuring the lashes fit into the pre-moulded base.

Cleaning and storage:

1. Synthetic lashes should be immersed in warm soapy water and rinsed well.

2. Natural hair lashes should be cleaned using the manufacturer's instructions or wiped with a diluted alcohol solution. Over time, the lashes may start to lose their curl.

To re-curl the lashes:

1. Wrap part of a full tissue around a pencil.
2. Place the clean strip lash onto the tissue-covered pencil, keeping the base of the lash straight to ensure the curl is even.
3. Roll the remainder of the tissue around the pencil.
4. Secure at both ends with adhesive tape or elastic bands and leave overnight.
5. Replace the newly curled lashes onto their pre-moulded base.

Semi-permanent (individual) lashes

The semi-permanent method is also popular with clients who participate in sporting activities. Clients should always be informed, however, of the limitations of the treatment and the expected duration of the application. The effect normally lasts up to six weeks with the individual lash being lost when the natural lash falls out.

Individual lashes can provide a subtle, natural effect and can be worn without eye make-up. They are available in a variety of lengths, colours and styles (for example, flared (several lashes from a single knot), or a single lash). The individual lashes are pre-curled and can be made from synthetic hair or natural hair. The special adhesive to be used is available in clear or black.

The timing for application of individual lashes is longer than that of strip lashes. Each individual lash is attached to the natural eyelash using very strong adhesive and great care is needed to ensure the adhesive does not enter the eye. Continually check for excessive watering of the eye. It is important to have an eye bath and distilled water available to enable swift irrigation of the eye if necessary.

 Health and safety

The fixing agent is very strong glue, which can be an irritant and can damage the delicate eye area if incorrectly used. It is therefore important to perform a patch test on your client 24–48 hours before treatment.

Preparation for treatment

Ensure that you have the following items prepared and available on the workstation.

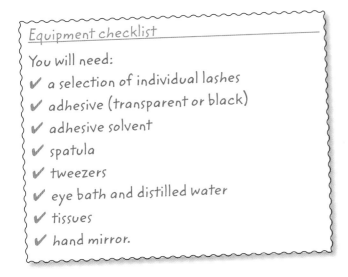

Equipment checklist

You will need:
- ✔ a selection of individual lashes
- ✔ adhesive (transparent or black)
- ✔ adhesive solvent
- ✔ spatula
- ✔ tweezers
- ✔ eye bath and distilled water
- ✔ tissues
- ✔ hand mirror.

Procedure for applying semi-permanent (individual) lashes

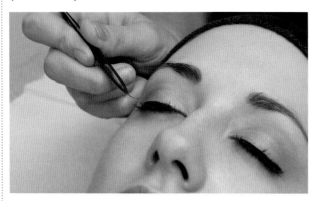

1. Ideally, apply the lashes from behind, with the client in a semi-reclined position.

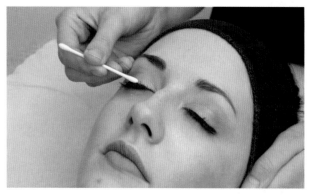

2. Ensure that the natural eyelashes are clean and free from oil.

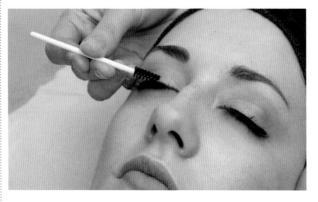

3. Comb the natural lashes.

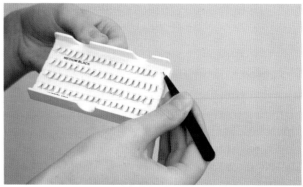

4. Select the individual lashes to apply by carefully removing the lashes from the display case. Firmly hold the lash using the tweezers, close to the knotted end (the bulb) of the lash.

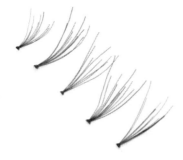

5. Place on a clean tissue (in the order of application where a mix of lengths and styles are being used).

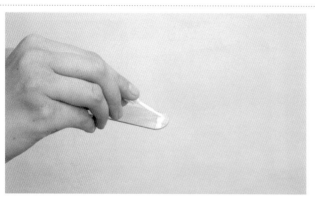

6. Dispense a small amount of adhesive onto a clean spatula.

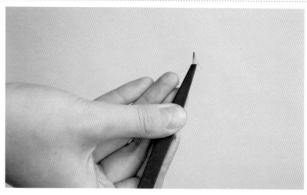

7. Hold the selected lash using the tweezers with the knotted end (bulb) exposed.

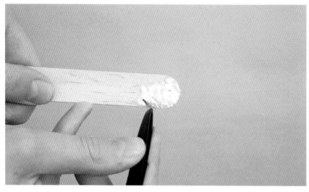

8. Gently dip the knot into the adhesive.

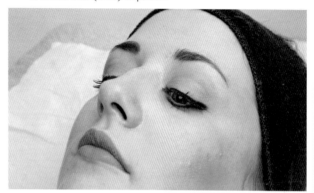

9. Advise the client to look down but without closing the eye.

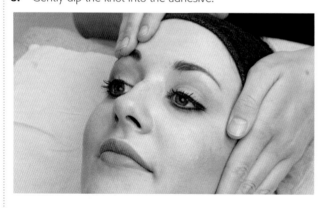

10. Gently lift the eyelid to ensure the natural lashes are clearly defined.

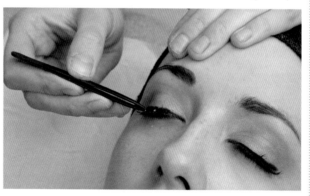

11. Working from the pre-determined area of the eye lid, i.e. from the centre of outer area of the lashes depending upon the desired effect, place the adhesive-coated bulb onto the root of the client's natural lash and stroke along the natural lash to distribute the adhesive, before securing close to the base of the natural lash. Always apply the shortest lashes first, working to the outer edge of the eyelid with the longest lashes.

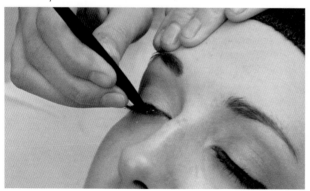

12. Using the tweezers, hold the lash in place for a few seconds until the adhesive has bonded.

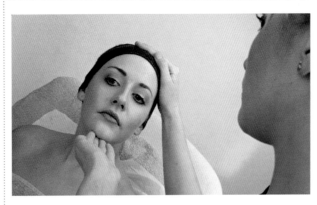

13. It is advisable to apply consecutively to both eyes to ensure the finished effect is balanced. When application is complete, ask the client to open their eyes gently. Check that the adhesive has not come into contact with lower lashes. Apply to lower lashes if desired.

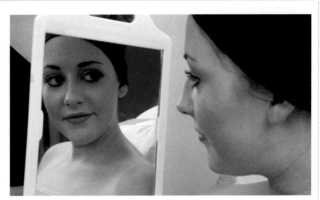

14. Allow the client to view the finished result using the hand mirror.

Removal of semi-permanent (individual) lashes

Semi-permanent lashes can be worn for up to six weeks although the client should be advised to expect some individual lashes to be lost as they will be lost when the natural lash falls out. Typically, the life cycle of an eyelash is up to six weeks hence it will depend on the stage of the natural lash growth cycle as to how long each lash will remain.

Procedure for removal of individual eyelashes

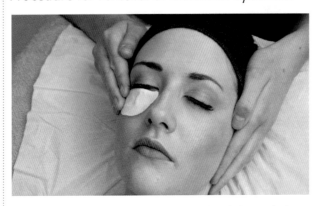

1. Place dampened shaped cotton wool pads beneath the lower lashes and advise the client to close her eyes.

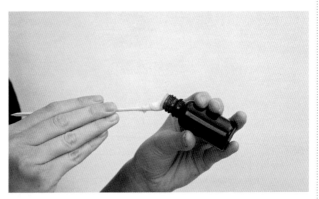

2. Using a cotton-tipped bud or cotton wool covered tip of an orangewood stick, soak in the special solvent supplied by the manufacturer.

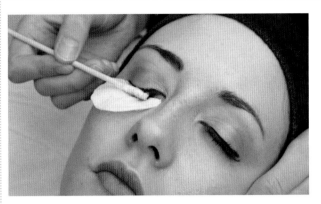

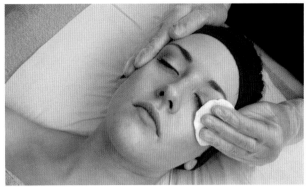

3. Apply the solvent to the base of the lash. Leave for a few seconds and then using a gentle, rolling movement, lift the lash away as the adhesive is weakened by the solvent.

4. Once all lashes are removed, wipe the eye area with clean, dampened cotton wool pads.

Outcome 6: Provide aftercare advice

To enable clients to maintain the benefits from their lash and brow treatment, provide them with the aftercare advice that follows for each treatment.

Aftercare advice for shaping

- Avoid use of make-up for 24 hours after the treatment.
- Do not touch the area as this can cause skin infections such as pustules.
- Slight redness after shaping is normal but should dissipate within hours.

Aftercare advice for tinting

- Avoid other chemical treatment such as lash perming for 24 hours.
- There is no need to wear mascara but use non-waterproof mascara if desired.
- If swelling, irritation or redness occurs, inform the salon. If severe irritation occurs, seek medical advice.

Aftercare advice for artificial lashes

- Treat the area with care and try not to rub the eyes as it may dislodge the lash.
- Use an oil-free eye make-up remover.
- Avoid excessive use of mascara. Only non-waterproof mascara should be worn.
- Return to the salon if you would like to have the lashes removed. This is important as any home-based attempt to remove the lashes could cause damage to the natural lashes.
- Return to the salon for infill/replacements as part of the service.

Recommended time intervals between treatments

It is necessary to repeat the services to maintain effects and the client should be encouraged to rebook appointments as follows:

- shaping: 2–3 weeks
- tinting: 4–6 weeks
- strip lashes: as desired
- semi-permanent lashes: 3–4 weeks.

> **Activity**
>
> Prepare a leaflet for the client that gives details about the home care of temporary or semi-permanent lashes.

 Want to know more?

Individual permanent lashes that adhere permanently to the natural lash and remain until the lash is replaced is a service used by celebrities that is now becoming popular with the general public. Application of this type of lash is covered in Level 3 Beauty Therapy qualifications.

More information can be found on the following websites:

www.habia.org

www.AHFrancis.com

Test yourself

Test yourself on eyebrow and eyelash services by answering the following questions.

1. What are the different uses of manual and automatic tweezers?
2. Explain the importance of patch tests.
3. What action can you take to minimise client discomfort during eyebrow shaping?
4. What may cause a poor outcome to an eyelash tint?
5. Give four contraindications to the application of false lashes.
6. Tinting colours the eyelashes and brows by a process called:
   a) hydration
   b) pigmentation
   c) exfoliation
   d) oxydation.
7. Give two benefits of lash tinting to a client who wears contact lenses.
8. How can a natural effect be achieved when applying strip lashes?
9. Why should personal protective equipment be worn during lash and brow treatments?

Are you ready for assessment?

 Remember...
Client consultation is essential to establish the natural appearance of the eyebrows and lashes and 'the look' the client is after.

Remember...
Always keep your logbook handy.

The following checklist will help you to be fully prepared for your assessment.

The range of clients/treatments you must cover:

- Various consultation techniques.
- Your actions if contraindications are present.
- Eyebrow shaping to include reshape and trim.
- Lash tint for eyebrows and lashes.
- Client's natural colouring.
- Artificial lashes and products used.
- After care advice.

 Remember...
Your assessor will observe your performance on at least three occasions, each involving different clients (not a fellow student or colleague) and carrying out different treatments from the range.

1. **Practical observation**
   Your assessor will look at how you:
   - prepare the treatment area, ensuring that you carry out safe and hygienic practice
   - carry out a patch test as required
   - consult with the client and prepare a record card
   - carry out eyebrow shaping on clients
   - carry out eyebrow and lash tint
   - apply artificial eyelashes
   - carry out each treatment in a commercially acceptable time
   - check with the client that the lash and/or brow treatment meets her expectations
   - provide aftercare advice
   - demonstrate professional practice throughout the service
   - carry out all treatments with regard to health and safety.

2. Knowledge and understanding

What you must know:

- ❧ Organisational and legal requirements.
- ❧ How to work safely and effectively when providing lash and brow services.
- ❧ Consult, plan and prepare for treatment with clients.
- ❧ Contraindications and contra-actions.
- ❧ Anatomy and physiology.
- ❧ Eyebrow shaping procedure.
- ❧ Lash and brow tinting procedure.
- ❧ Procedure for applying artificial lashes.
- ❧ Aftercare advice.

To ensure that you have the necessary knowledge and understanding of lash and brow services your assessor will:

- ❧ ask you questions before, during and after carrying out the treatment
- ❧ ensure that you have completed project work and written exercises relating to the unit
- ❧ check that you have recorded in a log/diary treatments you have carried out with signed record cards showing that you have completed at least three services competently
- ❧ check that you have covered the range in your candidate logbook
- ❧ require you to take a test.

 Remember. . .

Lash and brow treatments are often combined with other facial treatments and make-up.

Sources of evidence

- ❧ Completed client record cards indicating the range of clients and lash and brow treatments covered.
- ❧ Video or photographic evidence, preparing models for a show may involve the application of lashes, for example. Verification of this evidence through a signature and date by a senior member of staff will be necessary.
- ❧ Project work such as compiling photos and pictures of various brow shapes and fashion trends.

 Remember. . .

Several treatments can be carried out on one client.

Chapter 6
Unit B34: Provide threading services

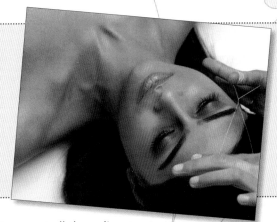

Learning outcomes

This chapter covers Unit B34 'Provide threading services'. This involves the temporary removal of unwanted hair from the face using different threading techniques, including the shaping and maintenance of different eyebrow shapes.

> There are four learning outcomes for Unit B34 and they are:
> 1 Maintain safe and effective methods when removing hair by threading.
> 2 Consult, plan and prepare for threading services with clients.
> 3 Remove unwanted hair.
> 4 Provide aftercare advice.

You will need to be competent in all of these outcomes to be competent in threading services, qualify for insurance and perform the treatment on members of the public.

Evidence requirements

Your assessor will need to observe you perform this treatment successfully on at least four occasions, each involving a different client. Two occasions must include a full eyebrow reshape. You must:

1 Demonstrate the use of consultation techniques:
- questioning
- visual
- manual
- reference to client records.

2 Carry out all threading treatments:
- eyebrows
- upper lip
- chin.

3 Take one of the following necessary actions:
- encourage the client to seek medical advice
- explain why the treatment cannot be carried out
- modify the treatment.

4 Use all methods of threading on appropriate parts of the face:
- mouth technique
- neck technique
- hand technique.

5 Perform threading on these eyebrow shapes:
- total reshape of the brows
- maintenance of original eyebrow shape.

6 Provide relevant aftercare advice:
- avoidance of activities which may cause contra-actions
- suitable homecare products and their use
- recommended time intervals between threading treatments.

Introduction

Threading is a method of temporary facial hair removal that has been practised for many centuries. It would traditionally have been a skill passed through generations of families to enable them to treat one another. The true origin of threading is hard to pinpoint, as many countries would take credit for it. However, it is often traced back to areas of the Middle East.

The treatment involves the use of a specific natural cotton thread that is resistant to wear and often slightly waxed. This allows a smoother movement against the skin. Some brands include a coating of an anti-bacterial product to promote a healthy skin reaction, and prevent infection.

Facial hair, including eyebrows and that found on the upper lip and chin, can be removed successfully by threading treatment, as can the external hairs on the ears and nose of male clients.

To perform the threading service a piece of thread is twisted into either one or two loops, depending on the technique being used. This twist is then rolled across the unwanted hair growth to grab and remove the hair from the follicle, in the same way as in a waxing or tweezing treatment.

Unit B4 'Provide Threading Services' is an optional unit for Level 2 Beauty Therapy General and Make-up routes and is worth four credits.

Meet the professional

"Threading is an ancient yet remarkable skill to master. Don't be disheartened if it takes a little time to fully master all the techniques; remember 'practice makes perfect!' Some people will prefer one of the methods over the others. However, with experience and patience you will soon master them all!

The consultation is always important: do not forget to inform your client during this time that they will be required to assist you with the stretching of the area. Although this is not required with other hair removal systems, it is necessary with threading to avoid catching the skin and causing discomfort. Always make sure clients are fully aware of what is required of them before commencing.

Last of all enjoy the precision and added benefits of this ancient mild hair removal technique that is delicate on the skin."

Sarah Sheridan

Outcome 1: Maintain safe and effective methods of working when providing threading services

Threading services are fast becoming popular in the West with both women and men of all ages. It is, however, like waxing, treatment where the hair is traumatically removed from the follicle. For this reason threading services should be treated with great care by the therapist and follow local and national legislation and the industry's Code of Practice guidelines.

The general national legal requirements for performing beauty therapy treatments can be found in Chapter 3 'G20 Make sure your actions reduce risks to health and safety'.

The hair and beauty sector's lead body, HABIA, have published guidelines for the safe and effective treatment of clients for services such as waxing and threading, and can provide general 'industry standards' regarding dress, sterilisation and infection control and other salon safety. Chapter 10 B6 'Carry Out Waxing Services' provides more detail.

The professional dress code and the expectations of the industry can be found in Chapter 1 'Professional Skills'. In addition, the Code of Practice suggests the wearing of a protective, disposable plastic apron and single-use latex-free gloves during the performance of threading services.

Treatment times for threading services

There are currently no guidelines given by HABIA regarding the service times for threading services. However, here is a guide for you to practise and develop your threading techniques. You can see they are similar to those for waxing the given areas of the body. In your salon, when treatments are combined, times are reduced because you will be setting up and performing the consultation only once for the combined service.

Service	Time
Eyebrows	15 mins
Lip	10 mins
Chin	10 mins

Hygiene and safety procedures when threading

Hygiene precautions specific to threading services include:

- Remove the fallen hairs with a clean cotton pad. Towels can be positioned over the client's shoulders to prevent the hairs falling onto their clothing.
- To prevent possible contamination when threading a fresh piece of thread should be used per area when treating the client and then discarded.

 Health and safety

Avoid touching the client's skin and wiping away the fallen hairs with the fingers — always use a clean cotton pad.

- Thread **can** be used more than once in the same area, but is unadvisable when a different area is to be treated.
- Complete hair removal from an area methodically. This avoids 'missing' hairs and leaving 'hairy patches'.

The hazards relating to the threading treatment are the risk of infection, bleeding and the formation of scabs. After the threading service the skin will be sensitised by the treatment. Specific safety precautions for threading include:

- Latex found in some disposable gloves is a known allergen and can result in contact dermatitis, a non-infectious skin condition. Clients with known allergies such as this should be treated with the use of a vinyl glove instead.
- The lifting of the skin away from the underlying tissues causes bruising. To prevent this, ask the client to stretch the skin to keep the area taught when removing the hair. The more 'loose' the skin, the more you need to stretch.
- Avoid over-treating an area by observing the skin colour and response during the treatment.
- Apply the correct threading technique and pressure, working in the correct direction
- After treatment apply aftercare lotion or oil, which soothes the trauma of the skin and reduces the possibility of infection.
- Explain aftercare procedures fully and ensure that the client understands them by giving the client the chance to ask questions.

Posture and positioning for threading

- The client needs to be comfortable and relaxed.
- For threading the client should be laid on the couch, either flat or semi-elevated. The angle of the backrest of the couch or the pillow needs to be adjusted for client comfort.
- The trolley must be close to the therapist while working to avoid undue stretching, which can cause fatigue.
- A height-adjustable chair can be used to allow the therapist to position themselves comfortably to prevent the risk of fatigue.
- The couch should be at a convenient height so the therapist does not have to overstretch or bend; this will eliminate the risk of injury to the therapist and minimise fatigue

> ☆ *Hints and tips*
> Other single-use items for the safe and hygienic performance of threading services include wooden spatulas, thread, disposable brow brushes, cotton pads, couch roll and tissues.

> ☆ *Hints and tips*
> If hands become sore gloves can be used to complete the treatment. The use of vinyl gloves are recommended as you would need to be aware of possible client allergies to latex gloves.

Test yourself

Test yourself on the related anatomy by answering these questions. Refer to Chapter 19 'Related Anatomy and Physiology' for answers.

1. The uppermost portion of the epidermis is made of several layers of dead keratinised skin cells. Is this statement true or false?

2. Which glands found in the skin are responsible for the slight natural acidity of the skin?

3. Secretion is the removal of waste products and water from the skin. Is this statement true or false?

4. Which glands found in the skin are responsible for excretion?

5. Which glands found in the skin are responsible for secretion?

6. Which of the following statements is true and which is false?
   a) Terminal hair is the fine hair found all over the body except on the lips, eyelids, palms and soles of the feet.
   b) Terminal hair is the coarse hair found on the scalp, eyebrows and lashes, arms, legs and pubic regions.

7. What is the name of the structure in which a terminal hair is seated?

8. Which of the following statements are true and which false?
   a) Anagen is the resting stage of the hair growth cycle
   b) Anagen can last from a few weeks to several years
   c) Terminal hair is known as a 'brush hair' when it is in telogen stage of hair growth
   d) Catagen is the transitional stage between anagen and telogen

Outcome 2: Consult, plan and prepare for threading services with clients

Consultation

A consultation should be carried out before every threading treatment and should involve:

- questioning techniques
- visual analysis of the area to be treated
- manual assessment of the area
- referral to the client's record cards.

Details of these techniques and why they are used can be found in Chapter 1 'Professional Skills'.

Contraindications to threading

The specific contraindications to the threading treatment can be grouped into those that prevent or restrict the threading service. Those that prevent treatment are:

- contact lenses
- infectious skin diseases and disorders
- infestations
- eye infections such as conjunctivitis
- recent scar tissue
- sunburn
- skin allergies.

Those that restrict treatment that lead to adaptations to the treatment include:

- the use of **AHA** products
- bruising
- open cuts and abrasions
- mild skin conditions such as eczema or psoriasis
- after recent deep skin peeling treatments, dermal fillers, laser or microdermabrasion, tattooing or semi-permanent make-up.

By this point of the consultation it is essential that the client fully understands the treatment process and the assistance required of them and any possible treatment contra-actions.

> **Key term**
>
> **AHA** – Alpha Hydroxy Acid products used for exfoliation of the skin.

Contra-actions

It is essential that the client is aware of the possible contra-actions that may develop during or after the threading service in order to make an informed decision whether to continue with the treatment or not. The client must also be made aware of the required aftercare advice suggested to prevent the chance of the contra-actions of the threading services from occurring.

Possible contra-actions are as follows:

- erythema
- swelling
- pain
- watery eyes
- sneezing
- nipping/cuts to the skin
- blood spotting
- allergic reaction
- ingrown hairs
- hair breakage.

 Hints and tips

Consider the skin reaction. If an excessive erythema is present or the skin feels hot to touch do not treat the area again.

Condition of the skin and hair

During the visual analysis of the treatment area not only should you check for the presence of any contraindications but also assess the client's suitability for the threading treatment. Assess the client's skin type, the hair growth direction and length in order to select the most suitable threading technique and plan the therapist's positioning for hair removal, allowing the therapist to follow the direction of hair growth.

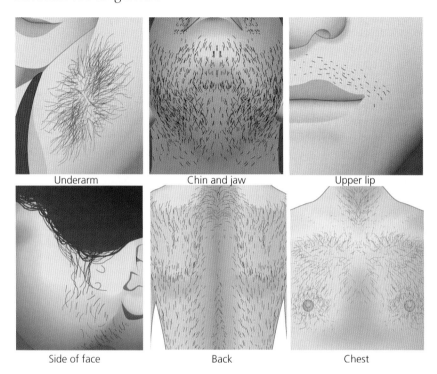

Underarm   Chin and jaw   Upper lip

Side of face   Back   Chest

◁ Direction of hair growth

Use of clients' records

Reference to the client's record card is a useful tool for the therapist. It can provide additional information about the client's previous threading and other related treatments, from which the therapist can make judgements regarding the adaptations necessary for safety and comfort of the client. Information on clients' records includes:

- information regarding the client's skin reaction to treatments, including degree of erythema
- other skin reactions such as swelling and warmth
- appearance of blood spots.

These can be classified as normal skin reaction for types of depilation treatment such as waxing and threading. The client should be made aware of the possible skin reaction to threading treatment before the service begins in order to decide whether to continue with the treatment.

Most normal skin reactions will reduce in a matter of minutes; however, some can last a few hours. This is usually affected by the skin type and any previous treatment in that area.

> ☆ *Hints and tips*
>
> The client may have a special occasion to attend that evening and may be concerned about the erythema in the area or may wish to wear make-up. If that is the case it may be wise to postpone the threading treatment until another time. Instead offer them another service that does not produce an erythema (for example a manicure) so as not to lose the income and the client.

Every client will react differently to the threading treatment and at certain times may feel more or less sensitive to the sensation of hair removal by threading.

It is important to obtain the client's signature after the consultation before the treatment begins as recognition of the accuracy of the facts recorded.

Preparing the client

Prepare the client by giving clear instruction of how to position themselves on the couch and any jewellery or accessories that will need to be removed.

Protect the client's clothing using disposable bed paper or a clean towel across their shoulders to catch the removed hairs as they fall. A headband must be used to protect the client's hair to prevent any accidental removal of the scalp hair which could fall into the working area.

Prepare the skin by cleansing the area with a specific pre-threading product, surgical spirit or rose water and, if required, once dry apply a light coating of talc to help to keep the hair away from the skin. While you complete the skin cleanse it is the ideal time to assess the hair growth direction and length, as it may be necessary to trim the longer hair growth to prevent pulling with the thread.

Now the area is thoroughly prepared and the direction of growth has been assessed the most suitable threading technique needs to be selected and the thread prepared accordingly.

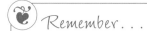 *Remember . . .*

The client's modesty, privacy and comfort must be maintained at all times throughout the treatment.

Preparing yourself for threading

Back to basics

Use the boxes to check your own personal appearance.

❑ A high standard of personal hygiene is presented.

❑ Fresh breathe free from cigarette or food odours

❑ Clean, pressed work wear.

❑ Clean, low-heeled, enclosed shoes.

❑ Arms and hands free from jewellery (plain wedding bands are acceptable).

❑ Any earrings or necklaces are discreet.

❑ Make-up is discreet and expertly applied.

❑ Long hair is tied neatly away from the face and shoulders.

❑ Nails are short, smooth, clean and free of nail enamel.

❑ Tights, or socks with trousers, are worn.

❑ Cuts or open wounds are covered with a clean dressing.

❑ Hands are washed immediately before and after a client.

❑ Adopt a calm and professional manner at all times.

Outcome 3: Remove unwanted hair

Threading techniques

There are three threading techniques that can be used; these are the **mouth technique**, **neck technique** and **hand technique**.

Mouth technique

To complete the mouth technique, one end of the thread is placed into the therapist's mouth and then a single loop is formed by holding parts of the thread in both hands. One point to remember is that with this technique it can be harder to communicate with the client with the thread in your mouth.

Neck technique

The neck technique is very similar to the mouth technique. However, instead of positioning the thread into the mouth it is tied around the therapist's neck.

Hand technique

The hand technique involves a double loop, which means the thread can work in two directions. To complete this technique a piece of thread is cut to length and tied at one end; the hands then hold the thread open at each end and by rotating one hand you will create the twist in the centre of the thread.

Threading has benefits that no other hair removal technique can boast as it involves no sources of heat, no use of strong chemical products or stretching of the skin. Due to these factors the treatment's effects to the skin are mild, which often means threading can be suitable for those who are too sensitive to use other hair removal techniques. The treatment is easy to prepare for and relatively inexpensive to start up as there is no need for any expensive electrical equipment and there is no waiting for equipment to heat up to a working temperature like with waxing.

The threading treatment is ideal for all facial areas as it is possible to remove groups of hairs in larger areas or to create clean, defined eyebrow shapes using the thread to offer precision by removing hairs individually. There is no need for tweezing at the end of this treatment as even the short hairs can be removed with the thread and you can rework over an area more than once without the worry of the skin's sensitivity or over exposure to heat like during a waxing service.

Threading could be performed on other body areas and it is recommended to practise on arms or legs to help when perfecting your techniques. It would not be recommended on the underarm or bikini line areas.

> **Health and safety**
>
> When treating clients you must use a fresh piece of thread for each of the facial areas that you work on. If blood becomes present on the thread this must be correctly disposed of and replaced immediately.

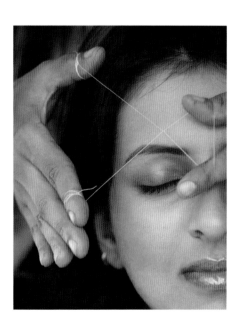

△ The hand technique

When performing the threading treatment the client is asked to assist the therapist by stretching the area to keep the skin taut during the hair removal. When working on the eyebrows the client is asked to hold one hand above the brow and one on the eyelid to stretch the area; with the other facial areas the client will be asked to tilt the head to one side or lift the chin upwards or even to blow out the cheek as the area is being worked over. When working on the upper lip the client is asked to position their tongue under the sides of the mouth and to pull down their lip as the therapist work across the central area, to enable the therapist to achieve a clean removal of the unwanted hair growth.

The therapist should advise a client undergoing a course of permanent hair removal, such as epilation, to avoid threading in the same facial area, as threading can have an adverse effect by increasing the blood supply to the area instead of reducing it. (For fuller details of epilation and other methods of hair removal, please see Chapter 10 'B6 Carry out waxing services'.)

If the client is likely to find it difficult to hold the area taut themselves it may be advisable that another person is available to stretch and support the treatment area on behalf of the client while the therapist performs the threading service for comfort and success of the treatment.

Once the client is positioned comfortably and the headband has been positioned the following procedure should be followed:

Eyebrow threading

To determine the shape of brow to be achieved, and one that suits the client, refer to Chapter 5 'B5 Enhance the appearance of eyebrows and lashes', and specifically the section on eyebrow shaping with tweezers.

1. Cleanse the skin with the chosen suitable cleansing product.

2. Confirm the areas to be treated and the desired brow shape.

3. Measure the eyebrow length and symmetry of the current shape and assess the suitability of the requested shape to be produced.

4. Ask the client to pull taut the eyebrow area and maintain this throughout the hair removal.

5. Begin to thread with the chosen technique from the outer point inward (against the hair growth) until all the required hairs have been removed, then repeat to the other brow. It is important to maintain the tension of the thread to allow an effective removal technique.

6. Check the shape that has been created and continue to tidy above the brow out towards the hairline to remove any stray hairs and provide further definition to the brow shape.

7. Brush the brows into position using a disposable brow brush and if any are growing out of line these can be carefully trimmed back into line with the use of sterile small scissors.

> ☆ *Hints and tips*
>
> *When selecting the different threading methods be aware of your own safety if you wear dental braces, false teeth or crowns as they may affect the suitability of the mouth technique being used. However, do think about adapting your techniques for the practitioner's and client's comfort.*

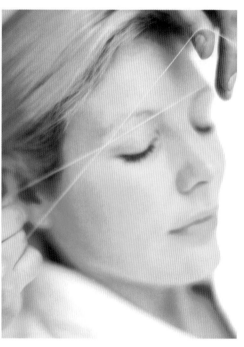

△ A client having an eyebrow thread treatment

8. Calm and soothe the area by wiping with the selected after-threading product, applied using a cotton pad. Remove the headband and allow the client to sit. Show them the results with a hand-held mirror. Check for client approval and continue to give aftercare advice.

Lip/chin or sides of face

1. Cleanse the skin with the chosen suitable cleansing product.

2. Confirm the areas to be treated with the client.

3. Explain to the client how to hold the area taut by stretching the chin upwards, blowing out the cheek, positioning the tongue under the sides of the lips or pulling down the centre of the lip. Explain that they should maintain this throughout the treatment.

4. Begin to thread with the chosen technique methodically against the hair growth until all the required hairs have been removed. Remember to maintain the thread tension to allow an effective hair removal technique.

5. Check by looking from either side of the face that all of the hairs have been removed effectively

6. Calm and soothe the area by wiping with the selected after-threading product, applied using a cotton pad. Remove the headband and allow the client to sit. Show them the results with a hand-held mirror. Check for client approval and continue to give aftercare advice.

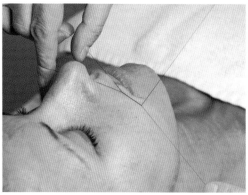

△ Lip, chin or side of face thread

Outcome 4: Provide aftercare advice

Completing treatment and aftercare

It is important to examine the area treated and to note the skin's reaction to treatment on the client's record card. Ensure that the treatment meets the client's expectations. Any remaining hairs that may be too short for removal by threading can be removed with sterile tweezers. If significant areas of hair remain in the area this could be for the following reasons:

- The hair was too short for the thread to grip properly.
- The area was not cleansed sufficiently to remove body lotion or natural oil on the skin.
- The client did not keep the skin taut during the treatment.
- The thread was applied incorrectly without following the natural hair growth.

Following treatment you should wipe over the area with after-wax lotion or a natural rosewater to cool and soothe the treated area.

Aftercare advice

During the 24 hours after treatment the client must avoid the following:

- Perfumed products and chemical-based products will increase skin sensitivity, prolonging the skin's reaction to threading.
- Wearing make-up over the area treated on the face as the follicles are left open and there is an increased risk of infection. A tinted medicated lotion can be used, such as that produced for use after epilation.
- Sunbathing or sunbed treatments, because the skin has been sensitised by the threading treatment and the effects of exposure to UV light will be increased.
- As the skin is sensitive it is wise to avoid any heated treatments such as steam facials, using a sauna or steam room or even taking a hot bath. This is more important the more sensitive the client's skin type.
- Avoid contact with strong chemicals such as those used in swimming pools.
- Avoid an intensive exercise session, as increasing the body temperature will lengthen the time the erythema lasts.
- Avoid touching the area treated as this will cause infections.

The client should be encouraged to purchase aftercare lotion or at least be told how to cool and soothe the treatment area at home. This is an ideal retailing opportunity!

As the hair growth begins to reappear (after two or three weeks), the client should be encouraged to exfoliate the area to avoid the formation of ingrowing hairs. They should be informed of the recommended interval between threading treatments to avoid over-treating the area. This interval will vary for each client but is usually between three and six weeks.

Clearing away after threading

Threading can be a messy treatment because of the hairs being removed falling on to the skin or surrounding areas. Ensure that the area and equipment are cleaned immediately.

Disposable items should be placed into a lined waste bin during the treatment after use, to make cleaning easier and to maintain the hygiene of the trolley.

The paper couch cover should be changed and the trolley should be wiped over.

Activity

Prepare an aftercare leaflet for use with your threading clients.

Want to know more?

The Code of Practice for hygiene and waxing are available from the HABIA website www.habia.org.uk.

Test yourself

1. What is the procedure for treating minors for threading services?
2. What Act of Parliament regulates the correct storage of client records?
3. How can you avoid repetitive strain injury during threading services?
4. What is the importance of using a new piece of thread for each facial area?
5. Name two contraindications that prevent threading.
6. From what is the thread used in threading services made?
7. How frequently should a client have a threading treatment?
8. How do you ensure a complimentary and symmetrical eyebrow shape?
9. How do you adapt the threading treatment to suit a male client?
10. What are the alternatives to threading for temporary removing unwanted hair?

Are you ready for assessment?

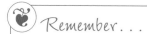

Remember . . .

Practice makes perfect! The more opportunities you have to complete threading services the more confident you will be when it comes to being observed by your assessor.

The following checklist will help you to be fully prepared for your assessment.

The range of treatments you must cover:

- Use various consultation techniques.
- Consider your actions if contra indications are present.
- Carry out the range of threading treatments.
- Use all the methods of threading on appropriate parts of the face.
- Use all the work techniques.
- Provide aftercare advice.

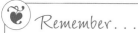

Remember . . .

Your assessor will observe your performance on at least four occasions, each involving a different client and two to include a full eyebrow reshape.

1. **Practical observation**

   Your assessor will look at how you:

   - prepare the treatment area
   - consult with the client and prepare a record card
   - carry out a threading service on a client (not a fellow student or colleague) using a range of methods
   - carry out the threading service in a commercially acceptable time
   - check with the client that the threading service meets her expectations
   - provide aftercare advice
   - demonstrate professional practice throughout the service
   - carry out all services with regard to health and safety.

2. **Knowledge and understanding**

   What you must know:

   - Organisational and legal requirements.
   - How to work safely and effectively when providing threading services.
   - How to consult, plan and prepare for threading services with clients.
   - Contraindications and contra-actions.
   - Anatomy and physiology of hair growth.
   - Tools, materials and equipment.
   - Threading services for different areas of the face.
   - Aftercare advice.

   To ensure that you have the necessary knowledge and understanding of threading services your assessor will:

   - ask you questions before, during and after carrying out the treatment
   - ensure that you have completed project work and written exercises relating to the unit
   - check that you have recorded in a log/diary treatments you have carried out with signed record cards showing that you have completed four threading services competently
   - that you have covered the range in your candidate logbook.

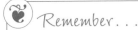 Remember . . .

Simulation is not a valid means of assessment for threading service.

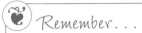 Remember . . .

Comply with the Personal Protective Equipment at Work Regulations 1992 when carrying out any waxing service.

Chapter 7
Unit B8: Provide make-up services

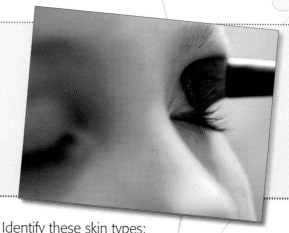

Learning objectives

This chapter is about day, evening and special occasion make-up and its application to a variety of skin types, skin tones and age groups.

There are four learning outcomes for unit B8 and they are:
1 Maintain safe and effective methods of working when providing make-up services.
2 Consult, plan and prepare for make-up services.
3 Apply make-up products.
4 Provide aftercare advice.

You will need to be competent in make-up services outcomes to qualify for insurance and perform the treatment on members of the public.

Evidence requirements

Your assessor will need to observe you perform this treatment successfully on at least three occasions, involving different clients with different skin tones. You must:

1 Demonstrate the use of consultation techniques:
   - questioning
   - visual
   - manual
   - reference to client records.

2 Apply make-up to these age groups:
   - 16-30 years
   - 31-50 years
   - over 50 years.

3 Identify these skin types:
   - oily
   - dry
   - combination.

4 Apply make-up for these occasions:
   - day
   - evening
   - special occasion.

5 Deal with one of these necessary actions:
   - encourage the client to seek medical advice
   - explain why the treatment cannot be carried out
   - modify the treatment.

6 Use these types of make-up product:
   - foundations
   - powders
   - facial contouring products
   - concealers
   - eyebrow products
   - eyeshadows
   - eyeliners
   - mascaras
   - cheek products
   - lip products.

7 Provide this advice:
   - suitable make-up products and their use
   - possible contra-actions and how to deal with them
   - suitable make-up re-application techniques
   - suitable make-up removal techniques.

Introduction

The effect of a professionally applied make-up should not be underestimated. In response to the growing demand for professional make-up application for weddings and portrait photography the service has become increasingly popular, with many salons including 'make-up lessons' as part of their service menu.

Unit B8 forms part of the Level 2 Beauty Therapy qualifications, as a mandatory unit for the 'Make-up route' but appears as an optional unit for the 'Beauty Therapy General' route. It is worth 6 credits.

This chapter is dedicated to basic make-up product selection and application. Once you have mastered these principles, they will form the foundation for the further development of your skills leading to a career in make-up. The art of make-up application is acquired through practice and experimentation with colour and different techniques.

Meet the professional

"When I apply bridal make-up, it has to be the most important make-up I apply and after doing make-up for over 20 years I still get a little anxious that I'll not make a bride look the way she really wants. If she isn't used to wearing make-up then I need to tread especially carefully and explain what's needed so she looks her best in photos. But team my unnecessary nerves along with all the attention of a celebrity wedding and you end up with Jade Goody's big day, which turned out to be the most fulfilling job of my career. What didn't bother me was the overwhelming media interest but that Jade was terminally ill with cancer, so I was especially concerned that I delivered the best results ever and supported her all day.

I knew I would have to tread carefully; she was known for speaking her mind, and I knew that her skin would be like paper and very dehydrated from chemotherapy plus she had lost all her hair. When Jade chose me, I jumped at the chance to be there for her because my own mum had recently been through chemo so I knew the horrid after-effects like nausea, tiredness and how grotty it makes the patient feel. My heart went out to Jade and the great thing now is that I am at a point in my career where I can help people with my services plus help raise awareness for so many good causes.

Anyhow, I met Jade on her big day at the venue and it was a really busy affair with media everywhere trying to get in, plus loads of people inside running around getting busy. A large room was provided for all the bridesmaids and Jade to have hair and make-up done. The lighting wasn't great, as is the norm in hotels, but you just have to make do and try to use daylight where possible. (Not all my jobs are in well-kitted studios.) I set my things up on a table then went to the bar in search of a high stool, yes, a high stool and not a large G&T, for Jade to sit on as it's better for my back after years of bending over doing make-up. Jade strolled in wearing just a bathrobe, with her nurse, and said 'Hi' to me and gave me a kiss. I could see she was tired but totally in control and determined that the day would be fantastic. I asked her how she would like her make-up. "Natural or smokey?" She replied, "Do whatever you think, Daniel, I trust you." I decided on lilac eye shadow with some shimmery white and pink with two sets of glamorous false lashes and some liquid liner, shimmery pink cheeks, soft pink glossy lips and bronzing lotion on her body. Her skin was really dry so I used formulas that nourished yet evened out her skin tone, even on her lovely, bald head. She looked sensational and presented me with a wonderful bottle of champagne as a thank you.

About three weeks later, Jade passed away, but I have amazing photos as a reminder.

For me as the make-up artist, doing someone's make-up is not just a job. We have a profound effect on how a person feels as well as how they look, so we must be sensitive and treat each client as special and be able to adapt to any situation. Case in question."

Daniel Sandler

Outcome 1: Maintain safe and effective methods of working when providing make-up services

Legal requirements

The following table gives a summary of the relevant legislation that applies to make-up services.

▽ Relevant legislation that applies to make-up services

The treatment room	Health & Safety at Work Act 1974	General safety of staff and visitors to the salon, including clients
	The Workplace (Health, Safety & Welfare) Regulations 1992	Governs the working environment, including ventilation, temperature and lighting, etc.
	Regulatory Reform (Fire Safety) Order 2005	The safe evacuation of the building in an emergency such as a fire
Equipment	Provision and Use of Work Equipment Regulations 1998	Governs the acquisition of safe and reliable equipment
Make-up products	Control of Substances Hazardous to Health 1988	Governs the exposure of persons to substances likely to cause harm, including flammability and the effect on the tissues
	Cosmetic Products (Safety) Regulations (2008)	Requires cosmetics to comply with correct labelling, to have safe formulation and be fit for the purpose intended
Disposal of waste	The Controlled Waste Regulations 1992	Governs the correct disposal of contaminated waste i.e. that contaminated with blood or other bodily fluids

Treating clients who are minors

Young people have always experimented with make-up, but with the advent of 'make-over parties', the age at which make-up is worn is getting lower and more parents find this acceptable. There are no legal guidelines about the wearing of make-up and it is entirely an individual's choice. However, there are legal implications for a therapist or a make-up/skin care consultant who offers make-up services to minors. A minor is a person who has not attained the age fixed for entering in to a legal contract or for making himself or herself legally liable for his or her actions.

The legal age at which a person is deemed a minor varies nationally. Therapists and consultants should check with their local authority and act accordingly. In England, a person under the age of 18 years is a minor. In Scotland, a person under 17 is a minor.

This means that for a client under 18 years of age, parental or legal guardian written consent is needed. For clients under 16 years of age, attendance at the salon during the service is required.

'Make-over parties' aimed at clients aged between 7 and 16 years of age or even younger are being added to a salon's treatment menu (alongside other treatments such as mini manicures and pedicures and nail art services). It is important that any therapist or make-up consultant offering these services is checked by the Criminal Records Bureau (CRB) and that this fact is stated on any literature promoting such events. In this case, it would still be necessary to obtain written consent for treatment from all parents or guardians of the minors attending the party.

Make-up services

The time taken to perform the make-up service must conform to commercially acceptable treatment times for the industry and should be shown on the salon treatment price list. Below is an example with the accepted timings for each service indicated.

▽ Make-up service timings

Service description	Service time	Price
Make-up application Simply, the application of make-up for those that want something special for a party or a family photograph.	30 mins	£15
Make-up lesson A more in-depth treatment that gives away some of the make-up artist's secret to a fantastic looking make-up.	60 mins	£25
Make-up package A two-stage treatment for a special event. First the 'trial' where time is taken to try out looks and products to find those that suit, and then the application on the day of the event itself.	Trial: 90 mins Event: 30 mins	Total for the package: £60

The prices quoted here are examples. A city centre salon may charge a lot more, due to the overheads (such as rent and rates) that accompany running a salon in a city. A mobile therapist may charge less. The pricing of a treatment is determined by many factors, but you should always consider your local competition.

Setting up for make-up application

Whether you are performing the make-up service within the salon or at the client's home you must always be professional and follow strict personal and treatment hygiene procedures. Your set up for make-up services should reflect these high standards. It is important to instil confidence in your client and you must ensure your appearance is appropriate. A client will expect you to be professional both in appearance and manner. It is particularly important to wear make-up. This should not be heavy but will indicate that you take care with your appearance.

Equipment checklist

It is important to ensure the work area is prepared prior to the client's arrival. Your workstation should be equipped with:

✔ cleansing, toning and moisturising products — a selection should be available to accommodate different skin types
✔ concealer products — colour corrective and flesh tone
✔ foundations — a selection of shades and types
✔ facial powders — translucent and coloured
✔ facial bronzing products
✔ contour cosmetics — highlighters and shader
✔ cheek products — cream and powder type
✔ eyeshadows — a selection of colours in cream/powder and matt/pearlised finish
✔ mascara
✔ eyebrow products — powders and pencils
✔ eyeliners — liquid, powder and gel products
✔ lip products — lipsticks, glosses and pencils.

In addition, you will need:

✔ disposable items - cotton wool, cotton wool buds, tissues, spatulas and brushes
✔ a selection of small bowls
✔ laundry — headbands or hair clips, gowns and towels
✔ mirror
✔ a selection of brushes — different sizes, shapes and densities and disposable
✔ a selection of sponges and velour powder puffs
✔ a covered waste bin
✔ client treatment plan or record card.

Brushes

A good set of brushes will last for many years. You will soon find that they are familiar tools that you can easily select to meet the needs of particular make-up techniques. Professional brushes should be long handled and made from sable or soft bristle.

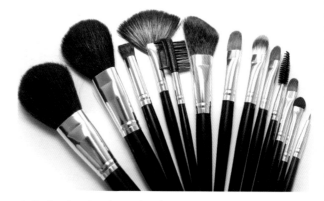

△ Professional make-up brushes

You will require a large-headed powder brush, a blusher brush, a contour brush and a selection of eyeshadow brushes. These should include a sponge-tipped applicator, an angled brush head, a dome-shaped brush head and a wider brush, which is useful for blending. You will find that most professional brushes have the suggested function identified on the handle. You may disregard these if you wish and use whichever suits the need of the application. A combined brush/comb is required for grooming the brows and for separating the eyelashes. A fine brush is essential for eyeliner application and a lip brush is vital for applying cosmetics to the lips with precision. You will also require a selection of sponges and facial wedges. Eyelash curlers can be also be used to enhance the eyes.

All tools and equipment should be sterilised in the appropriate way (see Chapter 1) and should not be brought to the trolley until you are ready to use them.

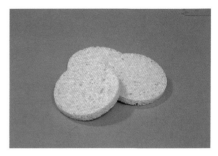

△ Make-up sponges

Positioning the client

The client should be comfortably positioned on the couch or in the make-up chair. They should be in a seated position and not lying flat for make-up application, due to the effects of gravity on the facial features. This is a vital point to note when performing make-up services on older clients.

The client's clothes should be protected with towels and/or a gown and their hair either pinned back carefully or protected with a headband. The therapist can be either seated or standing, depending on the working height of the couch or chair

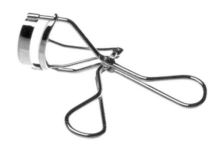

 Eyelash curlers

The treatment environment

One of the most important requirements for make-up application is good lighting. Ideally, this should be natural daylight. However, this is not always possible. You will need a good quality lamp, one that is capable of simulating natural daylight and that does not flood the face with bright white light. It should also be adjustable to accommodate client positioning. It is important to ask the client about the conditions in which the make-up will be worn and adapt it accordingly. For example, you will have to consider the effects of artificial light on evening make-up.

✋ Health and safety

The couch or chair should be height adjustable so that the client and therapist are at the same eye-level. This will help you to avoid fatigue and lower back pain from bending. The trolley or work surface should be conveniently positioned in front of you to avoid unnecessary twisting of the spine. You should work so that your favoured hand is closest to the couch when facing the client (so, on the client's right if you are right-handed).

Effects of different lighting conditions on make-up

Daylight

Daylight is a pure white light. It reflects off light-coloured walls and surfaces and therefore does not create shadows. It gives a 'true' representation of the colours of the skin and also of any make-up applied. It can, however, show up all make-up mistakes such as the wrong choice of tone in a foundation base or if the make-up is not blended. Special types of simulated daylight bulbs are available – these are designed to recreate daylight that gives out a warm white light, which, when placed either side of a mirror, give the ideal lighting for the application of make-up.

Fluorescent lighting

Fluorescent light should be avoided as it is usually delivered through strip lighting – tubes of blue-white light that remove the warmth from make-up colours. The light is normally directed straight downwards, creating shadows. However, modern fittings have diffusers, which soften the light and spread the light source. This has the effect of removing shadows.

Filament lighting

This is found in standard light bulbs and produces a yellowish light, which dulls any blue-toned colours and darkens any that are red-toned. The shades used with these bulbs create sharp shadows as they direct light down instead of allowing it to go outwards.

Hygiene procedures specific for make-up

General hygiene and sterilising procedures are discussed in Chapter 1. The section that follows here is about the application of general procedures to the tools and equipment used during make-up services and the maintenance of hygienic products during their application.

1. Avoid applying make-up when there are known infectious skin diseases present, such as conjunctivitis, sties or herpes simplex (cold sores).
2. Follow sterilising procedures for make-up tools and equipment as outlined in the table on page 162.
3. Avoid cross-contamination of products by using the 'cut out' procedures outlined on page 163.
4. Use disposable make-up applicators that once have been in contact with the skin must not be placed back into the product, but discarded.

> **Hints and tips**
> Ideally, the make-up room should be decorated in a soft neutral colour. Strong, bold colours with a definite hue on walls and furniture can reflect on the client's skin tone, giving the therapist the wrong information during consultation.

▽ Applying hygiene procedures to make-up tools and equipment

Tools/equipment	Use	Sterilising/hygiene method
Brushes	A universal make-up tool used to apply and blend cream, liquid and powder products from foundation through to lip gloss	A brush cleaner with at least 70% alcohol content will destroy most micro-organisms effectively. Simply dip into the liquid and blot onto a tissue, repeating until the brush is clean. For large brushes such as a blusher brush, place the cleaner onto a tissue and wipe brush bristles until clean. Useful for when washing and drying a brush ready for use is impossible due to time pressures but continued use of brush cleaner will dry out the bristles, so occasionally 'shampoo and condition' brushes to maintain condition. Alternatively, wash brushes in hot soapy water to remove make-up and place in sterilising fluid for time recommended by the manufacturer; rinse and remove excess water then dry overnight in a warm place that allows air to circulate around the bristles. Take care not to wet the 'join' between brush head and handle as this will result in their separation.
Sponges	To apply cream and liquid products such as concealers, highlighters, shader, blusher and foundation	Wash in hot soapy water to remove make-up and then submerge into a sterilising liquid for the appropriate time. Alternatively they can be washed and offered to the client as part of the make-up service.
Powder puffs	To apply face powders to 'set' the foundation base and to provide a protective pad for your hand when applying other products	Wash in hot soapy water and submerge into sterilising fluid or wash in a washing machine with other suitable laundry at a temperature of at least 60°C. They should be then re-shaped and placed in a warm place to dry.
Fingers	To apply cream products such as concealers, foundation, highlighters, shader, cheek and eye products	Wash hands thoroughly immediately before and after each client with an anti-bacterial or alcohol-based hand-wash. Cover any open wounds with a waterproof dressing.
Sharpeners/ spatulas/scissors/ palette	To maintain the hygienic state of the make-up products	Clean away make-up residue and sterilise in sterilising fluid.

▽ Cut-out procedures for hygienic use of make-up products

Types of product	Examples	Cut-out procedure
Liquid	Mascara, eyeliner, cheek or eye make-up	Use disposable applicators such as wand or liners, one for each application even on the same client or dispense product onto a sterile make-up palette.
Cream	Foundations, concealers, highlighters, shader, eyeshadows, blusher, lip gloss and lipstick	Remove from container with clean spatula or cotton bud onto a make-up palette before use. Replace lid or close pot immediately. Can use straight from the clean spatula if desired.
Pencil	Eyeliners, eyebrow and lip pencils, eyeshadow pencils	Sharpen before and after use with a clean sterile pencil sharpener.
Powder	Foundations, concealers, eyeshadows, blushers, face bronzers, highlighters and shader	Scrape from the container with a clean spatula, returning lids and closing container immediately.

For information regarding legal requirements for make-up services see page 157 and for general safe, effective methods of work including sterilising procedures see Chapter 1 'Professional Skills'.

Outcome 2: Consult, plan and prepare for make-up services

To obtain a perfect make-up finish, knowledge of the skin is essential. The beauty therapist must be able to make an accurate assessment of the client's skin in order to select the correct cleansing and make-up products, as well as the right application technique. You should have a clear understanding of skin structure, function, disorders, disease and damage. Learning about skin disease and disorders is important, as the presence of a condition can determine whether a treatment should be performed.

Details of skin structure and function can be found in Chapter 19 and disease and disorders of the skin and details of consultation techniques in Chapter 4.

It is vital to undertake a thorough consultation with the client to find out about their needs and wishes. A consultation also provides an opportunity to advise the client of the achievable outcomes. All findings from the consultation should be recorded on the client's treatment plan. Be aware that a client may feel sensitive about their personal appearance. You should show discretion and sensitivity when performing make-up services. You should respect the clients' modesty and privacy with personal information according to the Data Protection Act 1998.

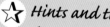

☆ *Hints and tips*

If your client is wearing contact lenses, take particular care when working around the eyes. Cream products may be a better choice than powder.

Contraindications to make-up

The specific contraindications to make-up services are divided into three groups. They are:

1. Those that require medical referral:
   - infectious skin conditions such as impetigo and herpes simplex
   - parasitic infections such as pediculosis and scabies
   - eye infections such as conjunctivitis
   - severe skin conditions such as acne, boils, herpes zoster, warts
   - severe medical conditions.

2. Those that restrict treatment:
   - recent scar tissue (less than six months old)
   - eczema
   - hyper-keratosis
   - skin allergies
   - bruising
   - styes
   - watery eyes
   - recent cosmetic surgery, tattoos or piercings
   - recent laser, microdermabrasion.

The client should also be made aware of the possible **contra-actions** that may occur after a make-up service at the time of the consultation and given time to ask questions. In this way the client can make an informed decision about whether to continue with the service or the therapist can adapt treatment procedures. You will find the contra-actions to make-up in Outcome 4 near the end of this chapter.

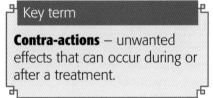

Key term

Contra-actions – unwanted effects that can occur during or after a treatment.

Outcome 3: Apply make-up products

Preparation of the skin before make-up application

To achieve a professional application of make-up, the skin must be clean and free from grease, stale make-up and cleansing products. It is important to prepare the skin correctly and this means choosing the correct cleansing products for the client's skin type. Details of cleansing, toning and moisturising products can be found in Chapter 4. Once the skin is cleansed and a suitable moisturiser applied the face and neck are ready for make-up application.

Make-up products

The foundation base is the basis of a successful make-up. It provides the ideal surface to receive other cosmetics and will even out the complexion. The key here is a flawless complexion that looks entirely natural. There are three stages to the perfect foundation base: the application of concealer, foundation and powder.

Concealers

Concealers are specially formulated to disguise minor imperfections and skin blemishes such as breakouts, scars, areas of pigmentation and red veins. They are usually cream-based, but stick, liquid and powder concealers are also available. They come in a range of specific colours or flesh tones and vary in texture depending on the amount of pigment present in the product. It is this that gives the variation in coverage.

Application

These products are applied with a brush, cotton wool bud or a clean fingertip, normally before the foundation, but they can be applied afterwards as long as there is a good colour match. Flesh tones are used to conceal areas where there is a change in colour pigment or dark circles under the eyes. Usually, a shade that is one or two shades lighter than the skin area will give the best results. Coloured concealers are used to disguise areas of colour, such as redness caused by erythema. Knowledge of the 'colour wheel' is necessary in these cases. Details of the use of the colour wheel in make-up application can be found in Chapter 9.

Foundation

A good foundation will even out differences in colour of the skin, conceal minor blemishes, correct any imperfections and act as a barrier between the skin and any atmospheric pollution. Many foundations contain sunscreens to protect the skin from the damaging effects of ultraviolet light. They are available as a liquid, cream, compact, stick, mousse, mineral-based powder and as a tinted moisturiser. Choose the correct type according to the client's skin type and condition to achieve a skin that gives a smooth, regular and lustrous appearance.

Application

A variety of tools can be used for the application of foundation.

1. Application with a sponge is the most widely used method with liquid, cream, mousse, compact foundations. Different sponges are available in varying shapes such as latex, latex-free, natural and synthetic, wedge and round. Dampen the sponge with water and remove excess water by squeezing in a tissue or towel before use. A sponge gives a medium, natural looking coverage when used in a 'stippling action' (a cross between a pat and a roll).

2. Application with the fingers is an acceptable method as long as the hands are free from open wounds and have been thoroughly cleaned. This method is suitable for almost all types of foundations except compact and enables the exact placement of the product. The application can be finished with a light stippling with a clean damp sponge to give a natural and durable result.

3. The use of a foundation brush gives a perfect application of a liquid or cream type foundation and can give a light covering or a well-covered effect, depending on the amount of product used.

⭐ *Hints and tips*

Less is more! A light application of a heavy cream can look better than a heavy application of a light cream concealer, particularly if there are fine lines and wrinkles in the area.

4. Airbrush techniques have increased in popularity for use in applying a flawless finish foundation. It is a technique that requires a great deal of practice but the results are excellent and allow for complete accuracy and speed in application for the therapist.

5. The 'Kabuki brush' has a special style and shape and is used after the application of a cream foundation with the fingers or foundation brush. It is used in a circular motion to 'polish' the base and gives an exceptionally natural finish. It can be used successfully with compact and mineral- based powder foundations and for the application of contouring make-up products.

Types of foundation

Liquid – a variety of liquid foundations are available with different ingredients for different skin types. Water-based liquid foundations dry to give a matt, natural finish. Oil-based foundations may have the addition of beneficial ingredients such as emollients, sun protection factors and free radicals to combat the effects of skin ageing.

Cream – cream foundations also vary, from a light mousse where the product is aerated, to a stick or compact. Cream foundations contain oils, fats or waxes and skin coloured pigments and it is the quantity of each of these that gives the product its different texture and coverage ability. A stick foundation has a high degree of waxes rather than oil, whereas a mousse will have more oils.

Mineral-based powder – these contain finely ground minerals to give a range of colours and tones and provide medium coverage for most skin types. They contain no 'fillers' (often found in cream and liquid foundations) that can cause allergies. Minerals such as zinc oxide and zinc dioxide also provide a sun protection factor (SPF) of 15–20.

Tinted moisturiser – these give a light coverage for skins that are blemish-free. They contain light oils (such as grapeseed), with copper light-reflecting pigments to give a 'shimmer' effect.

Selecting the right foundation type

When selecting a foundation you will need to consider the skin type, the coverage required and the skin tone.

Skin type – it is vital to consider this. If the wrong product is selected, the completed make-up may be poor and the effect may not last long. If the right product is selected and it is applied correctly, foundation should last throughout the day, should not change colour or need to be reapplied.

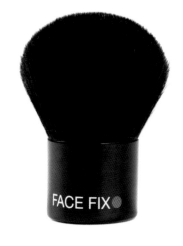

△ Kabuki brush

> ⭐ *Hints and tips*
> *When applying foundation, work systematically so as not to miss any areas. Finishing with the eyes will ensure an even coverage all over. Work up under the lower lashes and then over the eyelid ensuring you get right into the inner corner of the eye.*

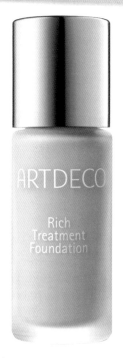

△ Foundation

▽ Choice of foundation type for skin type and condition

Skin type	Foundation type
Normal	Tinted moisturiser, mineral based, liquid or mousse
Oily	Water based liquid, mineral based or compact
Dry	Cream, stick or tinted moisturiser
Combination	Liquid, mineral based, compact or mousse
Mature	Cream, oil based liquid or stick
Sensitive	Hypo-allergenic liquid or cream or mineral based
Dehydrated	Mousse, mineral based or cream
Blemished	Medicated liquid or mineral based

Coverage – the different types of foundation will give varying degrees of coverage. Choosing the correct degree of coverage depends on the skin and the effect required. Care should be taken with mature clients that a light cream foundation is used, as heavy and powder products will emphasise lines and wrinkles.

▽ Coverage of foundation types

Coverage	Foundation type
Low	Tinted moisturiser
Medium	Liquid, mineral based, mousse, cream, compact
High	Stick, cream

Skin colour – when selecting a foundation, you should aim to match the colour as closely to the natural skin colour as possible. If the colour is not selected with great care, the result may be an unattractive, mask-like appearance. Consider not only how light or dark the skin appears (the shade) but also the 'tone'. This is described as either 'warm' or 'cool' and is the underlying colour within the skin. Skin tone does not change with age or exposure to ultra-violet light but skin 'shade' lightens with age and darkens in sunlight.

▽ Foundation colour for skin tone

Skin tone	Natural features	Foundation colour
Cool skin tones	Ash-blonde to black hair Blue, brown or black eyes Pale pink/beige to dark brown to ebony skin colour	Rose or beige tones in light to dark shades.
Warm skin tones	Golden/strawberry blonde to warm dark brown hair Green, hazel or warm brown eyes Cream, yellow, olive, or gold skin colour	Honey and golden tones in light to dark shades

> ☆ **Hints and tips**
> Water-based liquid and mousse foundations tend to 'dry' on the skin so blend edges in each area of the face as it is applied, paying particular attention to the hairline and the eyebrows.

> ☆ **Hints and tips**
> Always check around hairline and jawline for demarcation lines. Use a clean edge of a damp sponge to blend the foundation.

> ☆ **Hints and tips**
> A simple way of determining skin tone is to look at the skin on the inner forearm, if the veins here appear blue, the skin is 'cool' toned; if green, 'warm'.

Choosing a foundation is a particular problem when selecting foundations for black skins. The skin on the face can vary greatly in shade and the 'tone' is often difficult to determine due to the amount of pigment present. Aim to choose a foundation that matches in tone. View the lightest colour to determine the tone and a shade that complements the darker skin colour, as long as this is not too dark. Foundation is not always necessary on darker skins, if the colour is even. Instead, a light dusting of powder could be used to take off any excess shine and to provide a good base for the rest of the make-up application.

Face powders

The application of cream, liquid, stick and mousse foundation should always be followed by powder to set the make-up to make sure it will last and to reduce shine. Powders contain powdered talc and other minerals such as mica and silk proteins. Face powder also provides the ideal base on which to place powdered cheek and eye products and is perfect for a make-up retouch during the day.

Face powders can be loose (favoured by professionals) or compressed into a compact (convenient and avoids messy powder spillages in make-up bags and handbags). Types of face powders are translucent, mineral based, shimmered, and light reflecting. A good face powder should be easy to apply, smooth on the skin and allow the colour of the foundation to be seen, without changing the base colour. Some powders can be worn without a base and can be used to give a glow to the skin. Care should be taken when choosing a face powder for black skins – it should not contain talc or other white powder, as they will make a black skin grey in colour.

Translucent powder allows light to diffuse through without changing the underlying skin or foundation base colour. The main constituent of powder is talc, which gives slip and covering power. Compressed powders are often pigmented to offer dense coverage with a velvety finish all from one product. They are useful for touch-ups.

Metallic particles may be added to powder to give a pearly look or shimmer. They give the skin a healthy, ethereal glow. This type of powder is particularly effective for evening wear and could easily be added to adapt day make-up for evening. They should, however be used with caution: they emphasise breakouts on a blemished skin and during photography they can make the skin look moist as the metallic particles reflect light from the flash.

 Hints and tips
Foundation should always be tested on the face, not on the back of the hand. The skin on the hand is very different in both colour and texture and will not show the true effect of the product.

 Hints and tips
A simple rule to remember is 'powder on powder, cream on cream'. In this way the products such as cheek and eye products can be blended easily for a natural and professional finish.

☆ **Hints and tips**
Always apply a light dusting of powder to the lips and eyelids. This will help the eye and lip cosmetics adhere to the area.

☆ **Hints and tips**
Never apply powder that is darker than the foundation. Apply sparingly if the skin is excessively dry or if the under-eye area is wrinkled.

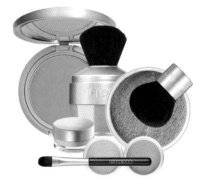

△ Face powder products

Application

There are two methods by which powder can be applied during a make-up application. In each case the powder should be removed from its container with a clean spatula and placed onto the make-up palette or a tissue.

1. To apply powder with a powder brush, place the brush into the powder and tap off the excess. Stroke the brush downwards over the face, concentrating on the eyes and nose and other areas where shine can be seen. This gives a natural appearance to the skin for day make-up or mature skins, where powder may emphasise lines and wrinkles.

2. To apply with a velour powder puff, press the puff into the powder and tap to remove excess. Starting with the eyes, press powder over upper lid and then under the eye. Gently press powder all over the face and remove excess with the powder brush in a downward direction. This method will ensure that the make-up lasts all day. However, it feels less natural to the client. It is suitable for clients with oily skins or for bridal or photography make-up.

> ⭐ **Hints and tips**
> Using the brush in a downwards movement ensures the tiny vellus hairs on the face are lying flat.

> ⭐ **Hints and tips**
> Take care when applying powder under the eye if the client is wearing contact lenses.

Bronzing products

Bronzing products are used to give 'sun-kissed' colour to the skin and can be used as an alternative to foundation, especially in the summer months. They are available in powder, gel and liquid form but all contain minerals such as iron oxide to give the bronze colouring. Powder bronzing products are similar to face powders and are available as a loose powder. However, they are more commonly found compressed in a compact or 'beads', which are more convenient and are applied with a large bristle brush like a blusher. Gel and liquid bronzers give a light coverage of colour and are best applied with the fingertips like a foundation, then blended with a sponge if necessary.

Due to the bronze colour of these products they are best suited for a client with a warm skin tone who requires a light coverage, such as those with normal or unblemished skins. Powdered bronzers can also be used successfully to correct a foundation that is pale, by brushing lightly over the face to warm the skin.

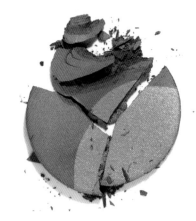

△ Bronzing products

Cheek products

Cheek products commonly known as blusher are the modern name for rouge. They are designed to add colour to the cheek area, simulating a natural cheek colour or adding warmth. They are available in cream, powder, liquid tints and mineral-based powder forms and the colours available vary from very pale pinks through to brick reds and dark browns.

Application

1. Powdered products should be applied with a large bristle brush. Take up from a tissue or palette and tap off the excess, then using a circular motion, apply from below the centre of the eye, working up to the top of the ear along the cheek bone. These types of cheek product are suitable for general use on normal, oily and combination skin types. Powder and mineral-based products are applied over foundation, after the powder has been applied.

2. Cream and liquid tints are best applied with the fingertips or a sponge and are suitable for dry, dehydrated and mature skin types and conditions. They are usually applied after the foundation but before the face powder.

> ⭐ *Hints and tips*
> *Do not exceed application beyond the centre of the client's eye. This can make the application look unnatural and can lead to the cheek having a clown-like appearance.*

Eye products

The eyes are a focal point on the face and therefore eye make-up is one of the most important aspects of a good make-up application. The shape of the eyes can be flattered or altered with an expert application of eyeshadow products. The main function of the application of eye products is to accentuate the eyes and to make them look brighter. On a darker skin the eyes will need to be given added definition by emphasising the eyelashes as well as the eyelids.

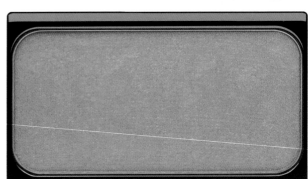

△ Blusher

There is a huge range of eye products to choose from. Care must be taken to discuss with the client their preferences and needs. If the make-up is for a special occasion, find out more about the function and the colour of the outfit to be worn. Ascertain the type of function – a different effect will be required for a wedding, party, family portrait or a job interview.

Mascara

Products to emphasise the eyelashes are waterproof and non-waterproof mascaras. Modern mascaras also contain a variety of beneficial and enhancing ingredients such as silk proteins and lash-building ingredients that lengthen, darken and thicken the lashes. Colour pigments and resins are contained in a base of water or alcohol and water with castor oil to prevent the mascara from becoming brittle. Filaments of rayon or nylon can be used to build and 'extend' lashes. Mascaras that contain such filaments should not be used on contact lens wearers, as the filaments can irritate the eye. Eyeliners include liquid, gel, kohl pencil, pencil and cake eyeliners.

Eyeshadow

Eyeshadows are available in powder, cream, mineral, gel and liquid forms. They can have a matt finish, or contain metallic particles that give an iridescent effect.

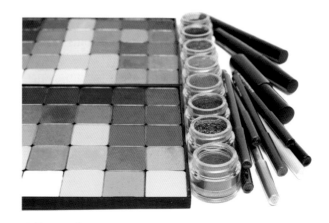

△ Eye products

Application

1. Cream, gel and liquid eyeshadow can be applied before or after the application of face powder onto the eyelid, depending on the effect desired. A brush, a sponge applicator or the fingertips are acceptable tools for application. The product needs to be removed from its container with a hygienic item – a sterilised or disposable spatula, for example – and placed onto a palette for use.

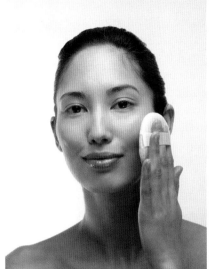

△ Using a powder puff

2. Powder and mineral-based eyeshadows are best applied after face powder to aid blending and can be applied with a make-up brush. Choose a brush that is the correct size and shape for the effect to be achieved: for example, a large flat brush if placing one colour over the entire eye lid or a round, narrow brush for use in the socket line. By using a wet brush a more defined effect can be achieved where a concentration of colour is needed. A hard edge can then be blended with a clean dry brush to soften if desired. To prevent the powder eyeshadow from falling onto the foundation on the cheek area it is advisable to use a facial tissue up under the lower lashes. This also provides a protective barrier between the face and your hand for you to lean on when applying eye make-up.

3. Loose-powder eyeshadows give a strong concentration of colour (perhaps for evening make-up) and are best applied with a brush by pressing the colour into the desired position on the eyelid. This prevents the colour from spreading onto areas where it is not desired.

Eyeliner

Eyeliner is used to encircle the upper and lower eyelids or just on the outer edges of the lids to add definition to the eye. Liquid gel and cake eyeliners are applied with a brush. Pencil and kohl pencil is applied directly to the eyelids after sharpening with a sterilised pencil sharpener before use. Kohl is soft and waxy in texture. It can be quite difficult to control because of its composition and the effect of the body heat on the waxes. Pencil eyeliner is easy to use and suitable for most skin types but care must be taken not to drag the skin, particularly if the skin type is mature. Liquid eyeliner takes more skill to use effectively. It gives strong definition and is more suitable for use in evening make-up application. Pen eyeliners are designed to apply liquid liner more successfully and modern versions give a more subtle effect and so are useful for daywear. The softer, non-setting formulations such as cake or pencil can be smudged using a sponge-tipped applicator or a cotton-wool bud. This gives a softer definition to the eyelid.

 Hints and tips
To prevent contact of your hand, the warmth of which may ruin the foundation application, use the velour powder puff to lean on by looping it over the little finger of your working hand.

 Hints and tips
A 'powder guard' also forms an effective barrier onto which powdered eye make-up products can fall without ruining the foundation and can be easily brushed away when complete. It is, however, not advisable to use this method on clients with dry, dehydrated or mature skin conditions.

 Hints and tips
Clients with contact lenses are advised to use compressed powder or cream eyeshadow to lower the risk of the product entering the eye. A range of products has been designed to suit the needs of contact lens wearers and could be considered when selecting a suitable retail range in the salon.

 Hints and tips
Vary the thickness of the eyeliner on the upper eyelid to suit the shape of the eye. Often, a narrow line at the inner and outer corners gives a natural look that suits most eye shapes.

Mascara is used to give definition to the eyes by thickening and darkening the lashes. These products come with an applicator wand within the product that should not be used in the salon as there is a risk of cross infection. Instead, a disposable applicator should be used for each eye and for each additional coat of product to prevent contamination of the product in its container. Curl the lashes prior to mascara application if required. Apply mascara to the bottom lashes of both eyes first and then ask the client to look down. Lift the skin of the eyelids from underneath the brow and apply to the top lashes. In this way you will not get mascara on your eyeshadow application. Use a zigzag movement to get lashes between the bristles of the brush to coat all of the lashes. Build up in fine coats, allowing each one to dry, rather than one thick coat. Separate using an eyelash comb if necessary.

Eyebrow products

Eyebrow products are available in grey, brown and black colours and in pencil or cake formats. They should be applied in light, feathery strokes, not in hard, defined lines. The cake type uses an angled brush with short, synthetic bristles. They are used to add definition to the eyebrow area and can also be used in corrective work to balance or to fill in missing brows. Take special care when using black eyebrow pencil to avoid dark, unnatural brow lines. The brows should be brushed into shape before application. Aim to create the appearance of natural hair growth by brushing through after application to soften the effect.

Lip products

Lip products are available in the form of lip liner, lipstick, lip gloss and lip balm: the choice of product will depend upon the finished effect required. They are each used to define, enhance and balance the lip shape. The main ingredients of lip products are oils, fats and waxes.

Lipsticks have a high percentage of wax, which gives it its stiffened form. They vary in terms of their staying power. A number of products claim to stay on all day. Softening ingredients such as petroleum jelly or mineral oil are also included in varying amounts depending on the formulation. Lip gloss is usually formulated with a high grease content. It can be clear or pigmented and is not durable. The introduction of a gel-based gloss has brought increased durability. These products can be very drying and can also stain the lips.

Lip balms are nourishing, moisturising and soothing products for the lips that can contain colour pigments, pearl essences and even flavourings. They are intended primarily to give beneficial effects. They can be used under another lip product or on their own to correct dry, chapped lips.

Lip pencils or liners are used for outlining the lips. Pencils are difficult to sterilise and therefore must be sharpened prior to every use. They are formulated with a high proportion of hard waxes. Pencils are good for corrective lip work because they can be used to balance and even to alter (temporarily) the alignment of the lips.

> ⭐ *Hints and tips*
> *A light application of a softer shade of eyeshadow can be used to good effect, if definition rather than correction is required.*

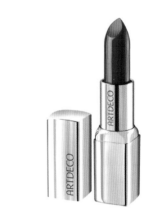

△ Lipstick

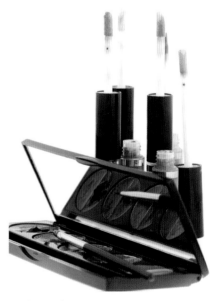

△ Lip products

Application

1. If using a pencil, outline the line of the lip evenly.
2. If using lipstick, gently scrape a small amount of the chosen colour onto a clean palette or spatula and, using a clean, sterilised lip brush, apply a clear outline to the lips. Then fill in the lips evenly with colour.
3. Outline the lips from the sides to the centre with the lips slightly apart to allow application into the corners of the mouth.
4. Protect the make-up by using a tissue on the client's chin to support the hand.
5. Blot after the first application and reapply. This prolongs the duration of the application.
6. Lipstick can be powdered through a single-ply tissue to set it and make it last longer.

> ☆ **Hints and tips**
> For uneven lip shape or colour, apply concealer and foundation over the lips at the start of the make-up application and then correct the shape with a lip liner. This technique will also allow the 'true' colour of the lipstick to be achieved without the natural colour of the lips altering the colour.

▽ Make-up products to suit different age groups

Age groups	Types of product
16–30 years	Foundation – water-based liquid, mineral based, compact, mousse, tinted moisturiser Cheek products – liquid tints, mineral based, powder, Eye products – gel, liquid, powder, mineral based Lip products – gloss, lipstick, lip balm
31–50 years	Foundation – oil-based liquid, mousse, light cream Cheek products – powder, mineral based Eye products – powder, mineral based Lip products – lipstick, lip balm, lip liner
Over 50 years	Foundation – cream, stick, tinted moisturiser Cheek products – cream, liquid tints Eye products – avoid highly pearlised colours; use cream, gel, waterproof mascara, pencil eyeliner Lip products – avoid high gloss; use lip liner to avoid 'bleeding' of lipstick

> ☆ **Hints and tips**
> It is particularly important to keep accurate records of the selected make-up products and application methods. These details must be entered on the client's treatment plan or record card.

Corrective make-up application

Face shapes

There are seven basic face shapes, which are formed by the shape and size of the bones under the skin. They are:

 oval
 heart
 oblong
 diamond
 square
 round
 pear.

Viewing the client face on from the front and then from the side will allow you to identify the shape of the face. It is important to remember that the client must be sitting upright and looking straight at you, and not lying down, which gives a false impression of the face shape. The hair should be taken away from the face with a headband or clips.

A variety of different products are available to correct face shape. They fall into two main categories: shader and highlighter.

Both come in the forms of powders, creams and even foundations. To correct eye shapes, eyeshadow is used in suitable colours and lip shapes can be altered with lip pencils and suitable lipsticks.

Corrections should be subtle and suitable for the type of make-up being worn. The aim is to create an illusion of a perfectly balanced face shape and features, but care must be taken not to apply too much or the finished make-up will look heavy and unnatural. Only correct the features that are unattractive and can be seen. Shading a heavy forehead when the client wears her hair with a fringe is a waste of time and product.

There are just two rules to remember in corrective make-up:

1. A colour darker than the skin tone (a shader) will diminish or hide a feature.
2. A colour lighter than the skin tone (a highlighter) will emphasise or bring a feature forward to make it more noticeable.

Choosing your shade and your type of product is where the skill comes in. For a day make-up, where naturalness is the aim, highlighters and shaders should be between one and two shades lighter or darker than the skin tone. For evening, the colours can be between two and three shades lighter or darker.

Your choice of product will also depend on the type of make-up to be worn. Powders are easy to use and give strong effects, so are most suitable for evening make-up. They should be applied *after* foundation and face powder. Creams and foundations are easy to blend to give a natural look so are suitable for day and bridal make-up. These are applied *before* face powder.

How to determine face shape

Consider the face in sections as shown in the diagram. Obviously, you cannot draw lines on a client's face, so to help you determine the face shape, consider the following:

- The distance between the tip of the chin and tip of the nose is equal to the distance between the tip of the nose and the eyes and the eyes to the hairline.
- The length of the eye from one corner to the next is equal to the distance from the side hairline to the outer corner of the eye
- There should be an eye's length between the eyes. So you should get five 'eye lengths' across the width of the face.

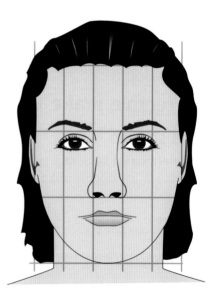

△ Method for determining face shape

The **oval face (a)** is generally accepted to be the 'perfect' shape in that the facial proportions are equal. No corrective work is necessary so blusher can be applied to the 'apple' of the cheeks and swept up over the cheekbones.

The **round face (b)** also appears short and wide but the width is apparent in the cheek area. The hairline and jaw line are rounded, not square.

To correct a round face, use shader at the cheekbones with the strength wide at the ear fading towards the apple of the cheek. Square the jaw line by using shader across the outer corners, fading towards the chin and underneath towards the neck.

The **square face (c)** appears wide and short with characteristic square jaw line and hairline.

To correct a square face shape, place shader at the outer edges of the widest areas and fade towards the centre of the face. On the jaw line, blend the shader under the bone until it meets the neck. Highlight the centre of the chin, nose and brow to give roundness to the face.

The **heart face (d)** is sometimes known as the inverted triangular face, with its wide-set eyes. The forehead is also wide but the jaw line is narrow and the chin pointed and/or receding. To correct a heart-shaped face, create width at the chin by applying shader over the point of the chin, blending under and outward on the jaw line. Apply highlighter to the sides of the chin just above the jawbone. (To narrow a wide forehead, see the instructions for a square face. Wide-set eyes will be dealt with later in this chapter.)

The **diamond face (e)** can be characterised by its broadness across the cheekbone area, often with wide-set eyes and a narrow forehead and jaw line, and often with a receding chin.

To correct a diamond face shape, consider the narrow forehead and receding chin if present. The narrow forehead should be highlighted at the temples and along the hairline fading towards the centre of the brow. A receding chin should be shaded directly under the jaw line with the strength under the chin fading outwards and downwards on the neck. Highlighter should be placed on the jaw line to give sharpness and definition.

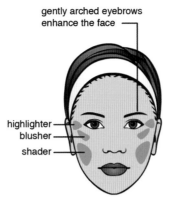

a) oval face

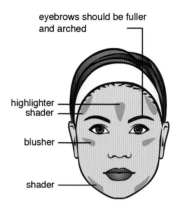

b) round face

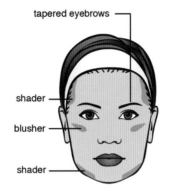

c) square face

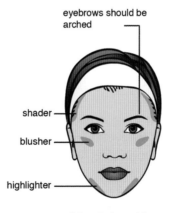

d) heart-shaped face

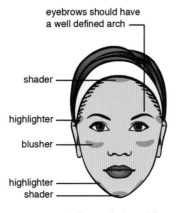

e) diamond-shaped face

The **oblong face (f)** is narrow across the width of the face. It is also long, often with a long nose and/ or tall forehead. Close-set eyes can often be seen with the oblong face.

To correct an oblong face shape, create width at the cheekbone area by placing blusher along the natural cheekbone. Place shader at the tip of the chin and centre hairline and highlight the jawline. (How to shorten a long nose, correct close-set eyes and reduce a tall forehead is dealt with later in this chapter.)

The **pear face (g)** is also known as the triangular face and is characterised by a wide jaw line and by being narrow across the eyes and/or forehead. Close-set eyes often accompany this face shape.

To correct a pear-shaped face, the wide jaw line can be treated as for the square-shaped face and the narrow forehead highlighted as with the diamond-shaped face.

Even though there are millions of people in the world, all our faces fit somewhere within the seven categories. Most faces are a combination of two or more face shapes. A characteristic of one face shape can dominate the face, making it appear to be another. This may sound confusing. However, if you decide first on the corrective make-up to disguise the face shape, and then concentrate on any features that are unattractive, you will achieve good results.

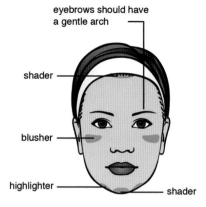

eyebrows should have a gentle arch

shader

blusher

highlighter

shader

f) oblong face

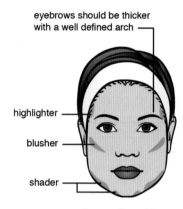

eyebrows should be thicker with a well defined arch

highlighter

blusher

shader

g) pear-shaped face

Recognising eye shape

When we discussed the oval face we talked about 'perfect proportions' and in particular the 'five eyes' across the width of the face. For a 'perfectly set' eye, the eye's height can be measured by the distance between the lower and upper lashes at the widest point when the eyes are open.

Close-set eyes (a) with a handle of a brush, measure the length of one eye from corner to corner. If the space between the eyes is less than an eye's length apart they are close set.

To correct close-set eyes, apply highlighter to the inner corners of the eyes from the lashes to the eyebrows, blending with a medium shade in the centre and a darker shade on the outer corners of the eyes. Line the outer corners of the eyes only on the top and bottom lashes, with a medium to dark soft coloured pencil.

Wide-set eyes (b) on measuring the eyes with a brush, if it is found that there is more than one eye's length between them, the eyes are said to be wide-set. To correct wide-set eyes, use a deep shadow on the inner corner of the eyes from lashes to brow for about a third of the eyelid. Fade through a mid to a light colour through the centre to the outer corner of the eye. Slightly extend the inner edge of the eyebrow into the centre to lessen the gap between them.

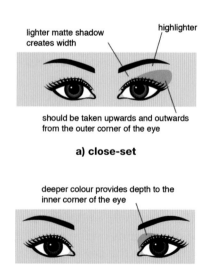

lighter matte shadow creates width

highlighter

should be taken upwards and outwards from the outer corner of the eye

a) close-set

deeper colour provides depth to the inner corner of the eye

b) wide-set

Round or prominent eyes (c) – these are eyes that show all (or virtually all) of the eyelid when the eye is fully open. To correct prominent eyes, apply a medium toned, matt eyeshadow all over the lid and brow area, fading the intensity towards the brows. A darker shade should be blended into the socket line and onto the outer half of the eyelid. Use a soft, dark eyeliner close to the roots of the top lashes to minimise the look of the lid and then coat the lashes in dark mascara to define and deepen the shape.

Overhanging eyelids (d) – these are also known as droopy eyes, where the brow or top eyelid hangs over the eye at the outer corner. To correct droopy eyes, blend light or mid-toned eyeshadows upwards and outwards to lift the outer corner of the eyes. Apply eyeliner to the outer third of the top and bottom lashes, taking the line towards the temples but not extending beyond the socket line. The outer top lashes should be curled and a light coat of mascara applied. The eyebrow can be used to great advantage for this eye shape. Lightly arch towards the centre of the eyelid and lift the outer corner.

Deep-set eyes (e) – these are set back into the eye socket so that little or no eyelid is showing when eyes are fully open. To correct deep-set eyes, use only light to mid toned colours placing the highlight colour on the eyelid all the way along by the lashes. Apply a light coat of mascara only, as too much will have the effect of closing the eye. Avoid too much eyeliner as this will make them recede further.

Small eyes (e) – these are small compared with the rest of the face. They may be set perfectly but sometimes they are deep-set. To correct small eyes, use light and/or frosted colours on the eyelid to open up the eye. Blend a medium tone into the socket line, blending outwards towards the temples to extend the eye. Apply a soft, smudged pencil line close to the lashes on the outer third of the upper and lower lids, extending the lines upwards and outwards. Highlight directly under the eyebrows. Curl the lashes before applying mascara and keep eyebrows high, thin and in a curved arch to make the most of the eyes.

Slanting eyes (f) – the outer corner of the eye slants downwards or upwards without an overhanging eyelid, and may appear very narrow. To correct downward slanting eyes, apply medium to dark tones upwards and outwards and mirror with the eyeliner. Two correction methods work well on this eye shape: 1. Use a medium-toned shadow at the outer and inner corners from lash to brow, then place a highlight in the centre to bring the centre forward. 2. Highlight the inner half of the eyes and blend into a mid or dark shade upwards and outwards at the outer half of the eyelid. Soft eyeliner can be used close to the lashes, lifting the outer edges, to mirror the eyeshadow.

Narrow eyes (g) – the eyes may be correctly set but appear narrow compared to the other facial features. To correct narrow eyes, place a medium tone eyeshadow along the socket line and blend above the socket so that it can be seen when the eyes are open and highlight under the eyebrow. Apply eyeshadow under the lower lashes and define with eyeliner.

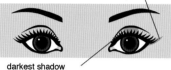

lift eyeshadow and eyeliner applicaton beyond outer corner of eye

darkest shadow colour to the centre of eyelid

c) round or prominent

highlighter

blended shadow working from applying darker colour over the lid area and blended

d) overhanging lids

dark shadow applied above natural socket line   highlighter

eyeliner applied above and below eyelid, softened with eyeshadow

e) small or deep-set

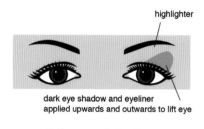

highlighter

dark eye shadow and eyeliner applied upwards and outwards to lift eye

f) downward slanting

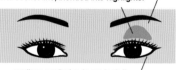

darken the socket line extending above   highlighter
natural socket line, blended into highlighter

eyeliner applied to lower lash line and softened with eyeshadow

g) narrow

177

Correcting lip shapes

The 'perfect' mouth should appear so that the corners of the mouth are in a straight line directly under the pupils of the eyes and the bottom lip should be slightly fuller than the top. The lip line should be easily seen all the way around the mouth and the 'cupid's bow' evenly placed under the tip of the nose.

The lips can be reshaped with lip pencil, lip brush and lipstick. Often, the colour choice and the intensity of colour is all that need to be considered to achieve the desired effect.

Thin lips are narrow in appearance with a shallow 'cupid's bow'. To correct thin lips, use a lip pencil in a matching colour to the lipstick. Then, trace a line outside the natural lip line and fill with light, frosted colours.

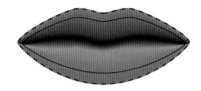

Thin lips

Full lips often have a deep cupid's bow and with the corners of the mouth appearing inside the line from the pupils of the eye. To correct full lips, use a lip pencil to trace a line inside of the natural lip line. Fill with dark, matt colour lipstick. Avoid the use of frosted, light and bright colours.

Full lips

Unbalanced lips can appear in a variety of forms, but the most common is the lower lip being narrower than the top. Correct unbalanced lips by using a lip pencil to trace a line inside of the 'heavy' lip and on the outside of the 'thin' lip. Then fill with coloured lipstick but a touch of matching gloss to the thin lip will create more fullness.

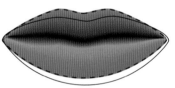

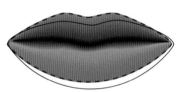

Uneven lip shapes

Drooping/asymmetrical lips: the corners of the lips appear to droop down, so the mouth also appears to droop, resulting in a sad expression. To correct drooping or asymmetrical lips, trace in the bottom lip first with a pencil, extending the corners upwards and outwards. Then draw the top lip line to meet the new corners. (With asymmetrical lips you will be only making this correction at the affected corner.) Fill with matching lipstick colour. As the new corners are liable to crease, blot the application, lightly powder and re-apply the lipstick.

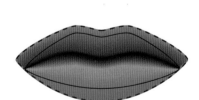

Drooping lips

Small mouth: the corners do not sit underneath the pupils of the eyes. To correct a small mouth, use light and frosted colour lipsticks and trace a line outside of the natural lip line, extending the corners as described in 'drooping lips'.

Wide mouth: the corners stretch further than the pupils of the eyes. To correct a small mouth, trace a new line with a pencil, inside the natural lip line. Use dark matt lipstick colours. Avoid glossy, bright and light colours.

Ageing lips have lines around the lip line, radiating outward. These lines lead to 'bleeding' of the lipstick into the surrounding skin. Avoid strong bright colours and use a matt lipstick colour. Blot the first

 Remember . . .
The lower lip should appear slightly fuller.

application and powder through a single-ply of tissue, then freshen the colour with a very light second application.

Other corrections

Wide noses can be corrected by placing shader down the sides of the nose fading out at the tip and down the sides. Highlight down the centre of the nose from between the eyebrows and off at the tip of the nose.

Flat profiles can be corrected if desired by use of highlighter between the brows at the bridge and the use of a medium to dark tone eyeshadow at the inner corner of the eyes if the shape allows it.

Colour corrections

Sometimes it is not possible to conceal blemishes or shadows with concealer alone, due to their colour. This is where knowledge of colour theory can help. Primary and secondary colours are arranged into a 'colour wheel', which has a number of uses in make-up. The colour wheel is discussed in Chapter 9.

There are a number of uses of the colour wheel in make-up services, including the following:

- Red cheeks or areas of broken capillaries can be hidden with green corrective cream mixed with foundation or concealer.
- Blueness in the corner of the eye can be taken away by the application of orange corrective cream mixed with foundation or concealer.
- Sallow skin (yellowness) around the mouth can be minimised by the application of a lilac (violet) corrective cream under the foundation.

Day make-up

Make-up for daywear should be well blended and natural looking. It will be observed in daylight, which means that all the colours will appear 'true' and any hard lines or mistakes will easily be seen. Lightweight products should be used in neutral, subtle shades. Follow these guidelines:

- Choose colours that are soft, natural colours such as peach, beige, brown, grey, and subtle blues and greens.
- The application must be perfect, with lines well blended.
- Corrective work should be restricted to the eyes and mouth and the concealing of blemishes.
- The foundation must match the client's skin tone.
- Concealer should be applied lightly on blemishes and shadows, such as those under the eyes.
- Colour correction and highlighting and shading should be avoided unless the facial feature concerned is very unattractive and then the corrective work should be subtle and look as natural as possible.

Procedure for application of day make-up

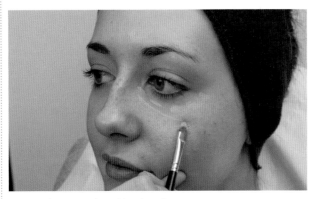

1. Apply concealer with a brush.

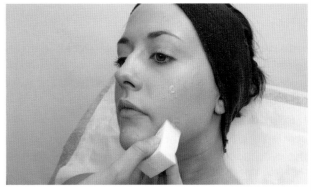

2. Apply foundation with a sponge.

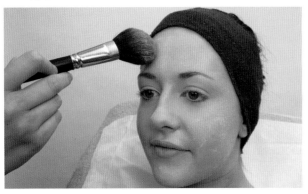

3. Apply loose powder with a brush.

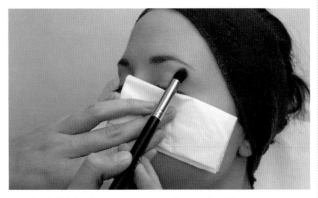

4. Apply highlighter eye colour all over the lid.

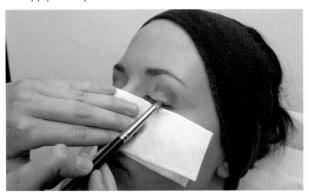

5. Apply a darker colour in the crease to define the eyes.

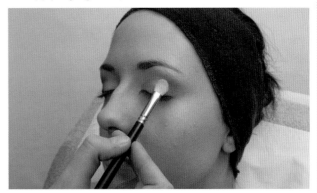

6. Blend all over the lid to make the shadow even.

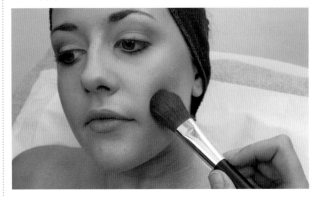

7. Apply powdered blusher with a brush.

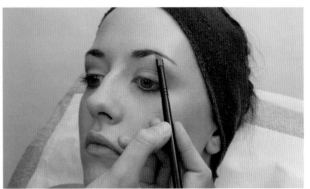

8. Apply eyebrow colour using a brush.

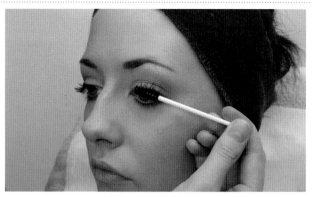

9. Apply mascara using a disposable mascara brush.

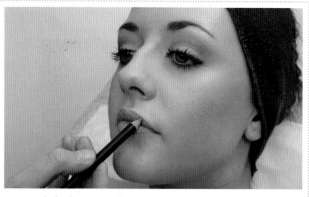

10. Apply lip liner pencil.

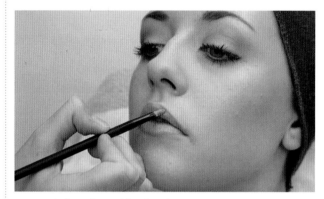

11. Apply lip colour with a brush.

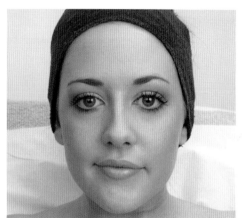

12. The finished look.

Evening make-up

In contrast to day make-up, evening make-up is viewed in either very bright or subdued lighting. These types of light absorb more colour and definition than daylight, so colours for evening can be bolder and more varied than those usually worn in the daytime. Shading and highlighting can also be used to accentuate facial features. Lip gloss, pearlised products, false lashes and eyeliner can all be used to create a dramatic evening effect. Consider the occasion, clothes, accessories and the personality of the client.

- **Foundation** can be darker for a tanned look, or lighter, which gives a dramatic appearance. Corrective techniques can be used to the full.
- **Concealer** can be used to cover every trace of blemish or shadow.
- **Eye make-up** – frosted, bold colours can be used, such as gold, silver, red, bright pink, black, blue and green. Definition to the eye can be given by the use of eyeliner, false lashes and/or mascara.
- **Cheek make-up** – should equal the eye and lip make-up in strength. Use colours such as rust, pink or red. Corrective work can be used to diminish unattractive features.
- **Lip make-up** – lip pencils in shades that are up to twice as dark as the lipstick can be used to accentuate the 'cupid's bow'. Suitable examples of colours are red, bright pink and burgundy. Lip-gloss is also effective.

Procedure for application of evening make-up

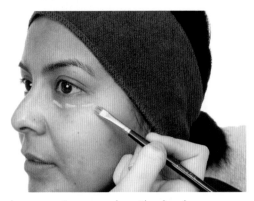

1. Apply colour corrective concealer with a brush.

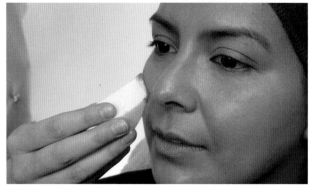

2. Apply foundation with a sponge.

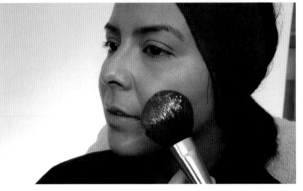

3. Apply loose powder.

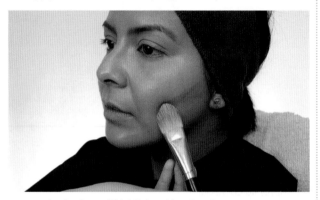

4. Apply shade and highlight with a brush.

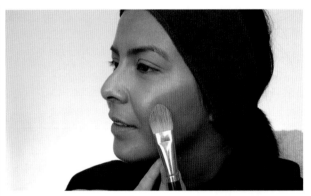

5. Apply blusher with a brush.

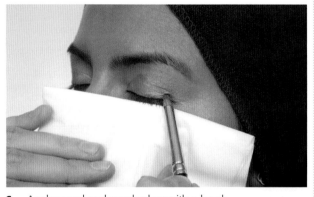

6. Apply powdered eyeshadow with a brush.

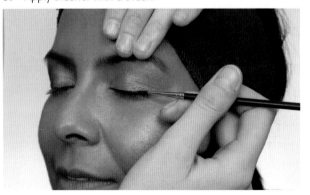

7. Apply liquid eyeliner.

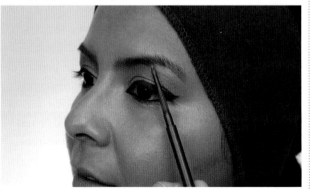

8. Apply eyebrow pencil.

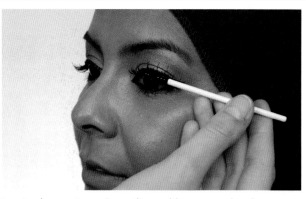

9. Apply mascara using a disposable mascara brush.

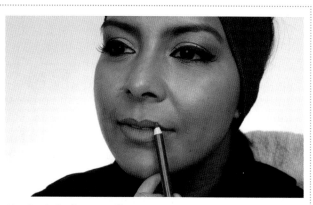

10. Apply lip liner pencil.

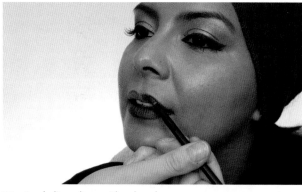

11. Apply lip colour with a brush.

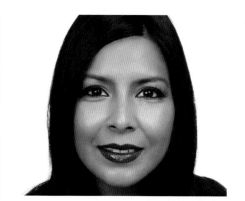

12. The finished look.

Special occasion make-up

There are many reasons for a special make-up application, from a family photograph to a Christmas party. Below are a couple of examples with make-up recommendations and suggestions, but ultimately good consultation techniques will determine the client's requirements.

Bridal make-up

Bridal make-up has special requirements to take into consideration. The make-up will be viewed in daylight for a large part of the day but needs to last well into the evening. A bridal make-up will also need to withstand being photographed, so consequently soft definition should be achieved with the use of lip and eye pencils.

Bridal make-up should be carefully planned and rehearsed prior to the big day as it is important that the bride feels confident with the look. This may mean several sessions with the bride to allow you to understand her needs and ideas. The bride may also require additional services such as manicure and nail art to compliment the look and a series of scheduled appointments for facial treatments leading up to the wedding so her skin appears radiant and blemish free. Sufficient time before the wedding day should be allowed for the skin to settle and before the make-up is applied.

- The make-up rehearsal should take place in similar lighting as the occasion, i.e. daylight for bridal make-up so that the same results can be achieved at the rehearsal as will be seen on the day.

- On the big day the ideal order for the hair and make-up application is to wash the hair before the make-up application and dress the hair afterwards so that the process does not ruin the foundation or make-up effect.

- It is important that the colour scheme of the bridesmaids, flowers, etc. are considered and reflected in the make-up where possible, particularly in the nail polish colour and the lipstick.

- Soft colours to match flowers or dress colours should be used on the eyes and should always be well blended to look soft and natural.

- The foundation needs to be powdered well to prolong the effect and to look matt in the photographs; special 'base' products can be used under eyeshadows also to prolong the look and keep them looking 'fresh'.

- The application of false individual lashes at the outer corner of the eye can give a bright and lifted look to the eyes and add that all important definition for photographs, yet look very natural.

Procedure for application of special occasion make-up

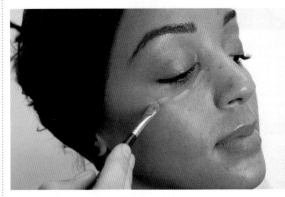

1. Apply concealer with a brush.

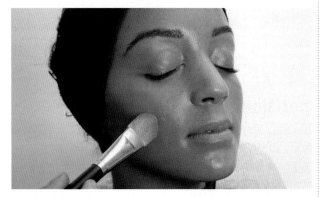

2. Apply foundation with a foundation brush.

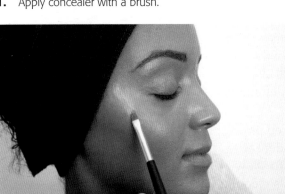

3. Apply shader and highlighter to contour the facial features using brushes.

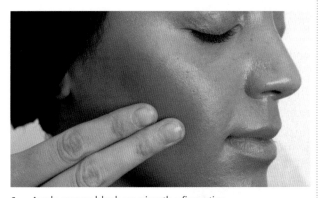

4. Apply cream blusher using the fingertips.

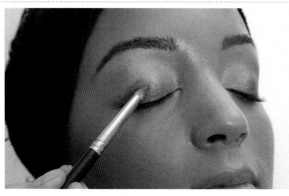

5. Apply cream eyeshadow using a sponge applicator.

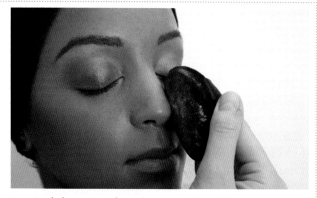

6. Apply loose powder using a powder puff.

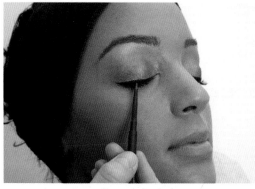

7. Apply eye pencil to define the eyes.

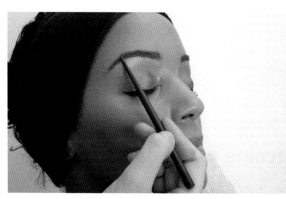

8. Apply eyebrow pencil to define the brow.

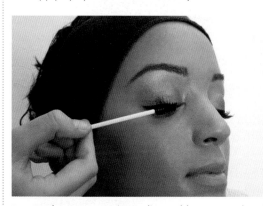

9. Apply mascara using a disposable mascara brush.

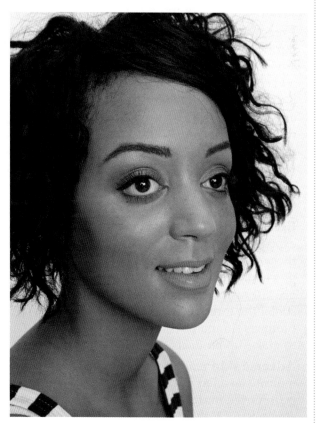

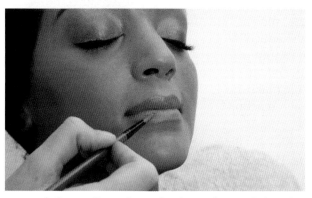

10. Apply lip pencil to enhance lip shape, then apply lipstick with a lip brush.

11. The finished look.

Photographic make-up

The effects created for make-up to be photographed can really allow the creative talents to come to the fore! The use of strong lighting, filters, diffusers and reflectors can create some wonderful effects on the image.

Highlighting and shading should be used when creating make-up to be photographed. A light foundation, which is suitable to cover the skin and mask imperfections, should be used. This will allow the defining effect of highlighting and shading to be seen to the best effect. Make-up must be blended well as the camera will pick out any imperfections.

The lighting used in photography can create a lot of heat. It is important to set the make-up with light translucent powder and to keep reapplying it throughout the shoot.

Be wary of using pearlised products for black-and-white imagery as it can cause 'kickback'. This is where the metallic particles in the make-up are reflected, causing the skin to look shiny. Matte products are preferable for black-and-white photographs.

Airbrushing is now commonly used on finished photographs to erase any flaws or imperfections that appear on the finished image.

Outcome 4: Provide aftercare advice

Contra-actions to make-up

Contra-actions are unwanted effects that can occur during or after the treatment. The contra-actions to make-up are:

- **Excessive perspiration** can occur through nerves and is common during bridal make-up application in particular or when the environmental temperature is very high. The use of waterproof and cream products can assist in combating excessive perspiration if the problem is known. However, if this occurs during application; the use of translucent powder in a light application with a velour powder puff, after blotting the affected area with a paper tissue, can minimise the effects.

- **Watery eyes** can also be treated with the use of waterproof and cream products that will resist the effect that watery eyes can have on a make-up application.

- **Excessive erythema** can be caused by touch, heat, products and exposure to the sun. Clients who are prone to redness, such as those with sensitive skin, should be treated carefully. Reduce procedures where touching the skin is necessary, for example use airbrush base application techniques and keep the client cool if the external environment is hot. Non-allergenic make-up products should be used on those clients with a known reaction to make-up products.

- **Adverse skin reactions** such as erythema, irritation and swelling indicate an allergic reaction to the make-up products. They must be removed immediately and the skin soothed with cold water compresses. If the effects are severe, the client should be advised to see a medical practitioner.

Homecare advice

It is likely that the client will show interest in the products you have applied. This provides retail opportunities that should be pursued. When advising the client on products, consider those that are suitable for their age, skin type and condition. It's also important to consider the difficulty of application. A client who does not normally wear make-up or who has a busy lifestyle will need to achieve the make-up effects quickly and easily and the best products are those that allow simple application techniques.

Clients often need help choosing the correct foundation and this is where you can advise on the best colour and texture to suit. A selection of eye and lip products in a variety colours may also interest the client.

Products needing a particular tool or application technique should usually be avoided. The client may not be familiar with them and may not achieve the same effect as is possible in the salon.

Make-up removal techniques

The client should be advised of suitable make-up removal techniques, including the following.

- The client should be encouraged to use eye make-up remover as the product is especially made for use on the delicate skin around the eye. They are formulated with a high degree of 'slip', which reduces unnecessary stretching, as well as being designed to dissolve the eye make-up effectively.

- A cleanser to suit the client's skin type and condition should be applied with the fingertips in circular movements and removed with damp cotton wool, sponges or rinsed off with cool water if the product allows.

- Cleanser should be followed by the use of a suitable toner. A spray applicator allows easy application.

- A suitable moisturiser should be applied that provides a protective layer onto the skin for the control of moisture loss, sebum control or sun protection as suitable for the client's skin type and condition.

Health and safety

Clients should be reminded to close their eyes when using spray applicators.

Want to know more?

Airbrush make-up

An airbrush is a tool by which a very fine spray of liquid make-up product, such as foundation, is 'sprayed' onto the skin, resulting in a flawless finish and a high degree of coverage. The technique has been used in the past to apply art products (for example in commercial art) and is now used to apply paints in nail art, spray tanning and make-up application. Airbrushing is popular in the television industry, with the development of high-definition and in digital photography. It can also be used to apply blusher, face contouring and eye make-up and is used in body painting competitions to apply body make-up.

Equipment

The equipment consists of a spray gun on which there is a trigger that controls the flow of product. Connected to the gun via tubing is a compressor that causes a vacuum and the movement of air within the equipment. The moving air picks up the make-up product, which is contained within a reservoir connected to the gun, spraying a fine and even application of the product.

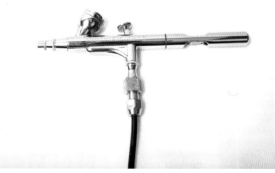

△ Airbrush make-up equipment

Test yourself

Test yourself on make-up services by answering the following questions:

1. How should day make-up be adapted for the evening?

2. What steps should you take to avoid the risk of cross-infection when using mascara?

3. What consideration should be given when selecting lipstick colour for black skin?

4. Eyeshadow should be applied with a disposable applicator:
   a) because it is easy to apply
   b) to avoid infection
   c) it makes the eyeshadow stay on longer
   d) it does not stretch the delicate skin round the eyes.

5. Why must the skin be kept cool during a make-up application session?

6. Why should a bride be recommended to visit the salon for a practice make-up before her wedding day?

7. Give two reasons for applying face powder.

8. What cleanser would you use on dry skin?
   a) soap
   b) cleansing cream
   c) cleansing milk
   d) cleansing lotion.

9. Eye pencils are sharpened before use because:
   a) they feel more comfortable on the skin
   b) a better effect can be achieved
   c) a more subtle effect can be achieved
   d) it is more hygienic.

10. Fluorescent light:
    a) shows the true colour of the skin and make-up
    b) dulls blue tones and darkens red tones
    c) creates a range of shades
    d) drains the face of colour.

11. Pearlised powder products should not be applied too close to the eyes of a mature client because it:
    a) would drag the features downward
    b) makes the eyes appear larger
    c) could cause dryness of the skin
    d) would emphasise fine lines and wrinkles.

12. Liquid foundations are recommended for:
   a) dry skins
   b) mature skins
   c) young oily skins
   d) sensitive skins.

13. Cream blusher is more suitable for:
   a) sensitive skins
   b) dry, mature skins
   c) dehydrated skins
   d) oily skins.

14. Bright and subdued lighting absorbs light so evening make-up needs to be:
   a) soft and subtle
   b) bold, with definition
   c) long lasting
   d) reflective.

15. Colours for a bridal make-up could be chosen to match:
   a) the groom's eyes
   b) the bride's mother's outfit
   c) the flowers and bridesmaid's dresses
   d) the décor at the reception.

16. What is the purpose of:
   a) shader
   b) highlighter.

17. Describe the corrective techniques that should be applied for each of the following.
   a) square face
   b) close-set eyes
   c) asymmetrical lips.

18. A lilac corrective product would be used on:
   a) a sallow skin
   b) a highly vascular skin
   c) very dark skin
   d) uneven skin.

19. What should be considered when selecting eye make-up for someone with small eyes?

20. What should be considered when correcting a diamond face shape?

Are you ready for assessment?

The following checklist will help you to be fully prepared for your practical assessment.

The range of clients/treatments you must cover:

🖎 Various consultation techniques.

🖎 Age groups.

🖎 Skin types.

🖎 Occasions.

🖎 Consider your actions if contraindications are present.

🖎 Make-up products.

🖎 Advice.

 Remember...
Always keep your logbook handy.

1. **Practical observation**

   Your assessor will look at how you:

   🖎 prepare the treatment area, ensuring that you carry out safe and hygienic practice

   🖎 consult with the client and discuss the client's requirements and the occasion

   🖎 establish the age group of the client

   🖎 establish skin types – oily, dry, combination

   🖎 establish skin conditions – mature, sensitive, dehydrated

   🖎 prepare a make-up chart

   🖎 apply make-up products

   🖎 carry out the make-up in a commercially acceptable time

   🖎 check with the client that the result is to the client's satisfaction

   🖎 provide advice on make-up

   🖎 demonstrate professional practice throughout the service

   🖎 carry out all treatments with regard to health and safety.

 Remember...
Your assessor will observe your performance on at least three occasions each involving a different client.

2. **Knowledge and understanding**

   What you must know:

   🖎 Organisational and legal requirements.

   🖎 How to work safely and effectively when providing make-up services.

   🖎 How to consult, plan and prepare for the make-up of clients.

   🖎 Contraindications and contra-actions.

   🖎 Anatomy and physiology.

   🖎 Make-up application using a range of products and colours.

   🖎 Advice on products, application and removal of make-up.

   To ensure that you have the necessary knowledge and understanding of make-up services your assessor will:

   🖎 ask you questions before, during and after carrying out the treatment

   🖎 ensure that you have completed project work and written exercises relating to the unit

- check that you have recorded in a log/diary make-ups you have carried out with signed record cards showing that you have completed three make-up services competently
- check that you have covered the range in your candidate logbook
- require you to take a test.

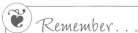 Remember...

Simulation is not a valid means of assessment for make-up service.

Sources of evidence

- Completed client record cards indicating the range of clients, skin types and conditions.
- Video or photographic evidence, for example preparing models for a show involving the application of make-up. Verification of this evidence through a signature and date by a senior member of staff will be necessary.
- Certificates of achievement from make-up courses (manufacturers hold courses for new products and fashion ranges).
- Following your attendance at a course ask your assessor to observe you showing your colleagues the skills you have learned by giving a make-up lesson.
- One-to-one tutorial with your assessor or salon supervisor to establish your progress and set targets. A copy of the tutorial report should be available for your portfolio.
- Client feedback.
- Project work to include photos and pictures indicating fashion trends in make-up.

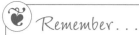 Remember...

The maximum commercially viable service time for a make-up application is 30 minutes.

Chapter 8
Unit B9: Instruct clients in the use of skin care products and make-up

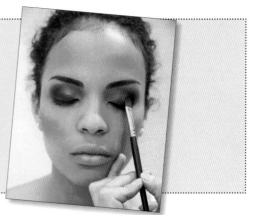

Learning objectives

This chapter covers Unit B9 'Instruct clients in the use of skin care products and make-up'. It provides you with the knowledge and skills required to give instructions about the use of skin care and make-up products to clients of all ages.

> There are four learning outcomes for Unit B9 and they are:
> 1 Maintain safe and effective methods of working when providing skin-care and make-up instruction.
> 2 Prepare and plan for skin care and make-up instruction.
> 3 Deliver skin care and make-up instruction.
> 4 Evaluate the success of skin care and make-up instruction.

You will need to be competent in skin care product and make-up instruction to qualify for insurance and perform the treatment on members of the public.

Evidence requirements

Your assessor will need to observe you perform this treatment successfully on at least three occasions on different clients, involving a different 'look'. You must:

1 Demonstrate the use of consultation techniques:
- questioning
- visual
- manual
- reference to client records.

2 Identify these skin types:
- oily
- dry
- combination.

3 Deal with one of these necessary actions:
- encourage the client to seek medical advice
- explain why the treatment cannot be carried out
- modify the treatment

4 Give this type of instruction:
- skin care choice and application
- day make-up
- evening make-up
- special occasion make-up.

5 Use these instructional techniques:
- skills demonstration
- use of diagrams
- verbal explanation
- use of written instruction.

6 Use these types of resources:
- skin care products
- make-up products
- make-up tools and equipment
- suitable mirror
- face chart.

Introduction

With images of celebrities everywhere we look, and many magazines carrying articles that list skin care and make-up 'must haves', the skills of the 'beauty consultant' are very much in demand.

Clients are sometimes not sure about how to express themselves with make-up. Make-up can give an unintended message about the wearer if they have made poor choices. Whether the client visits a salon, a department store or a demonstration in their thirst for knowledge and advice, the correct choice of skin care and make-up products ensures that they feel confident about how they look.

In the course of your work you may be asked to perform a demonstration or to give a talk on make-up and skin care. This requires confidence and a good understanding of the products being demonstrated and the range of treatments available in the salon.

Unit B9 appears as a mandatory unit of the Beauty Therapy Make-up route only. It is worth seven credits.

Meet the professional

"I love getting up on stage and showing off, it's the frustrated showman in me. Nothing gives me more pleasure than either being on stage demonstrating various fashion make-up techniques to a large crowd of beauty college students, or filming beauty videos that are shown online for Elle magazine or Boots the Chemist, or selling my make-up line live on the QVC home shopping channel. But it's taken years of practice to get to a point where I feel this confident. I still get nervous but tell myself it's just excitement and that I must really calm down and carry on.

The thing to remember is that when you're sharing knowledge and experience, you need to explain *why* you're doing what you're doing. If you don't, people won't understand what you're going on about and it'll be a waste of time. When I describe and demo, say, How to do Smokey Eye Make-up, I need to explain why I chose certain shades and formulas, plus why where I put them is so important. Within this, you need to explain how it affects eye shape, eye colour, skin tone and how it would look on an older lady, because smokey make-up isn't just for the under-30s. I don't just talk about make-up, I cover the importance of good skin care and prepping skin before make-up application. In fact, if you are giving someone a one-on-one lesson, it's just as vital they understand what you're teaching them in the same way that speaking to a hall full of people must grasp what you're harping on about. Keep things simple. Speak to people in a way they will understand. If you are chatting to fellow make-up gurus then they will get where you're coming from, but if you are teaching a total make-up novice then don't over-complicate things. Remember to go over things a few times, making sure they get it. It's a nice idea to follow up a lesson with a phone call just to find out if someone is getting on OK with your instructions.

Practise speaking loudly. I used to do this by reading text from any book out loud in the comfort of my bedroom. Daft as it sounds, it really works. Remember to speak clearly and don't mumble. Project your voice and imagine someone at the back of a theatre needing to hear you.

One important thing to remember is that watching make-up being applied can be like watching paint dry, so don't drag out your demo. Keep it upbeat and informative. Talk and work at the same time. People like to be amused so tell them funny anecdotes to keep them from falling asleep and always sound excited about what you're doing. And finally, people love to know my own personal reasons why I love what I do and how I do it, so offer up your own personal reasons in your presentation."

Daniel Sandler

Outcome 1: Maintain safe and effective methods of working when providing skin care and make-up instruction

Instructing in the use of skin care and make-up products is an exciting and rewarding part of being a therapist but there are challenges too. Within the salon it is relatively easy for a therapist to give a competent and safe make-up lesson to one client or to a small group. However, maintaining safe and effective methods of work in a variety of venues (from a church hall to someone's dining room) presents the therapist or consultant with a range of challenges.

Preparing for a demonstration in a venue

The following tips will help you overcome the challenges in maintaining safe and effective methods of working in a venue. They are all about preparing well.

Know your audience

Standing in front of an audience, particularly for the first time, can cause a great deal of anxiety. It is important to prepare well and to do your homework on the client group you are addressing. Knowing the age range of your audience ensures that you have the correct products and relevant information to hand.

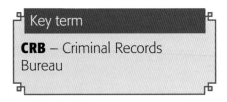

Key term

CRB – Criminal Records Bureau

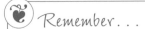 Remember . . .

If your audience are under the age of 16 they are classed as minors and you should follow the legal protocols ensuring that parents or guardians are present at all times. If demonstrating on one of them you will need written consent from the parent or guardian.

What are the audience's expectations from the demonstration or talk? Finding out about this will allow you to target the demonstration to the particular client group. Always give your audience plenty of what they want!

Know your venue

If possible, go to see the venue and find out about the facilities and equipment available to you. If you can't visit beforehand, contact the venue to ask. For example, is there hot running water available nearby? Check the lighting and the position from which you will be demonstrating. For example, is there a chair high enough so the client/model can be at your eye-level? If not, you may need to bring a suitable chair or a portable treatment couch to avoid fatigue or backache. If you are in a big hall, do not try to apply make-up so that the people at the back can see. Ask them to get up and take a closer look. It is also important to consider the disposal of waste products such as facial tissues and cotton wool. Pack a small bin liner into your demonstration kit.

In the salon environment the therapist has control of the working methods and environment with everything they need to hand, but when working at different venues this is not always possible.

It is essential to maintain hygienic working procedures to reduce the risk of cross-infection. Ensure that all equipment is clean and sterile before the event. The use of disposable make-up applicators is advisable. Take plenty of tissues, wipes and cotton-buds (useful for dispensing products on to the hands of interested clients). Take the make-up and skin care tester stands with you so that products and colours can be tried without contaminating your make-up and skin care supplies. The use of antibacterial hand wipes or alcohol-based gel to sterilise hands and equipment is essential for you and for wanting to try products.

 Remember...

Maintain professional standards if you are to create a good impression.

 Remember...

Daylight or simulated daylight is the best light in which to view make-up. However, these demonstrations are often in the evening and there will be artificial lighting giving warm yellow tones and your make-up application should reflect this.

Plan for the allocated time

It is also essential to be able to manage your time well. There will be a limited amount of time to demonstrate the products. Spending too long can become boring for the audience. They are interested in the finished result, not in a lengthy explanation. Limit the time spent on cleansing and preparing the skin.

Present yourself well

Remember you are representing the company for which you work and you should present yourself as carefully as if you were in the salon. The first tools of the professional therapist are: clean, pressed salon dress and appropriate shoes; hair neatly styled away from the face; clean hands with short, manicured nails; neatly applied make-up and fresh personal hygiene, including the breath. As you demonstrate, work neatly and tidily so that you can easily find tools and equipment.

 Health and safety

Strict hygiene procedures must be followed when working out of the salon at a venue by using disposable products, antibacterial hand wipes or gel-based products to sterilise equipment.

Make-up instruction services

The time taken to perform the make-up service must conform to commercially acceptable treatment times for the industry and should be shown on the salon treatment price list. Below is an example for each service indicated.

▽ Make-up instruction timings

Service description	Service Time	Price
Make-up lesson A more in-depth treatment that gives away some of the make-up artist's secrets for a fantastic looking make-up.	60 mins	£25
Make-up and skin care party An intimate meeting personalised for you and a small group of friends (maximum of 6 people).	90 mins	£60
Make-up or skin care demonstration For large groups with an interest in skin care and make-up.	60 mins	£60

Setting up for skin care and make-up instruction

The make-up and skin care demonstration kit should comprise a clean, well-organised box or holdall containing the following:

- examples of the skin care range, for example cleanser, toner and moisturiser and specialist skin care products
- a small box of facial tissues
- antibacterial wipes or alcohol-based gel
- cotton buds, cotton wool rounds, sterilised brushes and sponges
- a range of cosmetics with a good selection of colours
- tester stands of make-up and skin care products for clients to try
- a container of water (in case there is no water supply)
- a small disposable bag for waste
- disposable paper on which to lay out tools, equipment and products.

For information regarding legal requirements for skin care and make-up services see Chapter 3. For information on general safe, effective methods of work including sterilising procedures see Chapter 1.

Outcome 2: Prepare and plan for skin care and make-up instruction

When giving instruction on skin care and make-up, whether it is to an individual or a group of people, preparation and planning is the key to success.

A therapist should have a thorough knowledge of the cosmetic and skin care range in order to give useful and effective instruction. You should also develop instructional skills, such as:

- timing
- pace
- use of the voice
- use of visual aids, for example diagrams or charts
- use of written instruction.

These skills are important to appear professional and to be effective. They will ensure that the client or audience has a worthwhile experience and find your instruction informative and useful.

To ensure appropriate timing and pace means that you will hold the interest of your audience. It will also ensure that the instruction session does not overrun, which would inconvenience your next client or other users of the venue. Always allow time in your instruction for questions. Do not forget the importance of allowing time for the selling of recommended products.

You should use your voice in a suitable manner according to the audience. You will need to project your voice so that the audience can hear you. You may need to use a microphone for a larger audience. Use appropriate language for the age group and level of experience, but always keep it professional: do not use slang terms even when instructing younger people. However, avoid using terms that the audience do not understand (for example, use 'the outer layer of the skin' instead of 'the epidermis').

Using diagrams and charts may help to illustrate a point when you are talking but ensure that they are clear and large enough for the audience to see them. When instructing one person, as in a make-up lesson, charts can be used to indicate the placing of products as a reminder for when the client tries to recreate the make-up at home.

Written instruction that is given to the client or audience should be simple and contain appropriate terminology. Step-by-step instructions are easy to understand and give the order in which products should be used or applied. Instructions on how to use or apply a product should be simple, such as:

'Apply with the fingertips to the face and neck, twice daily.'

The type of resources required for skin care and make-up instruction include:

- skin care products
- make-up products
- make-up tools and equipment
- a suitable mirror
- a face chart.

Prepare for a range of clients (for example a range of ages and skin colour) by ensuring you take a good selection of colours and products.

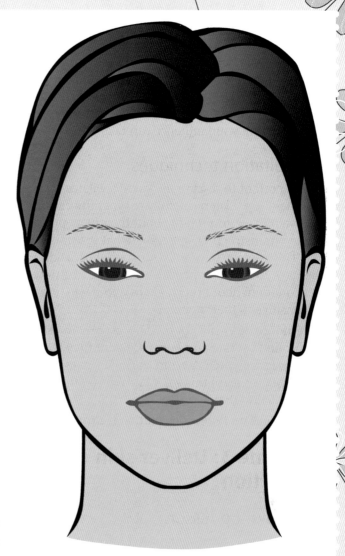

△ Typical make-up chart

⭐ *Hints and tips*

When writing instructions on how to use or apply a product, imagine that you are writing the information onto the back of the product or on its packaging. This will help you to write in an appropriate format that is clear and easy to understand.

Be organised. Carefully plan what you will need by rehearsing the demonstration in your head. Think about the information and present it using an appropriate method. Think about how best to present the information with images, charts or in words. Place the information into a logical sequence that matches your practical skills demonstration. Try to deliver small amounts of information at a time to ensure that your audience can take it in and understand it.

Consultation techniques

It is important to discuss the client's wishes when providing skin care and make-up. Listen carefully to what the client is saying. You can gain valuable information about their perceptions on what they want from your instruction, including what the finished make-up will look like. This is really important for special occasion make-ups or for clients who are having make-up for the first time. The client may not feel confident about their skin or about wearing make-up. You must be sensitive to their opinions.

Determine the client's or model's usual skin care or make-up application routine and how confident they feel and record their responses accurately. Record their skin type and condition and note their age group. All this will help you to provide skin care and make-up instruction that is suitable.

You will find more on consultation techniques in Chapter 1.

Activity

Design a promotional leaflet for a demonstration you are going to do at the town hall as part of a fashion show. Use a computer and include the salon name and a design that best represents your salon. Evaluate your leaflet by asking another therapist for their views.

Outcome 3: Deliver skin care and make-up instruction

The make-up lesson

The make-up lesson should be conducted in a private well-lit treatment area, with the client seated facing a large mirror. Ideally, the mirror should have lamps either side of the mirror.

There are a variety of make-up applications a therapist may be required to offer. These include

- day make-up
- evening make-up
- special occasion make-up.

Whatever the occasion, the effects of lighting on make-up must be considered. The client's clothes should be protected with towels and/or a gown and the hair secured from the face with either clips or a headband.

Discuss the client's usual skin care and make-up routine. This is also an opportunity to stress the importance of preparation of the skin before the application of make-up, for example, the use of cleansing and moisturising products and their application.

It is important to explain to the client the need to handle the skin carefully, without over-stimulating it. General hygiene should also be discussed, as well as the cleaning of brushes and sponges, the use of disposable applicators and mascara wands, care of the

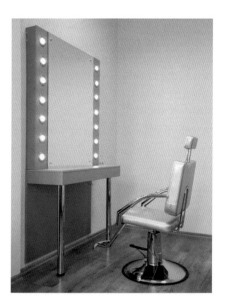

△ Make-up mirror

make-up and touch-up tips (such as using a dampened pad of cotton wool to 'freshen' the make-up).

It is important to keep each stage separate and to discuss each one thoroughly with the client. A record card in the form of a chart should be kept, clearly detailing the products and colours used and the effects achieved. The colours of make-up can be placed onto the chart in the areas of application and the colour name or number noted.

Clients who like the finished effect following make-up in the salon will often want to recreate the effect. This is also an opportunity for the therapist to sell items from the make-up product range.

SKIN
Cleanse _____

Hydrate _____

FACE Foundation Stick # _____
Corrector _____
Brush _____
Concealer _____
Brush _____
Foundation _Dewy Finish_
Brush _____
Powder _____
Brush _____
Bronzer _____
Brush _____

CHEEKS
Blush _____
Pot Rouge _____
Brush _____

EYES
Brows _Defined_
Brush _____
All Over _Gold Sparkle_
Brush _____
Lower Lid _Gold Metallic & Lavender_
Brush _____
Crease _Velvet Plum Metallic_
Brush _& Glitz Metallic_
Shadow Liner _____
Brush _____
Gel Liner _Violet Ink_
Brush _____
Mascara _Lash Glamour_

LIPS
Nugget Lip gloss

Brush _____
Lip System
Natural Match _____
Lip Wardrobe _____

Makeup Artist _Abbie Smart_
Store _Final Touches_
Phone _____

△ A completed make-up chart

The make-up demonstration

A demonstrator is also a salesperson. By demonstrating the range of products available and their application methods, the demonstrator is creating opportunities for selling the products. If you are representing the salon you should take price lists and details of any promotions or special offers and free samples, if available. Take product display stands with the full range on view. This will allow members of the audience to browse before and after the demonstration. For demonstrations to be cost-effective the aim must be to encourage members of the audience to come to your salon for treatment.

It is important at each stage to discuss what you are doing and why. It is also important to impart any hints or tips the audience may find useful. State your intentions at the beginning of the demonstration. Afterwards, you will be able to review how successful you have been in meeting your aims.

When you select a demonstration model from the audience it is usually a good idea to choose someone who appears not to wear cosmetics. You will then be able to demonstrate a noticeable effect to the audience.

The skin care lesson

With the advent of the 'skin bar' it is now popular to offer skin care advice separately from a facial treatment.

At a skin bar, a client may receive a thorough consultation and skin analysis to determine the skin care requirement and will be able to try the products on their skin to test their suitability and their preferences. This ensures that they purchase the correct product for their skin type and condition.

The therapist may be available to offer this service. However, it is often carried out by a receptionist or junior member of staff who has been fully trained in the selling and retailing of the product range.

A written document that lists the products recommended and their frequency of use is useful and serves as a reminder when applying the products at home.

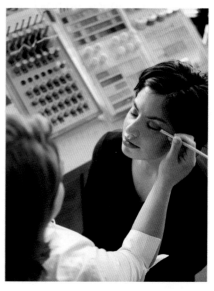

△ A make-up demonstration

Activity

Collect pictures and photographs from magazines and other sources that have interesting make-up designs. Examine your cuttings and analyse the techniques used. Look carefully at use of colour and continuation, and contrast of theme. Examine the use of accessories and backdrops. Put the pictures into a scrapbook and keep adding to it for future reference. This will become one of your most precious resources as a therapist.

☆ *Hints and tips*

Take samples of products for sale and offer 'goody bags' containing testers of the products and a salon price list. This is where a well-designed price list or promotional offer is essential. Take the salon appointment book to make appointments on the night of the event.

Client name:		
Date:		
Product	Application	Frequency
Cleanser	Apply using fingertips, apply to face and neck and remove with warm water	Twice daily, morning and evening
Spray toner	Hold 10–12" from face and neck and depress 2 or 3 times	Twice daily, morning and evening; or to freshen the face during the day
Day moisturiser with SPF	Apply using the fingertips to face, neck and chest area	Morning only under foundation
Night Cream	Apply gebnerously to face and neck with fingertips	At night after cleansing and toning
Eye and lip cream	Apply with ring finger to eye and lip area only using gentle patting movements	Twice daily, morning and evening
Moisturising mask	Apply a thin transparent coat to face, neck and chest avoiding eye and lip area	Twice weekly or when skin is feeling tight

△ Home care prescription summary

Outcome 4: Evaluate the success of skin care and make-up instruction

You can ensure that your clients are satisfied with the instruction by asking them appropriate questions and observing their body language. If you feel that a client is unsure, ask them directly. For example, 'Would you like me to go through the skin care routine again?'

Allow the client time to ask questions or check understanding. An evaluation questionnaire could be provided for the client to complete that requires them only to tick boxes rather than give written responses. Record client feedback with their record card.

Develop reflective practice procedures as a norm for all your treatments. Refer to the client's records and ask yourself:

❧ Were the client's objectives fulfilled?

❧ Were all the client's questions answered?

❧ Did you meet all of her objectives/requirements?

❧ If not, in what way?

❧ What will you do differently in similar circumstances?

Demonstrations can be time-consuming, particularly outside the salon. It is important for businesses to ensure that it is cost-effective. Gaining feedback from the audience about what they enjoyed or disliked about the demonstration will help with future planning of such an event.

Accurate figures on the take-up of any promotion will give an indication of how worthwhile it was in promoting the salon and creating further business.

A tally of the products sold at the event will show any profit from retail sales.

Catwalk and fashion show make-up

> **Want to know more?**
>
> Make-up artistry is also becoming increasingly popular as a career. For example, a person who has developed specialist make-up skills may work for a photographer, on film and promotional shoots, for fashion magazines or for a cosmetic company. Working for cosmetic companies will usually require the make-up artist to promote the product range through demonstrations.

Activity

Experiment with different make-up colours and application techniques and produce a series of photographs. Include evidence of corrective work. These will be useful for your portfolio of evidence and will also be of value to demonstrate your abilities to prospective employers.

This can be an excellent way to promote your salon. Working collaboratively with a fashion house or local businesses provides good promotional opportunities. Make-up for such events is usually based on the same application principles used in photographic and evening make-up. Emphasis should be placed on defining eyes and lips and the principles of highlighting and shading should be applied. In some cases, however, you may be required to work to a specific brief, particularly when working with fashion designers who may require a specific look. It is important to interpret the designer's brief fully, although it may not be in keeping with the look you had envisaged. Remember that models may have several costume changes and will require make-up to be touched up or refreshed. A fine spray of water will help to set the make-up and 'freshen' the look.

A make-up artist is not always concerned about skin preparation, as they do not want the skin to be over-stimulated or warm, which could affect the colour of the make-up. Models/actors will usually arrive for make-up having prepared their own skin.

Test yourself

Test yourself on instructing clients in skin care and make-up services by answering the following questions:

1. At what age is an individual classed as a minor in:

   a) England

   b) Scotland.

2. What actions should be taken before a 15-year-old can receive skin care or make-up instruction?

3. Why is the positioning of the client in relation to the therapist important when providing skin care and make-up instruction?

4. How should client records be stored to comply with the Data Protection Act?

5. Why is it important to complete skin care and make-up instruction within a commercially viable time?

6. Define the terms 'sterilisation' and 'disinfecting'.

7. What is the importance of lighting in make-up application?

8. Why is it important to speak clearly and in a way that suits the skin care and make-up instruction situation?

9. How can you vary the use of the voice for skin care and make-up instruction?

10. What are the main resources for skin care and make-up instruction?

11. What should you consider when preparing for skin care and make-up instruction?

12. How can you encourage clients to ask questions during the instruction service?

13. How would you adapt the skin care and make-up instruction if the client wore contact lenses?

14. How can you evaluate your skin care and make-up instruction service?

15. Why is it important to evaluate the success of your skin care and make-up instruction service?

Are you ready for assessment?

The following checklist will help you to be fully prepared for your practical assessment.

The range of clients/treatments you must cover:

- Various consultation techniques.
- Age groups.
- Skin types.
- Occasions.
- Consider your actions if contraindications are present.
- Make-up products and skin care choice and application.
- Instruction techniques.

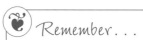
Remember. . .
Always keep your logbook handy.

1. **Practical observation**

   Your assessor will look at how you:

   - prepare the treatment area, ensuring you carry out safe and hygiene practice
   - prepare yourself to meet professional standards
   - consult with the client and discuss the client's needs
   - consult the record card and prepare make-up/face charts
   - deliver skin care and make-up instruction using resources, for example make-up throughout the session
   - encourage the client to ask questions and practise the application techniques.
   - provide written instructions on skin care and make-up
   - gain client feedback on the instruction technique
   - demonstrate professional practice throughout the service
   - carry out the service with regard to health and safety.

2. **Knowledge and understanding**

   What you must know:

   - Organisational and legal requirements.
   - How to work safely and effectively when providing skin care. and make-up instruction.
   - How to consult, instruct plan and prepare.
   - Instructional skills.
   - Contraindications and contra-actions.
   - Anatomy and physiology.
   - Resources.
   - Evaluation of skin care and make-up instruction activities.

   To ensure that you have the necessary knowledge and understanding in instructing make-up and skin care your assessor will:

   - ask questions before, during and after carrying out the instruction session
   - look at project work, which may include photographs and make-up/skin care charts
   - check you have recorded in a log/diary make-up and skin care instruction sessions and gained signatures from the client and assessor or supervisor
   - require you to take a written test.

Sources of evidence

- Make-up/skin care charts
- Videos/photographs
- Client feedback
- Project work
- Completed record cards indicating the range of clients, make-up designs and skin care routines covered

Chapter 9
Unit B10: Enhance appearance using skin camouflage

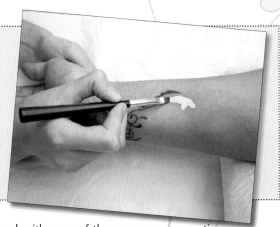

Learning objectives

This chapter covers Unit B10 'Enhance appearance using skin camouflage'. It is about applying skin camouflage make-up products, using simple techniques, to diminish the appearance of skin colouration and to match that of the surrounding skin.

There are four learning outcomes for Unit B10 and they are:
1. Maintain safe and effective methods of working when providing skin camouflage.
2. Consult, plan and prepare for skin camouflage.
3. Carry out skin camouflage.
4. Provide aftercare advice.

You will need to be competent in all of these outcomes to be competent in skin camouflage, qualify for insurance and perform the treatment on members of the public.

Evidence requirements

Your assessor will need to observe you perform this treatment successfully on at least four occasions involving a different client. You must:

1. Demonstrate the use of consultation techniques:
   - questioning
   - visual
   - manual
   - reference to client records.

2. Work on these camouflage needs:
   - tattoos
   - hyper-pigmentation
   - hypo-pigmentation
   - erythema.

3. Deal with one of these necessary actions:
   - encourage the client to seek medical advice
   - explain why the treatment cannot be carried out
   - modify the treatment.

4. Use these tools:
   - brushes
   - fingers
   - sponges
   - velour puffs.

5. Use these camouflage products:
   - camouflage creams
   - camouflage powders
   - setting products.

6. Apply camouflage products to these areas:
   - head or neck
   - chest or shoulders
   - limbs
   - back.

7. Provide this advice:
   - other products that can be used in conjunction with skin camouflage
   - products/substances/environments that should be avoided
   - durability and removal of skin camouflage products.

Introduction

Make-up can be used not only to improve and enhance, but also to correct minor imperfections and to balance the features. Skin camouflage for individuals with disfigurements (for example, a visible birthmark or a disfigurement resulting from an accident) is a specialised skill that requires the therapist to be understanding and thoughtful. Therapists can study the techniques after gaining experience and developing empathy with others.

Modern skin camouflage techniques were developed after the Second World War when pilots and soldiers were surviving with horrific burns and scars. Skin camouflage products and techniques were further developed for the film industry in the USA and now are available in the United Kingdom in hospitals, clinics and salons.

Specialised make-up products and methods of application may be used to camouflage pigmentation abnormalities and skin disorders effectively. In the salon, the therapist is expected to know the basics of effective skin camouflage in order to enhance their make-up services. They may be required to provide a complete service for clients on their wedding day or for a special occasion portrait photography session.

This unit appears as an optional unit of the Level 2 Beauty Therapy General and Make-up routes. It is worth three credits.

Meet the professional

"When faced with a birthmark, burn, scar or tiny blemish that needs disguising, I need to be equipped with the right formula and shade of concealer so my client's skin looks camera-perfect. On a photo shoot in a studio it's not such a problem, thanks to post-production and Photoshop, but if a client is walking down the red carpet or off to a glamorous, fashionable party I need to make them look flawless so they feel 100 per cent confident that they'll WOW.

And because celebs, like the rest of us, don't look perfect all the time, they are also prone to down days and mood swings. It's my job as the make-up artist to make them look sensational so they feel fantastic about themselves and forget about their troubles.

In my kit I carry camouflage make-up, bronzing lotions and sparkly potions. I don't carry every conceivable shade of concealer. That would be mad as there are over 200 shades available, but I do carry a mix of tones and shades that I can mix and blend to create the perfect cover.

It's a good idea to do a course in camouflage application because it really is an art form, but easy to do once you've got the knack. For example, what you'll learn is how a peach-toned corrector disguises blue marks such as a bruise, or how pink concealers neutralise yellow, green corrects high colour, etc., etc. Camouflage make-up is important as it changes people's lives. Severely disfigured people who use it become more confident and it can enable them to have a more active social life.

When I do shoots where models wear swimwear or lingerie, nine times out of ten they will have a little bruise somewhere or a small nick from a razor, so I need to dab on some waterproof camo make-up to make it disappear. Don't think you can apply a regular under-eye concealer to these areas as they will make a bruise look pale grey.

I have even had jobs where I need to make-up men to look like a woman. The problem here is the beard area is always dark even if the fellow is clean-shaven. If I used a normal foundation and concealer there would be a blue-grey cast showing through, so here again, camo formulas work a treat.

One added bonus of understanding camo make-up is that if you mix a little of it to normal concealers you can create the best under-eye disguisers and as soon as you apply it, it immediately brightens someone's entire face. Plus you can use it to contour or highlight and make someone who is relatively plain look super sensational."

Daniel Sandler

Outcome 1: Maintain safe and effective methods of working when providing skin camouflage

Therapists may need to restore the skin's colouration to that of the surrounding skin tone during a make-up application. This can be as part of another make-up service, such as 'bridal make-up', or can be offered as advice for a client with a particular problem. Sometimes this service is included within the price of the make-up, but if the service requires more time and specialised skills and products, the salon may need to charge a little more.

Setting up for skin camouflage

The setting up and hygiene procedures for skin camouflage are the same as for make-up services in Chapter 7. It is advisable for the lighting for effective skin camouflage to be natural or simulated daylight if the make-up is to look natural and undetectable.

Legal requirements are covered in Chapter 3. The basics of safe, effective methods of working are covered in Chapter 1. Hygiene procedures specific to make-up are covered in Chapter 7.

Outcome 2: Consult, plan and prepare for skin camouflage

The sensitive nature of providing skin camouflage treatments places additional demands on the therapist. Although the client's privacy should be respected when performing consultations for all services, the therapist must show particular respect for the client's modesty, privacy and any sensitivities regarding their personal appearance. A client with conditions needing skin camouflage may have low self-esteem and lack confidence. The therapist must show empathy and sensitivity to the client's position. In severe cases, clients may suffer from depression and may not function normally in social situations.

Contraindications to skin camouflage

For this service the therapist may be asked to treat skin conditions that are contraindicated. It is imperative that the therapist remains professional and sympathetically declines treatment when it would be inappropriate. For more information about the correct procedure to follow, consult Chapter 1.

The contraindications to skin camouflage are as follows.

1. Those that require medical referral:
    *   infectious skin conditions such as impetigo and herpes simplex
    *   parasitic infections such as pediculosis and scabies
    *   eye infections such as conjunctivitis
    *   severe skin conditions such as acne, boils, herpes zoster and warts

Activity

Answer these questions on health, safety, hygiene and professionalism.

1. Nail enamel should not be worn by the therapist during a make-up treatment because:
    a) It looks unprofessional.
    b) The client may be allergic to the nail enamel.
    c) The nail enamel may chip during the treatment.
    d) The nail enamel may contaminate the make-up.

2. Autoclave and chemical liquids are suitable methods of sterilisation for equipment. True or false?

3. Why is the physical position of a client important when performing skin camouflage?

4. Disinfectant is a substance that removes micro-organisms and destroys fungi and some viruses, therefore preventing infection. It will destroy most micro-organisms that are present but not the means by which they reproduce, allowing the disease to reappear. They are not successful in the destruction of viruses. True or false?

5. What are the benefits of good sterilisation and hygiene procedures?

Remember...

It is important to allow the client to indicate the area that they wish to be camouflaged and not makes any assumptions. It may lead to embarrassment if you are incorrect and the client may lose trust and not return.

* severe medical conditions
* undiagnosed skin changes in the area being treated
* moles that have changed colour, shape or size.

2. Those that restrict treatment:
   * recent scar tissue (less than six months old)
   * eczema
   * hyper-keratosis
   * skin allergies
   * bruising
   * styes
   * areas of sore or irritated skin.

The client should also be made aware of the possible contra-actions that may occur during or after the service and given time to ask questions. The most likely contra-action is an allergic reaction to the products due to the increased sensitivity of the skin, particularly with hypo-pigmentation conditions. If an allergic reaction occurs, the service should be halted and the products removed as quickly as possible and the area soothed with cold-water compresses.

Relevant anatomy and physiology

The structure and function of the skin is covered in Chapter 19. Diseases and disorders of the skin are covered in Chapter 4.

Photosensitivity of the skin

The Fitzpatrick classification system places someone's skin type into categories depending on how the skin reacts to sunlight. This system is useful to the therapist performing skin camouflage as many of the skin conditions requiring skin camouflage are exacerbated by exposure to the sun. The more photosensitive the skin, the more likely the need for skin camouflage. Using the system, the therapist can adapt the treatment and advise the client on adequate sun protection.

The categories of the Fitzpatrick classification system are described below.

Skin type 1 has very fair skin, usually with freckles and red or fair hair and blue or green eyes. Generally, they do not tan but burn in sunlight.

Skin type 2 has fair skin, blue eyes and fair hair. They burn easily and need to take care if trying to get a tan.

Skin type 3 has dark white skin, hazel or brown eyes and mid brown hair. They usually tan after burning initially.

Skin type 4 has light brown skin, brown eyes and brown hair. They tan easily and burn rarely in sunlight if care is taken by limiting exposure.

Skin type 5 has brown skin and brown eyes and hair. They do not burn and the skin darkens in sunlight.

Skin type 6 has brown to black skin, hair and eyes and the skin darkens easily in sunlight.

Activity

Answer these questions on skin structure and functions.

1. Name the pigment that determines skin colour.
2. Sweat is produced by the sebaceous gland. True or false?
3. How does the skin contribute to the regulation of body temperature?
4. The dermis is also known as the 'true' skin because it contains the main structures. True or false?
5. Sebum forms a protective layer on the skin's surface. True or false?

Key term

Photosensitivity – sometimes reffered to as sun allergy, this is an immune system reaction that is triggered by sunlight.

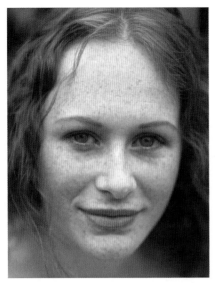

△ Skin type 1

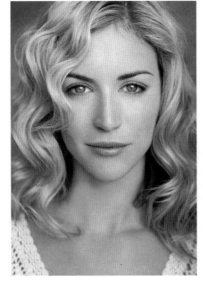

△ Skin type 2

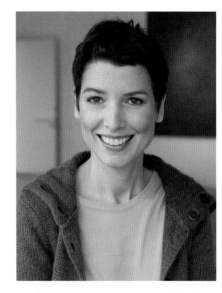

△ Skin type 3

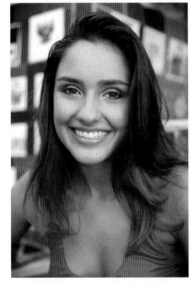

△ Skin type 4

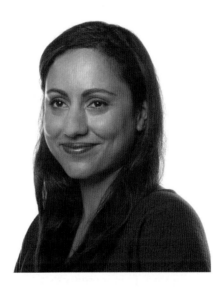

△ Skin type 5

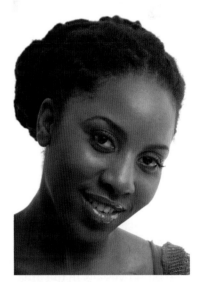

△ Skin type 6

Non-infectious skin conditions

There are a number of non-infectious skin conditions that need skin camouflage. They can be categorised into those associated with pigmentation (colour) problems and those with a **vascular** appearance.

Pigmentation disorders

Chloasma (hyper-pigmentation) appears as patches of increased pigmentation. It is very common in pregnant women or those taking the contraceptive pill, when there are large amounts of oestrogen in the blood stream. After delivery of the baby or coming off the pill, the lesions fade in time, but do not always disappear. If this is the case, exposure to UV should be avoided. Patchy, increased pigmentation

> **Key term**
>
> **Vascular** –'having or relating to blood vessels'. Avascular condition has a high degree of erythema.

may also occur on the face and neck, as a number of cosmetics are photosensitisers, which increase the pigmentation of the skin following exposure to UV.

Age spots (hyper-pigmentation) are irregularly-shaped areas of pigmentation present on areas of the body exposed to the sun, such as the hands, face and shoulders.

Leucoderma (hypo-pigmentation) is a congenital defective pigmentation: the melanocytes in the basal layer are unable to produce melanin.

Vitiligo (hypo-pigmentation) is an acquired condition of leucoderma. It appears in patches affecting the hair or skin. Due to the lack of melanocytes in the basal layer, the skin will never tan and should not be exposed to UV light. There is no protective melanin and so the patches of white skin will burn.

Stretch marks (hypo-pigmentation) or 'striae' are linear-shaped scar tissue caused by the tearing of the dermis after rapid stretching of the skin, for example from rapid growth, resulting in damage to the collagen and elastin fibres.

Vascular conditions

Rosacea is a chronic disorder of the blood vessels of the face. It usually affects people over the age of 30 and often menopausal women. It begins with a flushed appearance, particularly in response to alcohol, spicy foods and stress. This flushing becomes permanent as the blood vessels in the area become dilated. This increases the skin temperature and so stimulates sebum production, leading to papules, pustules and open pores.

Thread veins are fine red capillaries found on the face, cheeks, nose or legs that can be seen through the skin. They are caused by exposure to the sun, pregnancy or harsh handling of the skin. They are harmless but may cause distress because of their appearance.

Therapists are also frequently asked to camouflage tattoos.

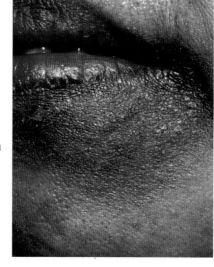
△ Chloasma

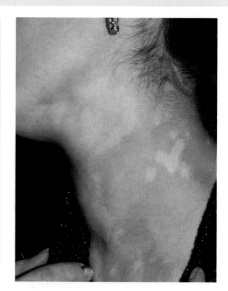
△ Vitiligo

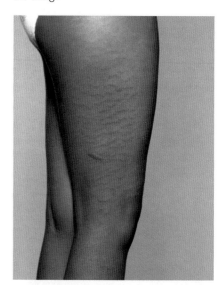
△ Stretch marks

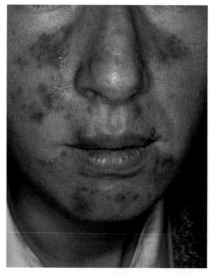
△ Rosacea

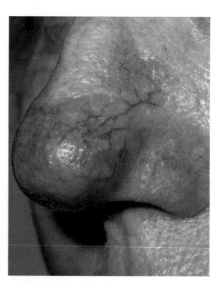
△ Thread veins

Tattoos have been fashionable for a long time and involve the permanent application of pigment into the skin. Many people regret having a tattoo or may need to cover the mark because of a request from an employer. Removal by 'laser' is available but is expensive and painful. Camouflage make-up is an alternative option to hide tattoos, for example for a special occasion, such as a wedding.

Outcome 3: Carry out skin camouflage

Skin camouflage products

Skin camouflage products are heavier in consistency than normal foundation and are usually available as a cream, either in a compact or stick form. The product also contains more of the flesh-coloured pigments, giving it a high degree of coverage and more suitable for the camouflage of skin disorders and conditions. The resulting make-up gives a heavy appearance so a therapist should aim for a balance between the coverage and the weight of application to achieve an appearance that is acceptable for the client.

Many skin camouflage products contain a high degree of sun protection factors, so they offer protection to hypo-pigmentation conditions such as vitiligo. However, care should be taken if the resulting make-up is to be photographed. Skin camouflage products containing titanium dioxide and iron oxide, which are often used in sunblock, give a very pale appearance to the skin in flash photography.

The principles of colour theory

An understanding of the theory of colour is important for effective skin camouflage services.

There are three primary colours: red, yellow and blue.

Primary colours cannot be achieved by mixing. Colours that can be achieved by mixing equal amounts of the primary colours together are known as secondary colours.

These colours can be arranged in a 'wheel' format, with the primary colours separated by the secondary colour, made by mixing them together as in the diagram.

A 'tertiary' colour is created by mixing a primary and secondary colour and the resulting hue is given a two-word name, such as blue-green, red-violet, and yellow-orange. Colours directly opposite to each other on the colour wheel are known as complementary colours because when placed next to each other they become extremely vibrant and are useful when you want to make something stand out. (Note the red circle in the diagram.)

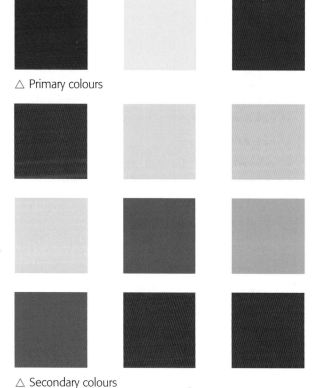

△ Primary colours

△ Secondary colours

However, if you mixed the complementary colours the result would be a neutral brown colour and it is this knowledge that is used to beneficial effect in camouflage make-up. By placing, for example, green corrective concealer onto a red blemish such as thread veins, the effect is to 'neutralise' the red so that it becomes less noticeable.

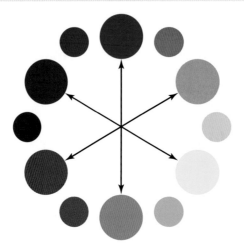

△ The colour wheel

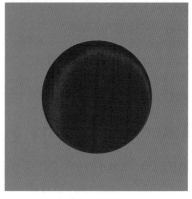

△ Complementary colours

Analogous colours are those next to each other on the colour wheel: red and orange, blue and green, and so on. They usually match extremely well, but create almost no contrast. This knowledge is useful when 'harmony' is needed in your make-up design. The terms **tint**, **shade** and **tone** are frequently used incorrectly, although they describe fairly simple colour concepts.

Skin camouflage application

> **Key term**
>
> If a colour is made lighter by adding white, the result is called a **tint**.
>
> If black is added, the darker version is called a **shade**.
>
> If grey is added, the result is a different **tone**.

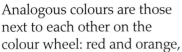

Equipment checklist

It is important to ensure that the work area is prepared prior to the client's arrival. Your workstation should be equipped with:

✔ cleansing, toning and moisturising products — a selection should be available to accommodate different skin types

✔ solid foundation base

✔ cake make-up

✔ powder

✔ a bowl of water

✔ disposable items - cotton wool, cotton buds, tissues, spatulas and brushes

✔ a selection of small bowls

✔ laundry — headbands or hair clips, gowns and towels

✔ mirror

✔ a selection of brushes — different sizes, shapes and densities and disposable

✔ a selection of sponges and velour powder puffs

✔ a covered waste bin

✔ the client's treatment plan or record card.

> *Remember...*
>
> Show empathy towards the client and explain the treatment as you go along.

Basic method of application

1. Check for contraindications.
2. Cleanse, tone, moisturise.
3. Study skin colour and disfigurement.
4. Apply creams using brush, finger or damp sponge.
5. Always explain the procedure to the client as you go along.
6. Apply finishing powder and allow to set for a few minutes before brushing off the excess in a downward direction.
7. Blot with damp cotton wool to remove excess powder.
8. If necessary, repeat steps 5 to 7.
9. Complete make-up application.
10. Explain homecare and removal procedure to your client.
11. Book a further consultation to answer queries and to check progress.

Procedure 1

This technique is used to disguise pigmentation disorders, particularly those that cover a large area, such as vitiligo or chloasma, or a tattoo, before applying densely covering make-up. When covering a large area, allow some time for the make-up to settle before going out.

1. Choose an appropriate colour by testing on a small area adjacent to the treatment area for a colour match.
2. Take up a generous amount of solid foundation base that matches the surrounding skin and apply with the fingertips to cover the entire blemished area with a light film.
3. Ensure even coverage by stippling the make-up with the tip of the third finger, which is the weakest and gives the lightest touch. Blend the edges by stippling or with a sponge squeezed dry. Dust with powder to set before application of cake make-up. Buff lightly with a puff to remove any surplus.
4. An application of cake make-up to restore even skin tone and texture. Wet the sponge thoroughly, so that the make-up flows evenly on to the skin. Work the dripping sponge into the solid cake and apply quickly with long, even strokes over the area covered with base.
5. Carefully blot the damp make-up with a tissue until completely dry and dust with powder to set, as in point 3 above.

Procedure 2

This technique is used to disguise vascular conditions where there is a need for 'colour correction' before the application of a flesh tone.

1. Prepare the area to be treated by cleansing, toning and moisturising.
2. Choose a base colour to correct the skin colouration and neutralise the blemish by considering the colour wheel.
3. Apply the base colour accurately with a brush on the area of discolouration only.
4. Apply a flesh tone foundation colour to match the surrounding skin.
5. Powder the area by pressing in the product with a powder puff.

 Remember . . .

Carefully analyse the area to be treated to establish the camouflage procedure required.

Procedure for the application of camouflage make-up to cover a tattoo

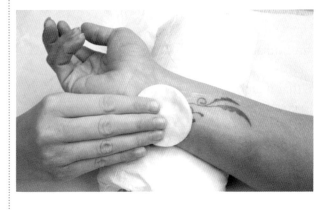

1. Prepare the area, including cleansing, toning and moisturising.

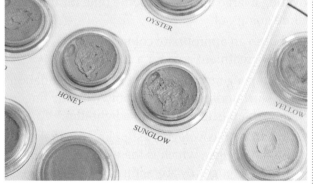

2. Choose colours to hide the blemish/tattoo.

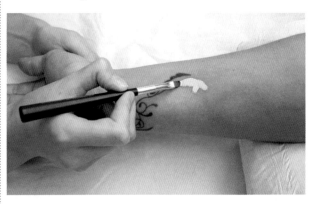

3. Apply the base colour with a brush.

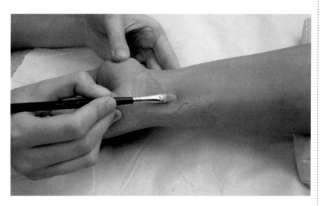

4. Apply the flesh colour to match surrounding skin.

Procedure for the application of camouflage make-up to cover a tattoo

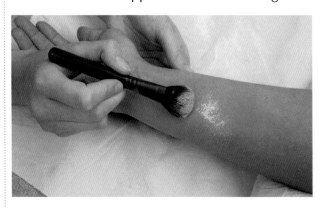

5. Powder on the area.

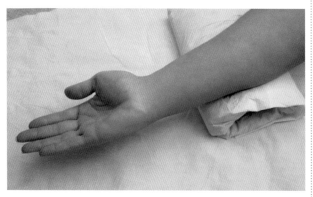

6. The finished result.

Outcome 4: Provide aftercare advice

To maintain the make-up effect in a hot environment or damp conditions, reapply the fixing powder in a patting action with a powder puff or dry cotton wool.

The client may need to recreate the make-up effect and it is very important that products for use at home are discussed with every skin camouflage client. This provides a good retail opportunity. Sell only the correct products for the client's need. The minimum requirement would be the skin camouflage cream in the identified shade to match the skin colour and the fixing powder, with the addition of a colour corrective cream if appropriate.

The removal of cosmetics should also be discussed and demonstrated to ensure that the client fully understands. Skin camouflage products should be removed thoroughly with an appropriate product such as a cream-based cleanser. The cleanser should be applied and massaged into the product and removed with damp cotton wool or facial sponges. Repeat the process until clean and pat dry. Do not rub the skin. Finish with toner and moisturiser to suit the client's skin type.

> **Activity**
>
> Design an information leaflet that describes the use of skin camouflage products and their removal at home.

 Want to know more?

For more information and specialist training, visit:
www.skin-camouflage.net
www.skincamouflagenetwork.com
www.redcross.org.uk (Use the 'search' box to find the information on skin camouflage.)

Test yourself

1. The choice of colour used in camouflage make-up depends on:

   a) the skin's natural colour

   b) the effect required

   c) what light the make-up is to be viewed in

   d) the client's choice.

2. What type of blemish requires 'green' as a corrective colour to camouflage?

   a) vitiligo

   b) chloasma

   c) rosacea

   d) moles.

3. Rosacea is identified by:

   a) tiny red papilla with red 'legs'

   b) a capillary naevi that is present at birth

   c) a flushed appearance, particularly in response to alcohol, spicy foods and stress

   d) a scar that is fibrous and lumpy.

4. Camouflage make-up product best adheres to:

   a) a wet surface

   b) a damp surface

   c) a dry surface

   d) any surface.

5. Camouflage make-up is best stippled with which finger?

   a) the index finger

   b) the third finger

   c) the little finger

   d) the middle finger.

6. Powder is used in camouflage make-up application to:

   a) dry the skin before application

   b) set the cake make-up

   c) set the camouflage product.

   d) dry the skin after application.

7. Camouflage make-up product is more opaque. This is due to the:

   a) high level of pigments in the product

   b) low level of pigments in the product

   c) high level of cream in the product

   d) low level of cream in the product.

8. Skin camouflage products are best removed with:

   a) soap and water

   b) cream cleanser

   c) milk cleanser

   d) soapless cleanser.

9. A complementary colour on the colour wheel is one that is:

   a) a primary colour

   b) made by mixing two primary colours

   c) next to another colour on the colour wheel

   d) opposite another colour on the colour wheel.

10. The Fitzpatrick classification system refers to the:

    a) opacity of the skin camouflage product

    b) photosensitivity of the skin

    c) cause and appearance of skin conditions

    d) recording of the client's treatment or service.

Are you ready for assessment?

The following checklist will help you to be fully prepared for your assessment.

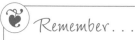

Remember...
Always keep your logbook handy.

The range of clients/treatments you must cover:

- Various consultation techniques.
- Your actions if contraindications are present.
- Work on a range of camouflage needs, for example tattoos, pigmentation.
- Use a range of tools and techniques.
- Use a range of camouflage products.
- Apply camouflage products to different areas.
- Provide advice.

1. **Practical observation**

   Your assessor will look at you:

   - prepare the treatment area ensuring that you carry out safe and hygienic practice
   - ensure the client is comfortable and relaxed
   - maintain safe and hygienic practices
   - consult with the client and discuss the client's requirements and prepare a plan
   - identify any contraindications
   - select products suited to the camouflage requirements

- apply skin camouflage products using a range of techniques
- check with the client that the result is to the client's satisfaction
- provide advice on skin camouflage aftercare, removal and reapplication
- demonstrate professional practice throughout the service
- carry out the service with regard to health and safety.

2. **Knowledge and understanding**

What you must know:

- Organisational and legal requirements.
- How to work safely and effectively when providing skin camouflage services.
- Consult, plan and prepare for the service.
- Contraindications and contra-actions.
- Anatomy and physiology, for example, of the skin, pigmentation conditions.
- Skin camouflage application using a range of products and techniques.
- Advice on products, application and removal.

To ensure that you have the necessary knowledge and understanding of skin camouflage services your assessor will:

- ask you questions before, during and after carrying out the treatment
- ensure that you have completed project work and written exercises relating to the unit
- check that you have recorded in a log/diary skin camouflage services you have carried out with signed record cards showing that you have completed four make-up services competently
- check that you have covered the range in your candidate logbook
- require you to take a test.

Sources of evidence

- Completed client record cards indicating the range of client need.
- Video or photographic evidence.
- Certificates of achievement from skin camouflage courses.
- Following your attendance at a course ask your assessor to observe you showing your colleagues the skills you have learned by giving a lesson to colleagues.
- One-to-one tutorial with your assessor or salon supervisor to establish your progress and set targets A copy of the tutorial report should be available for your portfolio.
- Client feedback.
- Project work researching skin camouflage needs and products available from manufacturers.
- Devise a consultation card that can be used for camouflage make up.
- Devise an information/aftercare leaflet.

Remember...
Skin camouflage service requires a sensitive caring approach to the client's needs.

Remember...
Simulation is not a valid means of assessment for skin camouflage service.

Remember...
Your assessor will observe your performance on four different occasions, each involving different clients (not a fellow student or colleague) and carrying out different treatments from the range.

Chapter 10
Unit B6: Carry out waxing services

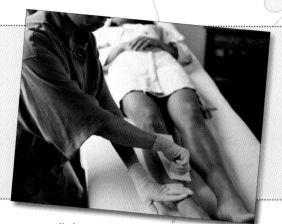

Learning objectives

This chapter covers Unit B6 'Carry out waxing services', that is the temporary removal of unwanted hair growth, including the skills and knowledge needed to perform the services.

There are four learning outcomes for Unit B6 and they are:

1 Maintain safe and effective methods when removing hair by waxing.
2 Consult, plan and prepare for waxing treatment with clients.
3 Remove unwanted hair.
4 Provide aftercare advice.

You will need to be competent in all of these outcomes in waxing services qualify for insurance and perform the treatment on members of the public.

Evidence requirements

Your assessor will need to observe you perform this treatment successfully on at least four occasions, each involving a different client. You must:

1 Demonstrate the use of consultation techniques:
- questioning
- visual
- manual
- reference to client records.

2 Carry out all the waxing treatments:
- eyebrows
- upper lip
- chin
- full leg
- half leg
- underarm
- bikini line.

3 Take one of the following actions if necessary:
- encourage the client to seek medical advice
- explain why the treatment cannot be carried out
- modify the treatment.

4 Use all types of waxing product on appropriate parts of the body:
- hot wax
- warm wax.

5 Use all the work techniques:
- stretching and manipulating the skin during application and removal
- speed of product removal
- direction and angle of removal
- on-going product temperature checks.

6 Provide relevant aftercare:
- avoidance of activities which may cause contra-actions
- suitable homecare products and their use
- recommended time intervals between waxing treatments.

Introduction

Smooth, flawless skin is much sought after, particularly during the summer months when the body is more exposed or when clients are going on holiday. It is then that waxing becomes a very popular salon treatment but there are also clients who have waxing all the year round.

Superfluous is the term used to describe any unwanted hair growth. For Western women this is usually the hair that is found under the arms, around the bikini line, on legs and sometimes on arms and face. It is regarded as unattractive and unacceptable on the female and there is a fast-growing trend towards the 'hair-free' male too. Many European women, on the other hand, do not regard hair in these areas a problem and do not remove hair from underarms or legs.

The amount and colour of superfluous hair will vary in individuals but is regarded as normal if it follows a normal growth pattern on the legs, underarm and bikini line, and can be seen as a hereditary characteristic. The skin and hair characteristics of different races also influence the colour and amount of body hair. For example, Asian clients have dark, fine hair on the body whereas people from the Far East have very little body hair. Hormones influence the amount of hair, with changes seen during puberty, pregnancy and menopause. Superfluous hair may be unsightly because it is dark or grows thickly. This can cause embarrassment to the client and they may look to you for appropriate treatment.

Unit B6 'Carry out waxing services' is a mandatory unit for Level 2 Beauty Therapy General route only and is worth seven credits.

> **Key term**
>
> The term **'superfluous'** describes unwanted hair growth.

Meet the professional

"Double-dipping is a No! Use a fresh spatula for each client and where blood is involved NEVER put your spatula back into the wax. Protect yourself and your clients. It may work out more expensive in the long run but it has its benefits too. I tell my clients we don't double-dip and the reasons why we don't and it's a big selling point, even if I charge slightly more than other salons."

Jacqui Bostock

Methods of hair removal

For hair removal, the client may use a whole range of home treatments including the following:

- **Shaving using an electric or wet razor** – these cut the hair at the skin surface, leaving a blunt end which will reappear at the skin surface as rough stubble within 24–48 hours.

- **Depilatory cream** – this uses a strong alkaline chemical that dissolves the keratin in the hair and skin. The hair is only removed to the surface of the skin so will reappear within 24–48 hours. The skin can become very sensitive during and after use.

- **Abrasive gloves** – these are rubbed over the skin in circular movements, which breaks off the hair at the surface of the skin. The hair reappears as rough stubble within 24–48 hours. The skin may become sore and sensitised by this method.

- **Cutting or clipping** – in this method, scissors are used to cut the hair close to the surface of the skin. It is time consuming for a large area so is usually used on single hairs from moles for example, which should not be waxed or plucked. Coarse stubble will reappear in less than 24 hours.

Depilation is the term used to describe the temporary removal of unwanted hair. The hair is 'plucked' from the hair follicle but the base of the follicle (the **papilla**) remains intact and can therefore provide nourishment for a new hair to grow. This method of temporary hair removal can last for two to six weeks, depending on the individual hair growth cycle and the area of the body being treated. If hair is removed permanently using an electrical current or laser, this is called **epilation**.

Below is a table that compares these methods of hair removal.

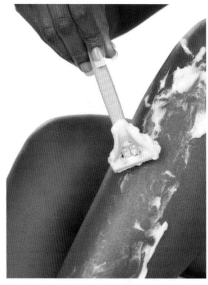

△ A wet razor is one method of hair removal

> **Key term**
>
> **Depilation** is the temporary removal of unwanted hair.
>
> **Papilla** is the name for the base of the hair follicle.
>
> **Epilation** is the permanent removal of unwanted hair.

Method	Description	Advantages	Disadvantages
Tweezing	A popular do-it-yourself treatment that removes the hair down to the root	Slow regrowth Low cost	Can treat small areas only. Can be painful so not for very sensitive clients
Shaving	Hair is cut off at the skin surface	Low cost	Fast regrowth Feels stubbly Can irritate or cut skin
Depilatory creams	Chemical that dissolves hair at or just below skin surface	Regrowth slightly slower than shaving but feels softer	Expensive for large areas. Smells unpleasant Not suitable for sensitive skins or coarse hairs
Electrical depilation	A battery or electrically operated device with rotary blades in which the hairs are gripped and pulled out from the root	Can treat large areas successfully and cheaply Slow regrowth if performed correctly	Expensive initial outlay Some find the process very painful

Method	Description	Advantages	Disadvantages
Cutting	Hair is cut at skin surface without irritating skin	Low cost Preferable to tweezing facial hair in between epilation treatments	Can treat small areas only Fast regrowth
Abrasive glove	Hair is rubbed away at the skin surface	Easy to use Low cost Suitable for use on fine hair	Fast regrowth Not for sensitive skins or coarse hair
Threading	A specialist technique that takes the hair out down to the root	Slow regrowth Quick and effective	Needs a specialist to perform the treatment
Waxing	Hair is removed down to the root, similar to mass tweezing	Slow soft regrowth Suitable for large areas Instant result Only slight discomfort for the client	Need to grow hair to a certain length before it can be treated Relatively expensive compared to tweezing. Removes vellus hair as well as terminal hair Can distort root, so if epilation is required later, treatment will be less effective. Some clients have problems with ingrown hairs Needs to be repeated at regular intervals. There is a belief that hair growth increases due to the stimulation of the blood supply to the follicle
Epilation	Electrical current is used to produce heat or a chemical reaction to remove hair down to the root	Permanent Slow regrowth as hair becomes finer and finer and then stops growing altogether Suitable for relatively small areas	Expensive, long treatment plan, especially for large areas Skin irritation may occur Can be painful in sensitive areas such as upper lip Treatment by incompetent therapists can lead to permanent skin damage and scarring
Intensive Pulse Light (IPL)	Use of light in intense short bursts to bring about the destruction of the hair follicle and permanent hair removal	Quick Can treat large areas of hair growth Effective on dark coarse hair	Expensive initial outlay Less effective on fair fine hair Skin is left with redness and raised wheals for a few days after treatment
Laser	Use of laser light to destroy the hair	Quick Can treat large areas of hair growth Effective on dark coarse hair especially if the skin is fair	Expensive There are questions surrounding its efficacy

When a client is using other hair removal methods at home or elsewhere it can cause problems for the therapist performing waxing services. The use of other temporary methods can affect the therapist's ability to give an accurate opinion about the possible success of the treatment. If the hair growth cycle is disturbed, the salon's waxing service may not last as long as normally expected.

The therapist should advise a client having a permanent method of hair removal such as epilation not to also have waxing in the same area of the body, as the treatment can undo the effect by increasing the blood supply to the area instead of reducing it.

Test yourself

Test yourself on the related anatomy by answering these questions:

1. What is the outermost layer of the skin called, which is most affected by waxing services?
2. Which glands found in the skin are most responsible for skin type?
3. Give four functions of the skin.
4. A healthy skin is slightly acidic. Is this statement true or false?
5. What structure of the skin is responsible for the discomfort sometimes felt during waxing treatments?
6. Give a definition of the term 'terminal hair'.
7. What is the name for the structure in which the hair sits?
8. Why might a client experience a few hairs with fine ends reappearing at the skin surface a week to ten days after a waxing treatment?
9. What structure of the skin is responsible for the contra-action 'bruising' during a waxing treatment?
10. What are the soft, downy hairs often found between terminal hairs called?

Outcome 1: Maintain safe and effective methods of working when removing hair by waxing

Waxing services are commonplace, popular with both women and men of all ages. The hair is removed traumatically from the follicle, causing minor damage to the hair follicle and dermal papilla. This takes time to repair before a new hair is formed and grows to the surface of the skin. For this reason waxing services should be treated with great care by the therapist and he/she must be aware of their responsibilities under local and national legislation and the industry's Code of Practice for Waxing.

It is important to perform waxing services to meet legal, hygiene and industry requirements not only to ensure safe and effective treatment but also to ensure the return custom of the client and therefore ensuring the success of your business.

The general national legal requirements for performing beauty therapy treatments can be found in Chapter 3 'Make sure your own actions reduce risks to health and safety'. On page 224 is a checklist that highlights the key legislation involved with waxing services.

▽ Key legislation involved in waxing services

The treatment room	Health & Safety at Work Act 1974	General safety of staff and visitors to the salon including clients
	The Workplace (Health, Safety & Welfare) Regulations 1992	Governs the working environment including ventilation, temperature and lighting, etc.
	Regulatory Reform (Fire Safety) Order 2005	The safe evacuation of the building in an emergency such as a fire
Waxing equipment	Provision and Use of Work Equipment Regulations 1998	Governs the acquisition of safe and reliable equipment
	Electricity at Work Regulations 1989	Governs the regular maintenance of electrical equipment including the recording of such
Waxing products	Control of Substances Hazardous to Health 1988	Governs the exposure of persons to substances likely to cause harm including flammability and the effect on the tissues
	Cosmetic Products (Safety) Regulations (2008)	Requires cosmetics to comply with correct labelling, to have safe formulation and be fit for the purpose intended
Disposal of waste	The Controlled Waste Regulations 1992	Governs the correct disposal of contaminated waste, i.e. that contaminated with blood or other bodily fluids

It is important for a business offering waxing services to have Public Liability Insurance and Professional Indemnity Insurance to protect the therapist against claims for damages and/or negligence by the client.

To reduce the risk of such a claim, the therapist should be aware of their responsibilities under health and safety legislation and perform the waxing services in line with the industry's Code of Practice. The Code of Practice was written by HABIA, the government approved standards setting body for the hair and beauty sector, and it gives information on the following:

- waxing systems
- client consultation
- dress code
- infection control and hygiene
- operational procedures
- salon safety
- prohibited materials/chemicals
- insurance
- training, education, CPD and qualifications
- mobile practitioners
- health and safety law
- blood-borne infections
- waxing national occupational standards.

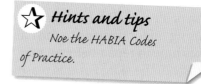

★ *Hints and tips*
Noe the HABIA Codes of Practice.

In order to promote professionalism, and a healthy and safe working environment, the therapist must be suitably attired. The professional dress code and the expectations of the industry generally can be found in Chapter 1. In addition to the wearing of a professional uniform, the therapist performing waxing services should wear a plastic apron to protect their clothing and disposable, single-use gloves for each client to prevent the spread of blood-borne infections through the release of serum and blood that occurs during waxing services. **PPE** is required under health and safety legislation.

Treatment times for waxing services

These times have been determined by the industry as standard commercial timings for waxing services and should be used during the practical assessment. When treatments are combined, times are reduced because you will be setting up and performing the consultation only once for the combined service.

Service	Time
Full leg wax	45 minutes
Half leg wax	30 minutes
Bikini line	15 minutes
Underarm	15 minutes
Eyebrows	10 minutes
Lip	10 minutes
Chin	10 minutes

Hygiene procedures when waxing

It is important to maintain high levels of hygiene when performing waxing services for the following reasons:

- It maintains client confidence, which will ensure her return for further treatment and ultimately the success of the beauty therapy business.
- Hygiene procedures protect the therapist and the client from cross-infection and in particular blood-borne infections such as hepatitis and HIV/AIDS.

Waxing is potentially also a messy treatment. Your attention to detail is necessary and strict hygiene procedures must be followed:

- Clean the wax heater of drips or minor spills of wax before and after use. This should be done at regular intervals depending on the number of clients, but once a week is suggested if in regular use. The wax pot should be emptied, cleaned and dried and any used wax discarded.
- Disposable wax pots that are not refilled are available and are recommended by the industry Codes of Practice.

 Health and safety

Surgical spirit or wax cleaner can be used to clean the wax heater. It should be applied with disposable paper and is easier to perform when the heater is warm but not plugged in, as surgical spirit and wax cleaner are flammable products.

- The waste bin should be such that the need to touch the bin is dispensed with (e.g. a pedal bin).

- The bin must contain a plastic bin liner for protection. Because of the presence of blood and serum on the waste materials, this liner must be removed after treatment, tied, and placed in a yellow bin liner for contaminated waste. The yellow liners are collected and incinerated by the local governing authority and there may be an additional charge for this service.

- The treatment area must be protected with plastic sheeting and disposable paper such as couch roll.

- The trolley should also be protected by sheets of disposable paper.

- Clean cotton wool, tissues, paper or muslin strips if being used and spatulas should be placed on the trolley.

- Tweezers should be sterilised by an appropriate method (see Chapter 1) and placed in a bowl with a square of cotton wool soaked in sterilising fluid such as surgical spirit. This will keep them hygienic until use.

- Bottles containing pre-wax cleanser, surgical spirit and after-care lotions should be cleaned and placed away from the heater, as some of these products are flammable. This also reduces the risk of dripping wax onto them during treatment.

- The appropriate client clothing must be removed before the treatment goes ahead, and placed safely so that wax cannot drip onto them. Disposable items such as underwear can be provided or the client's underwear protected by the careful placing of disposable paper.

- Wash your hands before and after wax treatment.

- PPE to reduce risk of cross-infection of diseases should be worn, such as disposable single-use gloves.

- The area to be treated should be examined for contraindications. If an infectious condition is suspected then treatment should not continue.

- The area should be wiped with pre-wax cleanser or surgical spirit, using a clean piece of cotton wool.

- To prevent possible contamination of the wax in the heater by blood, serum, skin cells and micro-organisms, wax applicators such as a wooden spatula should be used only once and then discarded if they have been in contact with the client.

- Wax strips *may* be used more than once in the same area but is unadvisable when a different area is to be treated.

- Wax strips should be folded to contain the wax on the inside. This prevents unnecessary soiling of the waste bin.

- When taking the wax from the heater to the area it is advisable to hold the strip or a tissue in the non-working hand, under the spatula to catch any wax that drips from it.

- If wax is inadvertently dripped on to the immediate working area, remove or protect it straight away to prevent the client from coming in contact.

Hints and tips
Creams, lotions and spray should be dispensed from containers with a spray or pump action, or a disposable spatula used to dispense the product from a pot or tub. The lid should be closed after dispensing.

Hints and tips
Other single-use items for the safe and hygienic performance of waxing services include wooden spatulas, orange sticks, cotton pads, disposable underwear, couch roll and tissues.

Hints and tips
Application methods vary: one method that avoids the excessive use of wooden spatulas is to use one spatula in the wax pot to take the wax, which is then 'drizzled' onto another that comes in contact with the client. This takes practice to maintain hygiene and commercial viability.

- Remove the wax from an area methodically. This avoids 'missing' hairs and leaving 'hairy patches' and also avoids placing the non-working hand in wax when stretching the skin.

- If tweezers are used to remove hairs left after waxing, the hairs should be placed onto a piece of cotton wool and disposed of in a lined bin.

- After treatment, the after-care lotion or oil should be applied with cotton wool to the area and if necessary, the client asked to massage in.

- The treatment area should be cleared of bed-roll, cotton wool, tissues, used strips and spatulas and placed in the lined bin along with the used gloves.

- Tweezers should be wiped with surgical spirit to remove wax and sterilised after use.

- The client, wax heater and treatment area should be clear of wax on completion of the treatment.

- If used, hot wax must be disposed of after each client to limit the risk of cross-infection.

- Clean towels and laundry by washing at a minimum of 60°C.

Safety precautions

There are several safety precautions that should be observed during wax depilation. The hazards relating to waxing are involved with the electrically run heater, which has the potential for electric shock and burning. Also, the trauma caused to the skin by the removal of wax could result in bruising, infection, bleeding and the formation of scabs.

After waxing the skin is sensitised by the treatment. All these hazards can be minimised by following these guidelines:

- Ensure the treatment area environmental conditions are suitable for the treatment.

- Have the heater checked for electrical safety yearly, or more often if in constant use.

- Do not use a heater where the flex is damaged or broken in any way or if any internal wires are visible either at the plug or near the heater.

- If the heater does not work, change the fuse and if still not working it will need to be sent to a reputable dealer for repair. Do not attempt to repair the heater yourself.

- Heaters must have a thermostat to control the heating of the wax. Check that the thermostat in the heater is working regularly by turning the control up and down. You should be able to hear the thermostat click on or off and/or see the indicator light switching on or off.

- You should test heated wax on your wrist before applying to the client. Remember to check the consistency of the wax. Overheated wax will be very runny and may emit strong fumes or give off smoke.

 Hints and tips

If gloved hands become sticky, apply a little surgical spirit or after-wax product before continuing the treatment.

Hints and tips

Safety and comfort must be ensured. Adjust the temperature of the work area so that it is not too cold, or too hot, which may result in heat exhaustion. Appropriate ventilation is necessary to protect against undesirable fumes from the wax products. Lighting should be sufficient to facilitate the ease and safety of the treatment.

- Test the client's tolerance to the heat of the wax (particularly when using hot wax) by applying a small amount with a spatula to an area of the skin on which you will be working.

- The temperature of the wax must be checked throughout the treatment.

- Wax heaters must be placed on a secure trolley. Position the heater securely on a trolley so that it cannot fall or tip over. Do not move the heater when the wax is hot.

- The wax heater should also be situated a distance away from the client, to ensure that it will not come into contact with the client.

- The heater's position should also be so that its flex is not trailing where you or the client can fall over it, or stretched to the socket where the heater can be pulled off of the trolley if moved.

- As the heater gets hot, do not place in contact with unsuitable materials such as glass or plastic, which may be affected by the heat.

- Do not place the heater near flammable materials, such as surgical spirit and paper.

- Check the heater does not overheat the wax.

- Explain the treatment procedure, contraindications and contra-actions to the client before beginning treatment and give the client the opportunity to ask questions.

- Obtain a doctor's permission for treatment if the client has a medical related contraindication, for example diabetes.

- To prevent cross-infection, do not treat anyone with a suspected infectious condition.

- To prevent infection, equipment must be sterilised, the area to be treated cleaned and disposable items thrown away after use.

- Disposable single-use items such as gloves prevent the transference of disease from one person to another, especially HIV and Hepatitis B viruses.

- 'Rosin' found in wax and 'latex' in some disposable gloves are both known allergens and can result in contact dermatitis, a non-infectious skin condition. Clients with known allergies such as these should avoid waxing treatments.

- The lifting of the skin away from the underlying tissues causes bruising. To prevent this, stretch the skin with the non-working hand when removing the wax. The looser the skin, the more you need to stretch.

- Areas of excessive **desquamation** or scabs are caused by the removal of the epidermis, usually by waxing over an area several times. This can be avoided by observing the skin before treatment commences and assessing the skin type and condition.

- Applying the correct amount of wax, pulling it off in the correct direction and *quickly* will also reduce the risk of excessive trauma to the skin (see the section headed 'Procedures for waxing' for details).

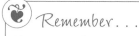

Remember . . .
Always test the temperature of the wax before starting treatment and throughout the treatment.

Hints and tips
Turning the thermostat control to a temperature higher than working temperature does not heat the wax any quicker. In fact, it wastes time waiting for it to cool.

Hints and tips
Fine, thin, dry skins are prone to desquamation, and therefore these types of skin must not be treated several times. Consider also the skin reaction: if an excessive erythema is present or the skin feels hot to touch (as with hot wax) do not treat the area again.

Key term

Desquamation is the loss or shedding of the epidermal skin cells at the skin surface.

Erythema is reddening caused by dilated blood capillaries in the dermis.

- After treatment apply after-care lotion or oil, which soothes the trauma of the skin and reduces the possibility of infection.
- Explain after-care procedures fully and ensure that the client understands them by giving the client the chance to ask questions.

Posture and positioning for waxing

- The client needs to be comfortable and relaxed.
- For waxing, the client should be laid on the couch, either flat or semi-elevated. The angle of the backrest of the couch or the pillow needs to be adjusted, for example, for leg wax the client can be in a sitting position. For underarm waxing the client needs to lie flat with arms held above their head.
- The wax heater must be close to the therapist while working to avoid undue stretching, which can cause fatigue, and also to ensure the wax does not drip on the floor.
- There must be no trailing wires, or wires that are being stretched that could in any way make the wax heater unstable.
- The couch should be at a convenient height so the therapist does not have to overstretch or bend. This will eliminate the risk of injury to the therapist and minimise fatigue.

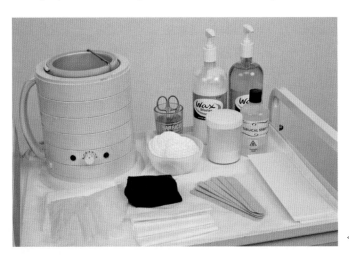

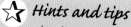
⭐ **Hints and tips**
The client may be required to lie in unusual positions to facilitate access to and removal of the superfluous hair. Pillows or rolled up towels covered with disposable paper can be used for support where necessary.

Remember...
Ensure the privacy and modesty of the client is maintained at all times.

◁ A clean and hygienic set up for the waxing trolley

Outcome 2: Consult, plan and prepare for waxing treatments with clients

Consultation

A consultation should be carried out before every waxing treatment to establish:

- the suitability of the client for the waxing service including the presence of contraindications
- the client's expectations of the treatment
- the details of the treatment, including the choice of products
- accurate records that reflect the client's personal details and that of the treatment.

When assessing the client for treatment, discuss their requirements and examine the area to be treated. Begin by checking for contraindications and examining the condition of the skin and hair. Note the length, texture, colour and growth pattern of the hair. This will help with the decision on the product choice, method of treatment and the direction in which the wax is to be applied.

> **Remember...**
> The Data Protection Act requires you to maintain confidentiality when gaining information from the client during the consultation.

Contraindications to waxing

The specific contraindications to waxing services are divided into three groups, as follows.

1. Those that require medical referral:
   - severe varicose veins
   - medicine-controlled diabetes.

2. Those that prevent treatment but do not require medical referral:
   - infectious skin conditions such as conjunctivitis (facial waxing) or ringworm (legs)
   - urinary infections/disease (bikini line)
   - thin skin
   - fragile skin
   - some medications, such as steroids
   - sunburn
   - known allergy to the products, such as 'rosin' found in waxes.

3. Those that restrict treatment:
   - mild varicose veins
   - oedema
   - epilepsy
   - sexually-transmitted infections (bikini line)
   - external haemorrhoids
   - vascular disorders
   - hypersensitive skins
   - moles
   - warts
   - recent scar tissue (less than six months old)
   - recent cosmetic surgery, tattoos or piercings
   - recent laser, **microdermabrasion**
   - infected, in-growing hairs
   - heat rash
   - skin tags
   - medication such as steroid creams
   - use of Retin A or Accutane
   - use of alpha or beta hydroxy-acids or skin peels.

> **Key term**
>
> **Microdermabrasion** – the cosmetic procedure by which mechanical exfoliation of the skin is performed with the use of vacuum suction and crystals of aluminium dioxide.

Treatment adaptation

For those contraindications that restrict treatment, the waxing service will need to be adapted to suit. Such adaptations include those shown in the table below.

Adaptation/actions	Contraindication
Avoid the area either by going around the affected area or missing out the area from the treatment	Suitable for small affected areas such as moles, warts, skin tags, in-growing hairs, etc.
Delaying the treatment for a period of time in order for the condition to heal or dissipate	Use of medication, both topical and oral, such as Retin A or the use of steroid creams, recent scar tissue, microdermabrasion, recent tattoo, etc.
Careful choice of product and technique to suit the condition	Hypersensitive skins, mild varicose veins, heat rash, etc.
Use of disposable items such as underwear, spatulas, etc.	STIs and infected hair follicles

At this stage of the consultation it is essential to check that the client understands the waxing service and in particular the contra-actions to treatment.

Contra-actions

The client should be made aware of the possible contra-actions to waxing services in order to be able to make a decision as to whether to continue with the treatment. The client should be encouraged to follow aftercare advice, which can effectively reduce the chance of contra-actions to waxing services occurring.

The contra-actions are:

- excessive erythema or red spots on the skin that persist for more than a few hours (bikini line may last 24–48 hours)
- bruising, which can occur when poor technique is used (for example, pulling the wax upwards, especially on the bikini line or on clients with loose, crêpey skin)
- pustules forming at the mouth of the follicles two or three days after waxing, indicating poor hygiene
- excessive blood spotting
- abrasions caused by waxing over an area many times, the excessive use of a waxing strip to remove wax left on the skin or waxing thin and fragile skin
- broken hairs that appear a few days after treatment, caused by removing the wax in the incorrect direction
- allergic reaction to the waxing products or their ingredients
- excessive hair growth, caused by the removal of the **vellus hair** among **terminal hair** that may have been 'sensitised' through hormonal changes in the body.

Possible causes of contra-actions

1. Failing to recognise skin reaction following the sensitivity test.
2. The client being sensitive to ingredients in the wax or preparation lotion.
3. Wax too hot, which can cause burns.

> ### Key term
>
> **Vellus hair** – the fine soft downy hair that covers the whole of the body, with the exception of the eyelids, lips, palms of the hands and soles of the feet.
>
> **Terminal hair** – the longer, thicker and often darker hair that covers the scalp and pubic regions and includes the eyebrows and eyelashes.

4. Wax left uncovered during storage allowing micro-organisms (such as airborne micro-organisms) to get into the wax, causing **folliculitis**. The wax is warmed, providing ideal conditions for the growth of bacteria that cause infection. Infection will appear as pustules at the mouth of the follicle caused by bacteria entering the open follicle. This indicates poor hygiene procedures by the therapist or incorrect home care by the client. May be treated by the use of antiseptic lotion.

5. Pulling the wax strip away from the skin during removal lifts the skin, causing blood vessels to rupture (bruising). This is a particular problem in the bikini line area or on the legs where skin might be thin and loose (as in mature clients).

6. Bruising may occur if the skin is not supported and held firmly when removing the strip or hot wax.

Condition of the skin and hair

The next stage of the consultation is a visual and manual check of the area to be treated. This involves getting the client suitably dressed (details are given later in this chapter) and looking at the skin type of the area to be treated (such as normal, dry or oily) and at the skin condition (sensitive, dehydrated or mature). The length, texture and colour of the hair should be noted and most importantly the direction of hair growth. The temperature of the skin is particularly important when using warm wax. The skin may feel cold to the touch, indicating poor blood circulation and this can cause the wax to cool sufficiently to make removal from the skin difficult.

> **Key term**
>
> **Folliculitis** – a bacterial infection of the hair follicle caused by, for example, poor hygiene.

> **Health and safety**
>
> If any skin reaction lasts longer than 48 hours or progressively becomes worse, for example irritation or erythema, then the client should return to the salon for advice. The most likely explanation will be an allergic reaction to something in the product used. This can be treated with antiseptic soothing lotion and the condition noted on the client's record card. Serious cases may need to be referred to a doctor.

> *Hints and tips*
>
> *Where there are areas of poor blood circulation the wax should be applied in small sections and removed straight away so the chance of the wax cooling are greatly reduced.*

> **Activity**
>
> It is essential that warm wax is applied with the hair growth and removed against the hair growth. Indicate with arrows, the direction of hair growth on the following diagrams.
>
>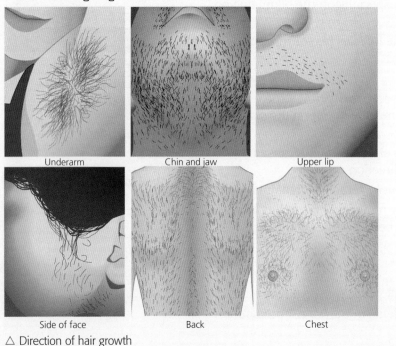
>
> Underarm   Chin and jaw   Upper lip
>
> Side of face   Back   Chest
>
> △ Direction of hair growth

Use of client's records

Some clients can be very sensitive to the products so it is important to check the record card to see if they have had hair removal previously and whether the skin reacted in any way. New clients should be questioned carefully to establish whether they have had any previous adverse reaction to any hair removal treatment administered at home or in another salon.

The treatment should be clearly explained to the client, giving some indication of how it might feel and how the skin may react and look for a short while afterwards. If this explanation is delivered before the treatment it will also improve the client's trust and confidence in the therapist when the normal reactions become apparent. The normal skin reaction can come as a shock to some clients, who expect smooth skin immediately.

The consultation techniques, questioning and listening skills and referral procedures to follow when performing a consultation for waxing services can be found in Chapter 1.

Normal skin reaction

The following may occur after waxing and are quite normal reactions:

- erythema in the area
- slight swelling
- tiny red spots around the hair follicles
- blood spots may appear during underarm or bikini-line waxing – this is due to the coarse nature of the hair and deep follicles, which have a rich blood supply and can lead to scab formation.

Normal reactions will last anything from a few minutes to several hours, depending on the area treated and the skin type.

Sensitivity

Each client will have different levels of tolerance to heat, pain and sensitivity to products. It is therefore essential that a sensitivity test, along with careful questioning of the client, is carried out before starting treatment.

- Skin sensitivity to heat – ensuring the temperature of the wax is suitable for individual clients is essential at the start of each treatment.
- Allergic reactions to products used in waxing – it is essential to ask the client about previous wax treatments and whether they experienced a skin reaction and to observe the skin's reaction during the early stages of the treatment to ensure there is no adverse reaction.
- Removing the hair can be quite painful – client sensitivity to pain (pain threshold) will vary considerably. Sensitivity can be increased when stressed or anxious or during menstruation.

Remember . . .

Refer to the most recent equality and discrimination law to ensure that salon literature concerning handling and treatment of clients comply with legal requirements.

Hints and tips

Different areas of the body will have different sensitivity. The skin around the bikini line area, for example, is very delicate and therefore will respond to temperature more quickly.

Hints and tips

Be careful not to overemphasise the pain involved in waxing for some clients. Instead, refer to it as discomfort. Always ask the client throughout the treatment if they are comfortable.

Thermal sensitivity testing

To test the temperature of the wax it is usual to test on the inside of the wrist initially and only then on the client, in a hair-free area close to the area being treated.

Product sensitivity testing

A patch test is recommended where a new client has a history of skin sensitivity or known allergies to products. It is performed at least 24 hours before the waxing service on a suitable area such as on the inside of the forearm and the results noted on the client's records.

How to identify histamine reaction to the skin

When the skin is injured, damaged or hypersensitive to a chemical, the mast cells release a substance called **histamine**. A histamine reaction causes the diameter of the blood vessels to increase (**vasodilation**) and the permeability of the blood vessel walls to increase also, producing a lowering of blood pressure.

A histamine reaction on the skin can be recognised by almost instant erythema, inflammation, localised swelling and irritation.

Erythema is reddening caused by dilated blood capillaries in the dermis. Blood flow increases and speeds up the removal of the irritant and brings antibodies to the area to repair the problem.

Inflammation is the body's natural reaction to infection or injury. The blood supply is increased, bringing extra white blood cells to fight the infection and promote healing Signs of inflammation are redness, swelling, area is painful to the touch and is hot.

Swelling is caused by extra blood being brought to the area by the capillaries, allowing fluid to seep into the surrounding tissue. Blisters may form, or swelling and puffiness of the skin. Swelling acts as a cushion to protect the area from further injury.

Irritation is caused by stimulation of the nerve endings. Severe itching can cause wheals and areas of broken skin.

Rarely, a potentially deadly allergic complication called anaphylactic shock can occur, which can kill if not acted upon immediately. The lips and tongue begin to swell and then the throat itself, restricting the airway. This abnormal reaction can be caused by allergens such as nuts, wasp or bee sting.

It should now be possible for you to choose the correct product and treatment procedure to suit the client's needs and expectations.

Depilatory waxing products

Hot wax (hard wax)

Hot wax has been popular for many years and there are still clients who prefer hot wax, particularly those with dark, coarse hair. There are, however, new 'hard waxes' on the market that have seen a resurgence in popularity of the use of this type of wax in salons, particularly in 'intimate waxing' treatments for both male and female clients.

Key term

Histamine – a chemical released by the mast cells within the skin as a response to exposure to an allergen and causes reddening, itching and swelling within the affected area.

Vasodilation – the increase in the size of the blood capillaries that allows more blood to the affected area.

Health and safety

Most clients who suffer from anaphylactic shock will be aware of it, and carry a device for injecting antihistamine by self-administration. You should be aware of the ingredients within your products to advise such clients effectively. If a member of staff or a client suffers from this condition it is wise to seek advice as to your legal position and to undertake training in the use of an epi-pen.

Traditional hot wax is bought in solid blocks or large 'chips', which when heated, become liquid and highly flammable. The hotter the temperature, the runnier the wax becomes. Hot wax melts at approximately 90°C and should be allowed to cool to a working temperature of 68°C. There have always been problems with this type of wax, due to it being brittle and breaking during removal.

Modern hard waxes (or 'non-strip' waxes as they are sometimes known) are sold as smaller granules or pellets or discs, which need a temperature of 37-45°C for use, which is similar to warm wax. These waxes vary in composition but are basically beeswax, rosin and other resins, soothing ingredients to minimise skin reaction and irritation, thickeners such as paraffin and other ingredients such as elastomers to ensure flexibility during use.

When placed on the skin and allowed to cool, the wax shrinks around the hair, gripping it tightly so that when the wax is removed the hair comes away too. No strip is needed to remove this type of wax. Hot wax is less desquamating to the skin than warm wax and more suited for the removal of coarse hair, making it suitable for use in treating the bikini line and underarm, although it can be used on any area of the body.

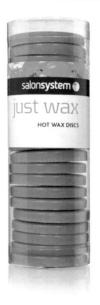

△ Hot wax in disc form

Warm wax (soft wax)

Warm wax, sometimes called strip wax or soft wax, is so named as it does not require heating to a high temperature. It is semi-solid at room temperature, which means it has a low melting point and working temperature (approximately 43°C) so it needs only to be 'warmed' to make it runny. This makes the wax more suitable for use on clients who are sensitive to heat. The wax is made from non-organic synthetic resins (man-made), or organic materials such as honey or sugar. They often appear transparent, like honey. They work by sticking to the hair (and skin) when applied to the area and then removed with a fabric or paper strip placed over the wax. When removed quickly, the hairs are pulled out of the skin with it. Many modern organic waxes are water-soluble so any excess can be removed with water. Non-organic waxes are removed with solvent-based cleaners such as surgical spirit. Warm wax is supplied in tins or tubs, which can be placed directly into a specially designed heater or dispensed into the heater.

Some warm waxes contain creams and moisturisers to moisturise the skin, making them suitable for dry skins. This gives them a cream colour. Others contain soothing ingredients such as lavender or calamine, which are often coloured pale pink or purple colour, others have antiseptic qualities (for example those containing tea tree oil) and are green in colour. Cream wax should be heated to a slightly higher temperature than resin waxes to achieve the required 'runny' working consistency but they work in the same way as the resin types – they are warmed, applied to the area and removed with a strip.

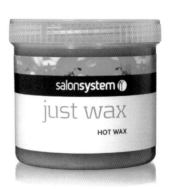

△ Warm wax in tub

All wax heaters must be thermostatically controlled. However, it is sometimes necessary to boost the temperature while working to keep the correct consistency of the wax. The consistency of the wax is an indication of the temperature. If the wax is thick like toffee it is not heated sufficiently and will be impossible to apply to the area evenly. If, on the other hand, the wax has a thin consistency, or is giving off fumes or smoke, it is an immediate indication of overheating and it cannot be used until cool. If overheated, the wax will be very runny and impossible to control on the spatula and it may burn the client's skin.

Roller or flat-head waxing systems

Roller waxing systems use special thermostatically controlled heating systems and disposable cartridges of wax containing warm wax. The heads of varying sizes, for use on different areas, are fitted to apply the wax once it has been heated to the working temperature of around 40°C. The heads should be disposed of after use. The disposable nature of the heads reduces the risk of infection and the equipment is easy to maintain. It is compact and, because of the sealed cartridges, very clean to use. There are a number of systems available from different manufacturers.

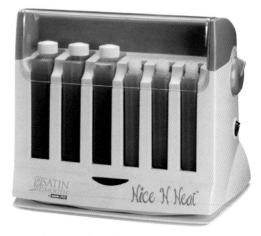

△ A roller or flat-head waxing system

Sugaring techniques

The art of sugaring to remove hair from the body has been passed down by generations from very early times. The technique originates in the Middle East where it was the tradition to remove all the hair from the body of the bride before her wedding day. All the female members of the family would gather to prepare the sugar paste from a recipe that included sugar, water and lemon juice boiled together to a caramelised paste. The sugar was applied as a ritual to ensure that the bride's skin was perfectly smooth.

Sugar paste is now made commercially and can be obtained from wholesalers at a reasonable price. Traditional practitioners of sugaring may make their own paste using a special recipe, but this requires considerable experience because of the dangers involved in boiling sugar.

Sugaring has gained recent popularity as many clients find this treatment kinder to the skin and is a less painful treatment. It can be used safely on all parts of the body, even sensitive skins, due to the natural ingredients of sugar, water and lemon juice. The product needs little heat to be of a working consistency and some may be (carefully) warmed in a microwave or placed in a hot water-bath, making them popular with mobile therapists. It has been noted that, with some hair growths, the hairs need not be as long as for warm waxing and as the product is water-soluble, the treated area and the therapist's hands can be washed with warm water, eliminating the use of harsh products. This also means that any accidental spills onto linens can be washed away.

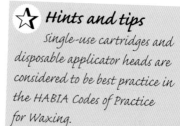

★ *Hints and tips*
single-use cartridges and disposable applicator heads are considered to be best practice in the HABIA Codes of Practice for Waxing.

Soft paste should be used in warm weather or if the therapist has warm hands. It needs little heating, usually a water-bath would suffice, but if heated further it is ideal for the strip sugaring technique.

Hard paste is darker in colour and needs more heating, making it ideal for use by therapists with hot hands and for use in hot weather. Used for the manual application technique only.

Suitability of waxing products

Below is a table that summarises the suitable use of waxing products.

Skin/hair type and condition	Hot/hard wax	Warm wax	Sugar
Dry skin	✓		✓
Oily skin	✓	✓	✓
Dehydrated	✓		✓
Sensitive			✓
Fine hair		✓	✓
Coarse hair	✓		
Short hair	✓		

Whatever the product or method, it is important that you follow the manufacturer's instructions. Wax can overheat and there is a risk of burning the client. The heating must be controlled carefully. There are safety precautions for heating and testing the temperature.

It is essential that the wax is heated well in advance of the client arriving. If the salon uses a range of products for different hair types or areas of the body then these must all be ready for a use. The client will be annoyed if they arrive for a waxing service to find they have to wait for the wax to heat to the correct temperature, or for it to cool to the working temperature because the heater has been left on.

Preparing the client

Prepare the client by asking them to remove the necessary items of clothing and jewellery in the area being treated. Clients should be allowed privacy and be provided with a gown or towels. Positioning the client for a bikini line wax is not very elegant, so you must ensure that some means of cover is available to maintain the client's modesty throughout the treatment. Disposable paper underwear is available for client use for bikini and intimate waxing.

Equipment checklist

Use the boxes to check you have all your equipment ready. To perform a waxing treatment you will need:

✔ large steady trolley
✔ couch prepared with plastic sheeting and/ or disposable bed paper
✔ heater with sufficient wax for the treatment (roller heads prepared)
✔ surgical spirit or anti-bacterial lotion or pre-wax lotion
✔ cotton wool
✔ tissues
✔ talc
✔ tweezers placed in disinfectant
✔ scissors placed in disinfectant
✔ fabric or paper strips for warm wax
✔ container for used wax strips and other waste
✔ disposable wooden spatulas for waxing
✔ after-wax lotion or other antiseptic soothing lotion.

Protect the client's clothing using disposable bed paper or old, clean towels (wax can spoil towels by getting into the fibres). Sugaring paste is easily removed by laundering the towels.

If you are applying wax to the face, protect the client's hair by placing disposable paper or a towel loosely over the hair. For the eyebrows the eyes should be protected with damp cotton pads and petroleum jelly used on the hairs of the brows that are to remain intact.

Prepare the skin by wiping over the area to be treated with cotton wool soaked in surgical spirit or specialist pre-wax lotion. This acts as an antiseptic to cleanse the skin and remove oil and perspiration from the surface of the skin. This must be done thoroughly or the wax will not stick to the hairs. An antiseptic solution may be used, especially if the client is allergic to surgical spirit, but it will leave the skin damp. The skin must be allowed to dry before applying the talc or blotted with a clean tissue. Surgical spirit evaporates immediately, making it a more efficient product to use.

Cleansing the skin should be done against the direction of hair growth to help to lift the hairs from the skin. At the same time, you can take note of the direction of the hair growth and plan how the wax needs to be applied. This is particularly important under the arm, where the hair can grow in a swirl (see page 232).

Talc-free powder is applied thinly to the area using a pad of cotton wool, against the hair growth to ensure that the hairs are lifted from the skin.

Excessively long hair should be trimmed with scissors or clippers but take care not to take the hairs too short for the waxing service to be successful. Leave at least 1.5cm of hair growth.

 Health and safety

Talcum powder is a known carcinogen similar to asbestos and has been linked to lung and ovarian cancer. For these reasons it should be avoided during waxing and other beauty therapy services.

Preparing yourself to give a waxing treatment

Use the boxes to check your personal appearance.

- ❏ A high standard of personal hygiene is presented.
- ❏ Fresh breath, free from cigarette or food odours.
- ❏ Clean, pressed work wear.
- ❏ Clean, low-heeled, enclosed shoes.
- ❏ Arms and hands free from jewellery (except wedding ring).
- ❏ Any earrings or necklaces are discreet.
- ❏ Make-up is discreet and expertly applied.
- ❏ Long hair is tied neatly away from the face and shoulders.
- ❏ Nails are short, smooth, clean and free of nail enamel.
- ❏ Tights, or socks with trousers, are worn.
- ❏ Cuts or open wounds are covered with a clean dressing.
- ❏ Hands washed immediately before and after treatments.
- ❏ Calm and professional manner is maintained at all times.

Outcome 3: Remove unwanted hair

Remember...

Double-dipping is a NO! Use a fresh spatula for each client and where blood is involved NEVER put your spatula back into the wax. Protect yourself and your clients. It may work out more expensive in the long run but it has its benefits too. You can tell your clients that you don't double-dip and the reasons why you don't – it will be a big selling point.

Treatment methods for different areas of the body

The majority of hair removal is from the legs and bikini line on the female client, and chest, back and arms on the male client, although the client may request removal of unwanted hair from other areas of the body. This will require a different approach to application and support for the skin.

Leg waxing can be a full leg or up to and including the knee, which is termed half leg. The toes and tops of the feet may also be included. A system of application must be used to avoid missing areas and to work cleanly and efficiently.

Procedures for waxing

Procedure for warm wax (application to half leg)

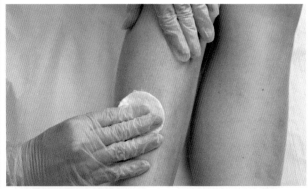

1. Cleanse the area with pre-wax or antibacterial lotion.

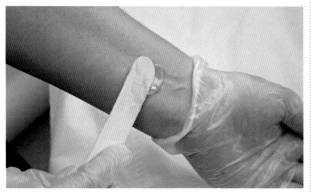

2. Check the consistency of the wax before testing it on yourself. Remember, if the wax is allowed to overheat, it will become very runny and will give off fumes. If the wax is the correct consistency, test the wax on the inside of your wrist.

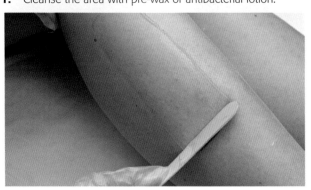

3. If it feels comfortable, you can apply a small amount on the client's skin in the area to be treated.

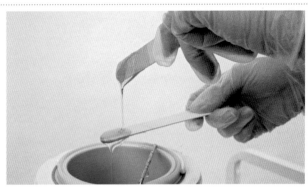

4. Take sufficient wax onto the spatula, then scrape one side of the spatula on the bar of the heater and hold flat as you move towards the client to avoid drips

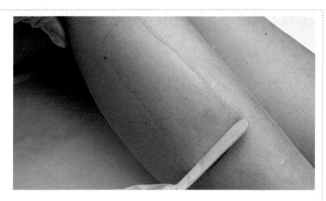

5. Apply the wax with the edge of the spatula following the hair growth to give a thin layer. The skin must be supported with the free hand to prevent overstretching the skin.

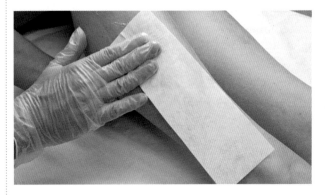

6. Take a fabric or paper strip and press it over the wax. Smooth over firmly with the hand to ensure the wax is sticking to the strip.

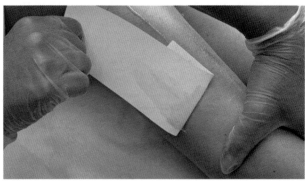

7. Grip the bottom edge of the strip with the fingers and pull the strip away very quickly against the direction of the hair growth. Stretch and support the skin with the other hand. The strip must be removed parallel to the skin. If the strip is lifted up away from the surface of the skin, it will cause bruising and considerable discomfort to the client. The same strip can be used again until it becomes thick with the wax and does not remove the hair. It can be disposed of by folding the wax sides together and placing in a suitable container away from the client.

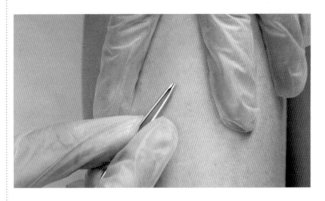

8. Any remaining hairs can be removed with sterile tweezers.

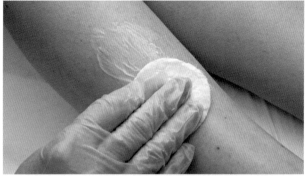

9. Repeat over the area, working methodically and cleanly. When complete apply after-care lotion.

Roller systems

1. Prepare the heater.
2. Remove the cap from a wax cartridge and attach the roller head. Screw down firmly but not too tightly, so the head can be removed easily.
3. Place the cartridge in the heater.
4. When sufficiently heated (check manufacturer's instructions) hold the cartridge upside down to allow the wax to flow to the roller head. The cartridge is now ready to use.
5. Hold the cartridge by its sides at about 45 degrees and roll *in the direction* of the hair growth.
6. Apply *one thin layer* of wax.
7. Return the cartridge to the heater to keep it at the working temperature.
8. Select a wax strip and place on the wax. Press firmly.
9. Pull the strip off *against the direction* of hair growth.
10. The routine and aftercare procedure is the same as for warm wax.

Techniques for other areas of the body that can be waxed (arms and abdomen) but that are not included in the range for this unit are described below.

Activity

Compare the heating systems for each of the depilatory wax treatments. Give advantages and disadvantages of each. If your salon does not use all the waxing methods, visit your local wholesaler and look at the equipment for waxing.

Arms

The arm can be rested on the couch with the client sitting on a stool. The hair may be quite long and often fine in texture with a tendency to break off if a good technique is not used. Take care also to apply and remove in small sections as the arm is smaller than a leg and because the hair growth isoften across the curvature of the arm, bruising can easily occur without care.

Abdomen

The area is soft as there is no supporting bony tissue underneath, making stretching the skin more difficult. The client should lie flat on the couch to stretch the area as much as possible. Work in small areas at a time following the hair growth which is often angled towards the centre of the body making application awkward.

Bikini line

The skin in this area is very delicate and prone to bruising if too much pressure is applied. It is possible that there will be some bleeding from the follicles. This is because strong coarse hairs have deeper follicles. Make sure that any cuts or open wounds on your hands are covered by waterproof dressing and disposable gloves are worn to protect yourself from infection. Wipe the area to be treated with cotton wool and antiseptic. Dispose of the soiled cotton wool in a closed waste bin. Correct positioning of the client and the use of disposable paper underwear will assist in the easy removal of the hair.

Procedure for warm wax (bikini line)

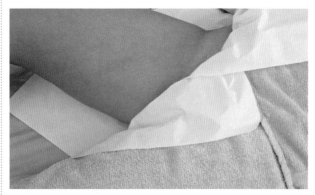

1. Prepare and protect the client to maintain modesty.

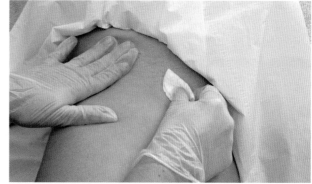

2. Cleanse the area.

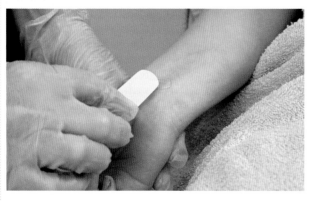

3. Test the temperature on a hair-free area nearby.

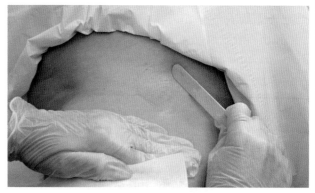

4. Apply the wax in the direction of hair growth.

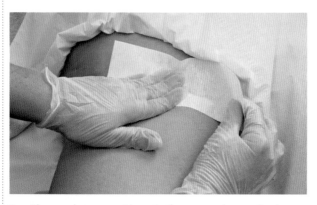

5. Place a clean wax strip onto the wax and press firmly.

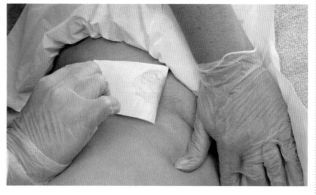

6. Remove the wax strip against the hair growth using the stretching technique.

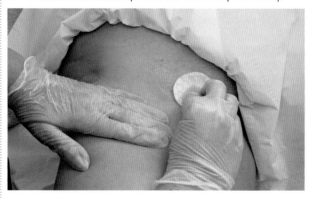

7. Apply waxing aftercare lotion with cotton pad.

Underarm using warm wax

Positioning of the client to reveal the whole of the axilla is important.
Take special note of the circular direction of hair growth. Follow
normal preparation and aftercare procedures.

Procedure for warm wax (underarm)

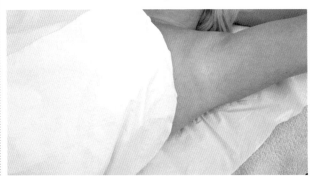

1. Prepare and protect the client to maintain modesty.

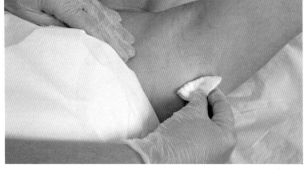

2. Cleanse the area.

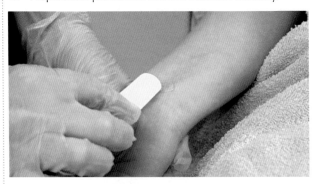

3. Test the temperature on a hair-free area nearby.

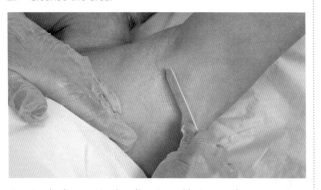

4. Apply the wax in the direction of hair growth.

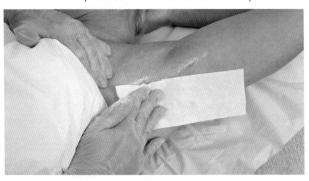

5. Place a clean wax strip onto the wax and press firmly.

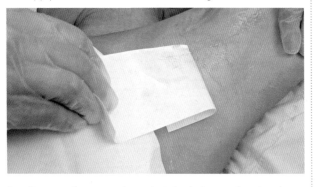

6. Remove the wax strip against the hair growth using the stretching technique.

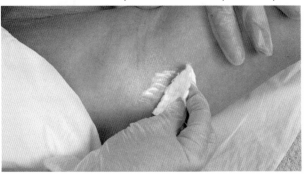

7. Apply waxing aftercare lotion with cotton pad.

243

Eyebrows

The areas to be treated are small, so application must be very careful and neat. Hair to remain in the eyebrow should be protected with petroleum jelly and cotton pads placed over the eyes and eyelashes.

Procedure for eyebrow wax

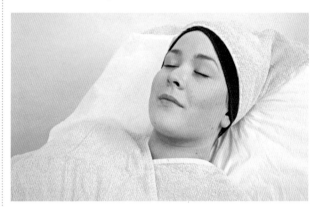

1. Prepare and protect the client.

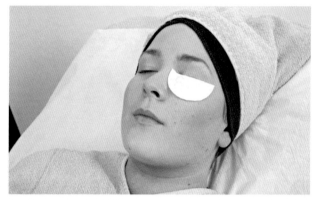

2. Cover the eye with shaped cotton pad.

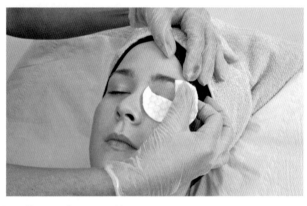

3. Cleanse the area with pre-wax

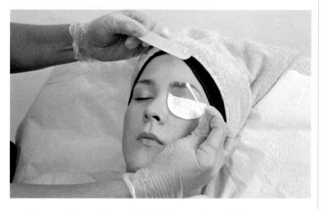

4. Protect the eyebrow hair with petroleum jelly.

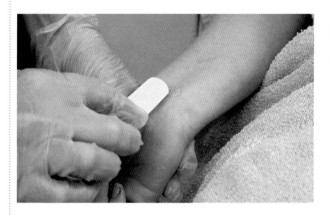

5. Test the temperature on a hair-free area nearby.

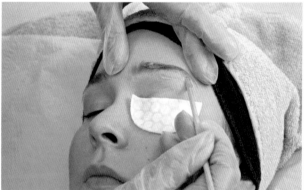

6. Apply the wax in the direction of hair growth with an orange stick or small spatula.

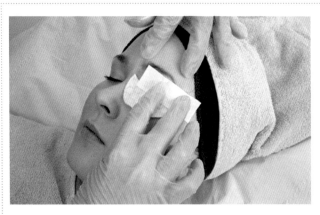

7. Place a clean wax strip onto the wax and press firmly.

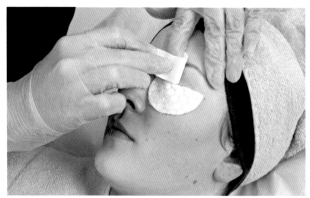

8. Remove the wax strip against the hair growth using the stretching technique.

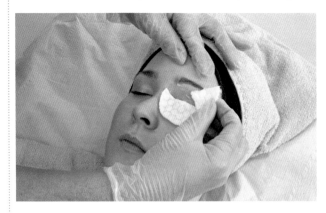

9. Apply waxing aftercare lotion with cotton pad.

Lip and chin

When working on the face, the client's clothing and hair must be protected.

Procedure for lip wax

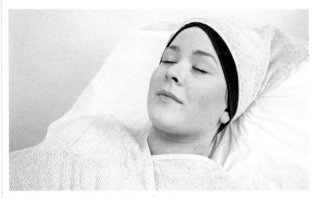

1. Prepare and protect the client.

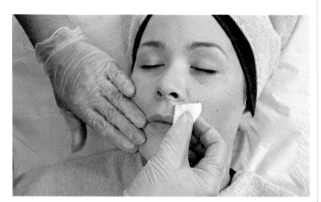

2. Cleanse the area with pre-wax.

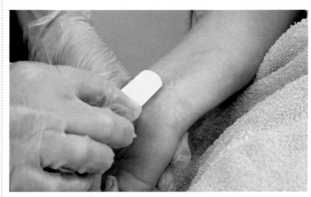

3. Test the temperature on a hair-free area nearby.

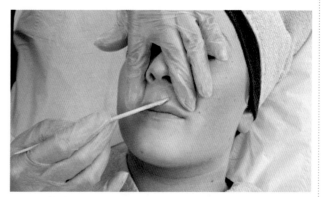

4. Apply the wax in the direction of hair growth with an orange stick or small spatula.

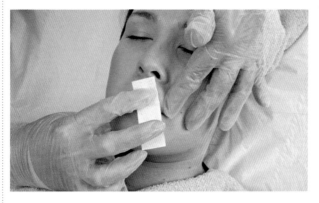

5. Place a clean wax strip onto the wax and press firmly.

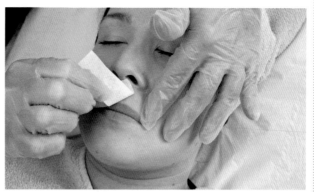

6. Remove the wax strip against the hair growth using the stretching technique.

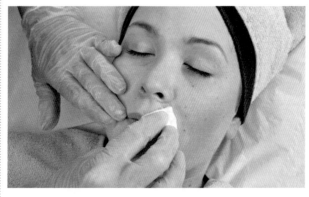

7. Apply waxing aftercare lotion with cotton pad.

Procedure for hot or hard wax application to the bikini line

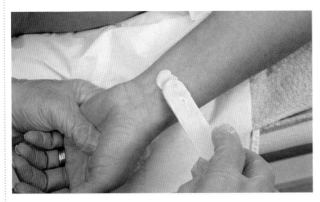
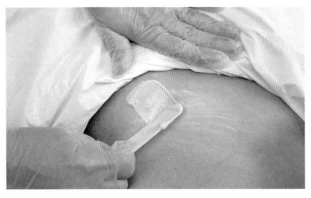

1. Check the consistency of the wax before testing the temperature on your wrist. If it feels comfortable to you, apply to a small area on the client's skin and check the client's tolerance to the temperature.

2. The correct consistency of wax will enable you to control it on the spatula and apply it to the skin without dripping. Twisting the spatula will control the wax as you take it from the heater across to the client. It is essential that the heater is close by on the side of the couch nearest to your working hand. Do not reach across the client for the wax as it may drip wax on their clothing.

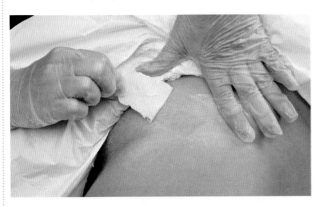

6. To remove the wax, flick up the bottom edge of the strip, gripping the wax between the thumb and first finger, with the free hand supporting the skin. A long, quick movement is needed to remove the wax. It can be very uncomfortable for the client if it is done slowly. If the hand is lifted, pulling the skin upwards, this can cause bruising, particularly in the bikini line area.

7. Pressure should be applied to the area immediately after the wax has been removed. This helps to reduce the stinging effect.

8. As you gain confidence in applying the wax, you will be able to apply a few strips at a time, removing them in sequence. This will ensure that the treatment is carried out in a commercially acceptable time of 30 minutes for a half-leg wax, with an additional 15 minutes for other areas. Variations to timings depend on how coarse and dense the hair growth is.

3. Apply the wax *against the direction of hair growth* in organised strips, following the growth pattern of the area. Ensure that the application of the wax is systematic. A disorganised approach will take longer and possibly leave hairs behind.

4. Hot wax needs to be applied thickly. This is done by building up one or two layers quickly, before the wax on the skin is allowed to cool. The aim is to achieve thick edges that can be picked up between the fingers, making it easy to pull off. If the application is too thin, the wax will cool rapidly and be too brittle to remove.

5. The wax can be gently pressed onto the skin as it cools to increase its attachment to the hairs.

9. Any small pieces of wax that remain on the skin can be lifted by using a piece of wax that has just been removed and pressing it onto the area. If small pieces of wax are particularly stubborn, dip your finger into the hot wax pan and press it onto the wax remaining on the skin. This should lift it off.

10. If the wax has cooled and become difficult to remove, another layer of hot wax from the heater will soften it sufficiently to aid its removal.

11. Check that the area is free of hair. Odd hairs can be tweezed, but large areas will need a further application of wax. This must be done carefully because the skin will be more sensitive and warm from the previous application. Check with the client that the temperature of the wax is still comfortable before continuing.

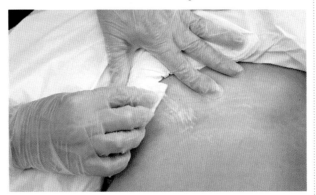

12. Apply after-wax lotion either by using gentle effleurage massage or by soothing onto the area with the fingers, or with cotton wool for bikini and underarm areas.

Procedure for hot wax (underarm)

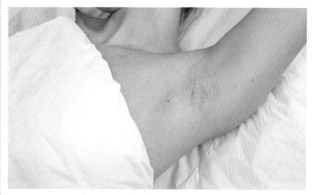

1. Prepare and protect the client to maintain modesty.

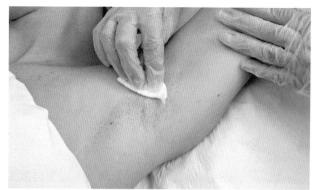

2. Cleanse the area with pre-wax.

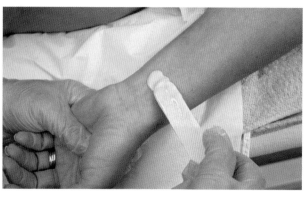

3. Test the temperature on a hair-free area nearby

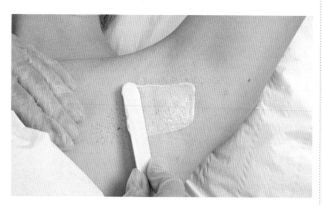

4. Apply the wax *against the direction* of hair growth.

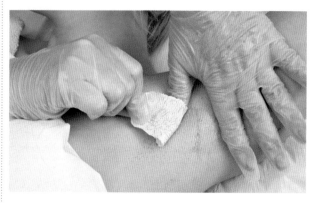

5. Remove the wax strip *against the direction* of hair growth, using the stretching technique

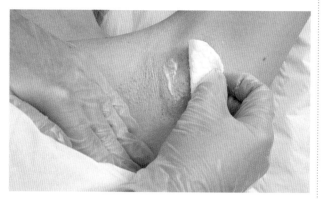

6. Apply waxing aftercare lotion with cotton pad.

It is important to develop a technique that leaves the minimum of wax on the skin. This is achieved by:

- applying several layers of wax
- leaving thick edges to enable the wax to be lifted off in one go
- not allowing the wax to overheat and become brittle
- removing the wax when it is still slightly warm and pliable
- working in a methodical way over the area.

Hand sugaring

1. Test the temperature of the paste.
2. Take sufficient paste from the container with a spatula and transfer to the fingers. It should be warm and pliable so work the paste into a ball.
3. Spread the ball of paste on the skin using the middle three fingers, in a strip about 6 inches long. When working on the legs or using less paste in smaller areas, spread to a more appropriate length.
4. The skin must be supported using the free hand (clean hand) by stretching the skin.
5. Remove the paste by flicking back along its length without lifting upwards. The process is repeated quickly on the next area until the paste loses its pliability, becomes full of hair, and cools.

Strip sugaring

There are many similarities between warm waxing and strip sugaring techniques.

1. Apply the strip sugar very thinly using a spatula in the direction of the hair growth.
2. Remove the strip sugar with fabric strips against the hair growth, supporting the skin below the strip to be removed.
3. Press the hand on the treated area immediately to help reduce any stinging.

Outcome 4: Provide aftercare advice

Completing treatment and aftercare

It is important to examine the area you have treated to ensure that all the hairs have been removed and that the treatment meets the client's expectations. If there are just odd hairs that have been missed, these can be removed with tweezers. Larger areas may need a second application, so do not apply any lotions to the skin until you are absolutely sure that the client is satisfied.

Reasons for poor hair removal

If the wax has not removed the hair successfully it could be that:

- the hair was too short for the wax to grip properly
- the area was not cleansed sufficiently to remove body lotion or natural oil on the skin

☆ Hints and tips

The art of sugaring relies on the ability of the practitioner to adjust the paste to the correct consistency. This depends on several factors, such as the heat of the hands, the temperature in the room, and the climate. Adding a few drops of water using a water spray can alter the consistency dramatically. Selecting a soft paste in winter or a hard paste in the summer can help to achieve the right consistency.

Activity

Look closely at the hairs you remove on the waxing strip and you will see some with a silver sheath. Others have no sheath, but a black blob on the end. Some hairs may appear straight across at the root as if they have been cut. They may have broken off. The way the root looks can identify the stage in the life cycle of each hair. Identify the stages of hair growth in a used wax strip.

- warm wax was applied too thickly or allowed to build up on the paper strip
- the wax was applied incorrectly without following the natural hair growth.

Following treatment you should wipe over the area with after-wax lotion, depending on the product used:

- Oil-soluble wax will require an oil-based after-wax lotion to remove any traces left on the skin.
- Water-soluble wax or sugar paste can be removed by wiping over the area with wet cotton wool and drying with disposable paper or tissue. Some practitioners recommend that sterile water is used (boiled water) to avoid any infection entering the open follicles.
- Hot wax tends to leave small particles of wax behind, so the area will require thorough cleansing with suitable after-wax lotion or surgical spirit, although this can be very harsh on the skin. A soothing cream is massaged onto the skin to cool and moisturise.

This is an ideal opportunity to explain home care advice.

Aftercare advice

Explain the skin reaction to the client and that it will take several hours for the skin to return to normal. During the 24 hours after treatment they must avoid the following:

- wearing tight clothing over the treated area, especially the bikini line, as bruising may occur
- perfumed products and chemical-based products such as deodorant which will increase skin sensitivity, prolonging the skin's reaction to waxing
- wearing make-up over the area treated on the face as the follicles are left open and there is an increased risk of infection. A tinted medicated lotion can be used such as that produced for use after epilation
- sunbathing or sunbed treatments because the skin has been sensitised by the waxing treatment and the effects of exposure to UV light will be increased
- heat treatment such as sauna, steam or taking a hot bath will also sensitise the skin and prolong the reaction to the waxing treatment. A warm shower is recommended, followed by an application of soothing after-wax lotion
- swimming also prolongs the skin's reaction to waxing
- exercise will increase the body temperature and the risk of friction from exercise clothing can exacerbate the skin's reaction to waxing
- touching the area increases the risk of infection.

The client should be encouraged to continue to use aftercare lotion for a few days after the waxing service and moisturise the skin regularly between treatments to keep the skin soft and supple and avoid excessive dryness. They should be discouraged from using harsh chemical-based products due to the risk of increased skin sensitivity associated with such products.

As the hair growth begins to reappear after two or three weeks, the client should be encouraged to exfoliate the area with an abrasive mitt or loofah to avoid the formation of in-growing hairs. They should be informed of the recommended interval between waxing treatment to avoid over treating the area. This interval will vary for each client but is usually between four and six weeks.

Clearing away after waxing

Waxing can be a very messy treatment because of the sticky products used. Ensure that the area and equipment are cleaned immediately.

Disposable collars are available for some heaters, preventing unsightly drips during treatment and making cleaning easier.

The wax heater must be thoroughly cleaned before returning to the store cupboard. Special cleaning products are supplied by the manufacturer, or use warm water for water-soluble wax, oil for oil-soluble wax and surgical spirit for hot wax. Sugar paste is water soluble and easily removed with hot water.

The roller system is particularly easy to clear away as heads are disposable or may be cleaned with after-wax cleaner.

Wax heaters should be covered by a lid when cool to ensure that the wax is not left exposed to the air. The warm conditions in the salon can encourage growth of micro-organisms and dust can settle on the surface of the wax. Ensure that there is sufficient wax in the heater before storing. This will save valuable time when you come to reheat the wax for the next client. Wax strips must be disposed of in the waste bin. The plastic bed cover and trolley should be wiped over.

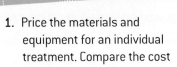

Activity

1. Price the materials and equipment for an individual treatment. Compare the cost of using:

    ❖ roller system

    ❖ warm waxing products

    ❖ hot wax.

    Remember the time for treatment will be influenced by the amount of hair, the client's tolerance to the treatment and areas to be treated.

2. List the advantages and disadvantages of each method.

Want to know more?

The Code of Practice for Waxing is available from the HABIA website www.habia.org.uk

Intimate waxing

Intimate waxing for both male and female clients should not be undertaken without experience of normal waxing and maturity as there is a risk that the client may take your actions when performing the treatment as sexual assault. There is no legal requirement for age to perform or receive this treatment but guidelines as described in Chapter 1 should be followed for those under the age of 18 years of age.

Intimate waxing services include:

- Brazilian, where the hair is removed from the pubic area leaving a strip an inch or so wide over the pubic mound.
- Hollywood, where the hair is removed from the pubic and anal areas entirely leaving no hair.
- Bollywood, where the hair is removed entirely as in the Hollywood but where the pubic mound is decorated with henna.

- Playboy, the hair is removed from the pubic and anal area but leaving a thin strip over the pubic mound
- Las Vegas, where the hair is removed as in Brazilian or Playboy but with the addition of diamante decoration.
- Californian, where the hair is removed as in Brazilian and then the remaining strip of hair is coloured.

Other intimate waxing services include shaping of the pubic hair such as in a heart shape and then coloured and for males there is the removal of hair from the lower back, penis, scrotum, buttocks and anal areas.

For more information on courses and their content visit the HABIA website www.habia.org.uk

Test yourself

Test yourself on hair removal by answering the following questions:

1. State two safety measures that must be carried out before applying wax to a client's skin.
2. Give two contraindications to waxing the:
   a) eyebrows
   b) top lip
   c) legs.
3. What PPE should be worn for waxing?
4. What is erythema?
5. What are the ingredients of warm and hot wax?
6. What are the alternative methods of hair removal to waxing?
7. What are the advantages of sugaring over other waxing methods?
8. Explain why shaving leaves the area feeling bristly.

Are you ready for assessment?

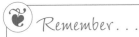 Remember...

Practice makes perfect! The more opportunities you have to complete waxing treatments the more confident you will be when it comes to being observed by your assessor.

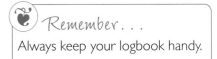 Remember...

Always keep your logbook handy.

The following checklist will help you to be fully prepared for your practical assessment

The range of clients/treatments you must cover:

- Use various consultation techniques.
- Consider your actions if contra indications are present.
- Carry out the range of waxing treatments.
- Use both hot and warm wax.
- Use all the work techniques.
- Provide aftercare advice.

1. Practical observation

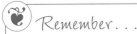 Remember...

Your assessor will observe your performance on at least four occasions, each involving a different client.

Your assessor will look at how you:

- prepare the treatment area for waxing
- consult with the client and prepare a record card
- remove unwanted hair using methods of application following manufacturers' instructions
- carry out various waxing treatments in a commercially acceptable time
- check with the client that the hair removal meets her expectations
- provide aftercare advice
- demonstrate professional practice throughout the service
- carry out all waxing treatments with regard to health and safety, including minimising waste and disposing of used wax correctly.

2. Knowledge and understanding

What you must know:

- Organisational and legal requirements.
- How to work safely and effectively when providing waxing services.
- Why minors require consent from a parent or guardian before being offered waxing services.
- Consult, plan and prepare for treatment with clients.
- Contraindications and contra-actions.
- Anatomy and physiology of hair growth.
- Waxing treatments for different areas.
- Aftercare advice.

To ensure that you have the necessary knowledge and understanding of waxing services your assessor will:

- ask you questions before, during and after carrying out the waxing service
- ensure that you have completed project work and written exercises relating to the unit
- check that you have recorded in a log/diary treatments you have carried out with signed record cards showing that you have completed four waxing services on different clients competently
- check that you have covered the range in your candidate logbook
- require you to take a test.

Remember...

Simulation is not a valid means of assessment for waxing service.

Remember...

Comply with the Personal Protective Equipment at Work Regulations 1992 when carrying out any waxing service.

Chapter 11
Unit N2: Provide manicure services

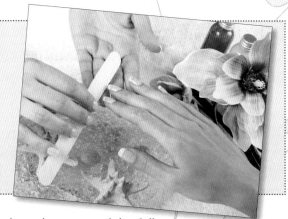

Learning objectives

This chapter covers the skills and knowledge required for Unit N2 'Provide manicure services'.

> There are four learning outcomes for Unit N2 and they are:
> 1 Maintain safe and effective methods of working when providing manicure services.
> 2 Consult, plan and prepare for the manicure service.
> 3 Carry out manicure services.
> 4 Provide aftercare advice.

You will need to be competent in all of these outcomes in manicure services, qualify for insurance and perform the treatment on members of the public.

Evidence requirements

Your assessor will need to observe you perform this service successfully on at least three occasions on three different clients. On each occasion you must perform a different hand and nail treatment from the range. You must:

1 Demonstrate the use of consultation techniques:
 - questioning
 - visual
 - manual
 - reference to client records.

2 Take at least one of the following necessary actions:
 - encourage the client to seek medical advice
 - explain why the treatment cannot be carried out
 - modify the treatment.

3 Demonstrate the use of four of these five hand and nail treatments:
 - paraffin wax
 - hand masks
 - thermal mitts
 - exfoliators
 - warm oil.

4 Demonstrate the application of all these types of nail finish:
 - dark colour
 - French
 - buffed.

5 Provide treatment advice:
 - suitable aftercare tools and products and their use
 - avoidance of activities that may cause damage or contra-actions
 - recommended time intervals between nail services
 - home care routines.

Introduction

Manicure treatments are popular services offered in beauty therapy clinics, hairdressing salons and nail salons. The treatment can be offered as part of other salon services, such as hair styling, or as part of a make-over in the beauty clinic and as preparation for nail extensions. The word 'manicure' comes from the Latin *manus* (hand) and *curo* (care). It involves treatment to improve the appearance of the hands and nails.

The unit is a mandatory unit in the Level 2 Beauty Therapy General and Nail Services routes. It is worth six credits.

The purpose of manicure is to:

- recognise common nail disorders and disease
- provide a range of treatments to improve the hands and nails
- offer the client advice on nail care.

The manicure will include:

- filing and shaping the nails
- cuticle treatment
- hand massage
- nail polish application or buffing
- special conditioning treatments.

The manicurist has an ideal opportunity during the treatment to advise the client on other services available in the salon and to build a relationship with the client through conversation.

Meet the professionals

"To some clients, manicure services are luxuries and for others their manicure is a routine treatment carried out once a month. Make your treatments different and interesting, even for a basic manicure. Offer something that your local competitor salons don't, like acupressure point massage or hand reflexology. You will need to stand out from your competitors. It may be a basic beauty treatment but don't treat it like one.

Keep up to date with the newest colours and treatments.

These services also offer the perfect opportunity for you to slip-up! In conversation, the client doesn't need to know how late you stayed up last night at a friend's party or that you haven't had chance for lunch yet, or that you've had an argument with the boss. This just tells your client you are tired, hungry or unhappy and are probably not doing your job properly and it may make them feel uncomfortable. Clients want to feel relaxed and comfortable.

When doing a manicure, make sure to ask your client what shape and length they would like their nails. Remember your job is to advise; it's not your decision."

Jacqui Bostock

To enable professionally informed and effective manicure treatments it is essential to have a thorough understanding of the relevant anatomy and physiology: the structure of the nail unit and the process of nail growth, the bones, muscles and blood circulation of the hand and lower arm, and the structure and function of the skin. This is covered in Chapter 19.

Outcome 1: Maintain safe and effective methods of working when providing manicure services

Health and safety is of the utmost importance in the salon and must be a priority when preparing and carrying out any treatment.

When assessing possible hazards, consideration must be given to:

- the salon environment/work area
- hygiene procedures
- equipment and manicure products
- the necessary competence to carry out the manicure safely.

Manicure service times

The table below provides the commercially accepted service times for manicure services.

▽ Manicure treatment times

Service description	Service Time
Manicure with polish including French	45 mins
Manicure without polish (buffed)	30 mins
File and paint	15 mins
Specialist hand and nail treatment	60 mins

Preparing the work area for manicure services

With the increase in popularity of nail services, special nail salons have emerged. Here, the environment and equipment are designed to allow easy positioning, good light and ventilation, for both client and therapist.

However, a manicurist in a beauty or hairdressing salon may be called upon to treat a client in a whole range of different situations: for example, while the client is having other treatment. It may be necessary to move to the client. This will require portable equipment: perhaps a movable manicure station (which is a specially designed stool with a small table and drawers to hold products and implements), or if this is not available, a lightweight stool with products and implements carried in a basket.

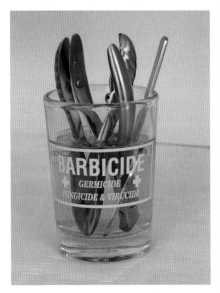

△ Disinfectant jar for small implements

Wherever you work, you should ensure that:

- the manicure table and stool are at the right height
- seating for the client and yourself is comfortable – you should not be in a slouching position as this can cause back problems over a period of time and will certainly cause fatigue
- there is good lighting – it may be necessary to have a magnifying lamp or an angle-poise lamp to hand
- there is adequate ventilation – when working with solvents it is essential that fresh air circulates freely (this applies particularly when using artificial nail systems)
- manicure implements are clean, sterilised and arranged in a neat and organised manner with everything to hand
- hot and cold water with liquid soap is available for washing your hands before and after treatment, for soaking the client's nails to soften the cuticle and to remove preparations from the nails during treatment
- there are plenty of clean towels available
- you have on hand disposable materials such as paper towels, tissues and cotton wool.

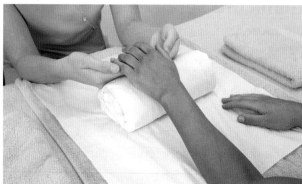
△ Manicurist ready for the client

Client care and preparation

Before examining your client's hands, ensure that you have washed your hands thoroughly using a medicated hand wash to minimise the risk of cross-infection.

Check that your client is seated comfortably. Ask them to remove rings, bracelets or watches, which may hinder the manicure treatment, particularly the massage, when hand cream could become lodged between the settings of the jewellery. The client's jewellery should be kept nearby, in a small bowl on the trolley.

The client's cuffs or sleeves need to be turned back and protected with tissue during massaging to avoid clothing coming into contact with manicure products, which may stain.

Remember...

Before carrying out a manicure treatment you must consult the client to establish any contraindications to the treatment and complete a record card.

Preparation and hygiene procedures

Preparation and hygiene procedures are an essential part of all salon treatments. Manicure implements are small items that can be cleaned and sterilised quite easily and some are disposable.

The trolley must be wiped over with disinfectant. Sterilised and clean tools need to be set out in an orderly way that allows the manicurist to have them close at hand while working. A mobile therapist may use a manicure basket with sterilised tools. A covered bin should be available for waste. This bin must be emptied into the main bin after every treatment.

Products, tools and equipment

Tools used in manicure

- **Nail scissors** – small curved blades for reducing the length of the nails.

- **Cuticle knife** – small, flat blade used to remove cuticle attached to the nail plate.

- **Cuticle nippers** – small scissor-like implement with a spring action to allow small movements, used to remove excessive, torn or damaged cuticle. Metal tools can be washed in hot soapy water and sterilised using an autoclave. They can be stored in an ultraviolet cabinet after sterilising. During the manicure small implements should be placed in disinfectant on the trolley.

- **Buffer** – an implement that has a surface covered with chamois leather. It is applied to the surface of the nail plate to create a shine using brisk rubbing (friction). The chamois leather cover can be wiped over after use with a damp cloth. The leather covers need changing regularly.

These items of small equipment can be washed in hot, soapy water and placed in the ultraviolet cabinet for storage. The orange stick, spatula and hoof stick (see below) should be placed in disinfectant during the manicure.

Emery boards are made of fibrous board and therefore cannot be washed. After use, they should be offered to the client for use at home, or thrown away.

- **Hoof stick** – orange-wood or plastic handle with a rubber end shaped like a hoof, used to gently push back the cuticle from the nail plate.

- **Nail brush** – used to remove all manicure products before the application of nail polish. May also be required to clean dirty nails.

- **Orange stick** – disposable wooden implement with one end slanted and the other pointed, which should be tipped with cotton wool before use. The orange stick has a number of uses: to push back softened cuticles with the cotton wool-tipped end soaked in cuticle remover, to clean under the nails with pointed end tipped with cotton wool and to remove small amounts of preparations from their pots.

- **Spatula** – used to dispense products from pots (may be made from plastic material that can be washed easily or wood that can be disposed of after use).

- **Emery board** – has a dark side that is coarse and used when nails are to be shortened in length or for filing very strong nails. The light side is fine and used for shaping and smoothing the nails. The emery board should be flexible and 12–15cm long to allow for good technique during filing of the nails.

> ⭐ **Hints and tips**
> Disposable emery boards used on the client can be included in the price of the manicure and given to them to take home Ensure that you explain to the client how to file correctly.

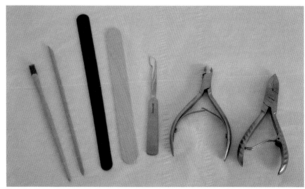

△ Tools and equipment

Products used in manicure

- **Polish remover** – a solvent that removes nail polish. Amyl acetate (acetone) is the main ingredient in polish remover, with a small amount of oil added to help counteract the drying effect of the solvent on the nail plate.

- **Cuticle massage cream** – an emollient used to soften and nourish the cuticles. Lanolin or mineral oils are the main ingredients. Cuticle oil may be used in the same way.

- **Cuticle remover** – an alkaline substance that softens the keratin in the skin, allowing the cuticle to be lifted from the nail plate and the excess to be removed using cuticle nippers. Potassium hydroxide is the main ingredient, which is caustic and very drying if not removed thoroughly after use. Cuticle remover also has a mild bleaching effect and can help to remove stains from the nails.

- **Buffing paste** – a mild abrasive substance which, when combined with the friction action of the buffer, gives the surface of the nail plate a shine. Pumice, silica or stannic oxide (jeweller's paste) is the main ingredient. Buffing may help increase the circulation to the nail bed and smooth ridges in the nail.

- **Hand cream/lotion** – an emollient that softens and nourishes the skin and assists in the application of massage. **Lanolin**, **glycerol** or **vegetable oils** are used to make an oil-in-water emulsion. Other ingredients include perfume, colour and some natural products such as aloe vera.

- **Nail polish: base coat, top coat and coloured varnish** – a plastic film that is applied to the nail plate. Nitro cellulose and a solvent such as amyl acetate are the main ingredients of all nail polish, with various pigments added to give colour, or guanine from fish scales to give a pearlised effect. Good quality nail polish lasts longer, has a good range of colours, has a good consistency for smooth application and dries quickly and evenly.

- **Base coat** – provides a smooth base for the application of coloured varnish, protects the nails from staining (which can be caused by colour pigment), minimises ridges or irregularities in the nail plate and prolongs the life of polish by helping to prevent chipping and peeling

- **Ridge filler** – provides a more even surface for polish when nails have ridges.

- **Top coat** – is used to give extra gloss to cream polish and to help the polish last longer by providing a hard surface, protecting the polish from chipping. Top coat is not required for crystalline polish as it can dull the finish.

- **Nail polish thinners** – a solvent used to thin down nail polish that has become thick. Ethyl acetate is the active ingredient. Thinner should be used very sparingly or the polish will not harden. Nail polish remover should not be used for thinning polish, as the oil it contains will prevent the polish from drying.

Activity

Familiarise yourself with the products used in your salon by reading the labels and manufacturer's instructions, checking the colour, consistency and smell. Make a list of the products needed for a manicure. Visit a department store or chemist shop and look at the range and cost of products and tools available to your clients.

Remember . . .

Product use and storage should be considered under the Control of Substanes Hazardous to Health (COSHH) Regulations.

- **Nail strengtheners** – a product that hardens the keratin in the nail plate. Formaldehyde is the active ingredient in these products. Nail strengtheners may also be an acrylic substance that provides a hard plastic coating to reinforce the nail.

- **Nail white pencil** – a pencil that is dipped in water before applying to the underside of the free edge. This whitens stained nails. Titanium dioxide is the main ingredient.

- **Quick-dry spray** – the cooling effect can speed up the drying process. A solvent aerosol spray that evaporates quickly is the basis of this product, although polish that is allowed to dry naturally is longer lasting.

- **Exfoliants** – a product containing abrasive ingredients that remove dead skin and help to smooth calluses and rough skin.

- **Masks** – can be adapted from facial products to draw impurities from the skin, soften and improve the texture of the skin.

- **Nail glue** – for minor repairs to the nail plate.

- **Nail bleach** – to whiten stained nails caused by smoking, gardening, hair colouring and so on. Contains citric acid or dilute hydrogen peroxide plus glycerine to combat the drying nature of the product.

 Health and safety

COSHH regulations are outlined in Chapter 3. Refer to the chart on page 72 and look at the substances listed. Identify those used in manicure and note the hazards in each case.

General items of equipment and materials

As well as specialist items of equipment and products, you will need some more general equipment and materials. These include:

- **Surgical spirit** – for cleansing the client's hands prior to examination and for disinfecting implements and surfaces.

- **Jar of sanitising fluid** – to hold manicure implements during treatment. This may be disinfectant or sterilising fluid.

- **Cotton wool** – for wiping over the hands when soaked in surgical spirit, for removing nail polish when soaked in polish remover and for tipping the orange stick before use.

- **Tissues** – for wrapping sterilised implements before use, for covering the towelling cushion during polish application to protect the towel.

- **Towels** – for drying client's hands during the manicure. A towel should be placed on your lap during the manicure for drying your hands.

- **Finger bowl** – filled with hot water and a few drops of medicated liquid soap for soaking the client's hands. (The water will have cooled sufficiently by the time the client needs to immerse their hand.)

- **Small receptacle** – for holding the client's jewellery safely while carrying out the manicure.

- **Waste bin** – for immediate disposal of waste materials. A small pedal bin is ideal.

- **Thermal mitts** – used to keep hands warm during paraffin wax or mask treatments.

Hygiene procedures and care of small implements and manicure products

Small tools

Always buy good quality, stainless steel manicure tools such as cuticle knife and nippers, so that they can be sterilised without damaging them. Make sure blades are sharp, particularly the cuticle nippers, to avoid tearing the cuticle. Ensure that the hinge moves easily on the nippers to allow for the correct technique to be used.

All small tools must be sterilised after use, whether by autoclave or chemical sterilising fluid, as appropriate (Refer to Chapter 1 for sterilising methods.) The items should be dried and stored either in an ultraviolet cabinet or placed in a tool roll.

Manicure products

Many manicure products contain solvents and must, therefore, be handled and stored carefully.

It is important that tops are secure on bottles to avoid evaporation of polish remover and solvent in polish.

Particular attention is needed when caring for nail polish. Your clients will want to choose from a wide range of polish colours. Polish should be of excellent quality to ensure a long-lasting finish and good colours.

The necks of the bottles should be wiped after use to ensure that the top fits securely. When the solvent is allowed to evaporate from the polish, it becomes thick and impossible to apply to the nails. Polish will require thorough shaking before use to ensure a smooth, well-mixed colour. Small beads are placed in some bottles to ensure thorough mixing. Slight separation may occur in cream polishes, leaving a white deposit. Sometimes, dark layers form at the top of the bottle.

Coloured polish needs to be stored upright, away from direct sunlight to avoid fading of colour pigments and thickening of the polish due to changes in temperature.

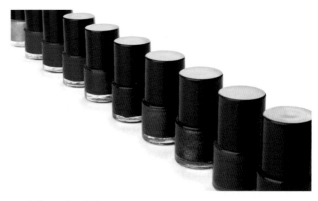

△ Coloured polishes

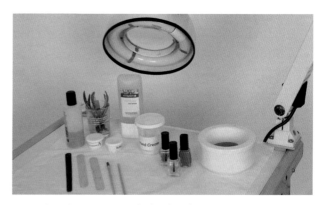

△ Workstation set up ready for the client

<u>Equipment checklist</u>

Check the following as you prepare for your first manicure.

✔ Is the manicure area warm and tidy?

✔ Have all used towels been placed in the laundry and replaced with clean ones?

✔ Has the waste bin been emptied?

✔ Have all used implements been replaced with clean sterilised implements?

✔ Do you have clean towels available?

Do you have the following tools?

✔ cuticle nippers

✔ cuticle knife

✔ emery board

✔ buffer

✔ orange stick

✔ hoof stick

✔ spatula

Prepare the following materials and equipment:

✔ manicure trolley/table

✔ stool

✔ water bowl

✔ waste bin

✔ cotton wool

✔ tissues

✔ manicure cushion

✔ jar of sterilising fluid

✔ bowl for client's jewellery.

Prepare the following products:

✔ polish remover

✔ cuticle massage cream

✔ nail scissors

✔ buffing paste

✔ hand cream

✔ base coat

✔ coloured polishes

✔ top coat

✔ ridge filler

✔ nail strengthener

✔ nail-whitening pencil

✔ quick-dry spray

✔ French manicure products

✔ mask

✔ exfoliant

✔ nail bleach.

Outcome 2: Consult, plan and prepare for the manicure service

Client consultation

Client consultation is a very important part of the service offered to a client. A client's health and circumstances can change between visits to the salon so it is important to go through the consultation process every time, whether the client comes for treatment regularly or for a one-off visit. You may also need to check progress against the treatment plan.

Remember...

The therapist should ask the age of the client, as you are required by law to gain parental or legal guardian's consent in writing before treating a minor (someone under the age of 18 in England and under 17 in Scotland). The parent or legal guardian should also accompany any minor under the age of 16 for the duration of the service. Treating a child of pre-school age is legal with parental or guardian consent, though some salons refuse to do this as part of their own salon policy.

Full details of client consultation and treatment planning can be found in Chapter 1.

Assessing the client's hands and nails for manicure

First, clean the client's hands with cotton wool and surgical spirit or another antiseptic. This will give you the opportunity to make a quick assessment of the overall condition. To enable thorough examination of the hands and nails it is necessary to remove nail polish.

Procedure for removing nail polish

1. Apply nail polish remover to a pad of cotton wool. Hold between your first two fingers to avoid the remover smudging polish on your own nails.
2. Press the pad firmly onto each nail and hold, allowing the solvent to dissolve the cellulose coating on the nail.
3. Slide off the nail in one movement, from the base of the nail to the free edge, to prevent the colour spreading over the finger.
4. It is sometimes necessary to repeat with fresh cotton wool or to apply remover to a cotton wool-tipped orange stick and remove colour from around the cuticle.
5. Ensure that there are no traces of old polish, as this will spoil the benefits of treatment and the final appearance of the nails.
6. Remember to place the top on the bottle of remover to prevent the solvent evaporating.

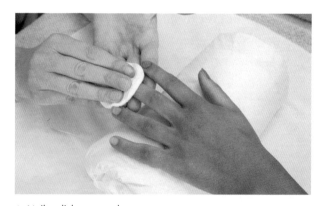

△ Nail polish removal

Assessing the client for treatment involves:

- **Visual** – looking at the hands.
- **Manual** – touching the skin.
- **Question** – questioning the client.
- **Reference** to the client's record card.

Look and touch (visual and manual assessment)

To carry out this stage, go through the following steps.

1. **The palms and backs of both hands**. Check for rough, dry patches of skin, any cuts or broken skin, sore areas where rings are worn and the colour of the skin, whether red and chapped or with pigmentation marks. The age of the client will affect the texture of the skin. Conditions such as arthritis may be apparent.

2. **The cuticles**. The condition of the cuticles will immediately indicate whether the client cares for their hands and has regular manicures. Overgrown, torn and dry cuticles will require extra work during the manicure and home care advice to the client. 'Hangnail' is a common condition where the cuticle becomes attached to the nail plate and it tears as the nail grows. Infection may then result. Biting the nails and cuticle also leads to thick and torn cuticle.

3. **The nails**. Inspect each nail for:

   - **shape** – there are many different shapes. A distorted shape may be the result of nail damage

   - **colour** – slightly pink colour is an indication of healthy nails. Discoloured nails may be the result of smoking or may be caused by the client's work, as in the case of the hairdresser who works with products that colour the hair. (As hair and nails are of a similar composition, that is, made from the protein keratin, the nails will take on the colour in a similar way to the hair)

   - **strength** – nails will vary in thickness, flexibility and strength. This is normally a hereditary factor, although illness, disease and certain drugs can severely affect the condition of the nails. Flaking and splits in the nail should be noted.

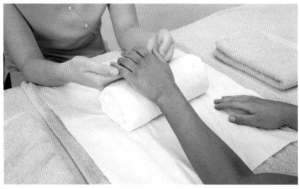

△ Therapist examining the client's hands and nails

Question

Discussion with the client at this stage is a very important part of the consultation. If there are any conditions of the hands or nails that are contraindications and prevent you continuing with treatment, this must be handled in a very sensitive manner. You must explain to the client about the condition and why it prevents you from continuing. This will usually be because there is infection present that could be passed on to other clients or therapists. It may be appropriate to explain to the client how the condition could spread and infect others in the home or workplace.

Gentle questioning will enable you to establish the lifestyle, habits and occupation of the client, all of which will have an effect on the condition of the client's hands and nails. You may be able to establish the cause of a condition by asking an open question, for example:

- How do you look after your hands and nails at home?
- What kind of work do you do with your hands?

By talking to the client you will be able to identify their needs and expectations. You will be required to advise them on what the treatment entails, what the end result will be and whether you can meet their expectations. It is important that you discuss the cost of the manicure, especially if you have agreed to include a special treatment that will take extra time.

The questioning phase of the client assessment will allow you to build a rapport with the client and help them to relax, making the treatment more enjoyable.

All the details that you discover through looking, touching and questioning should be included in the treatment plan or record card. The client record card is an important source of information and should state previous treatments the client has had.

Healthy nails

Healthy nails appear firm but flexible, smooth and slightly pink in colour. The surrounding cuticle should be unbroken, flexible and should not be stuck to the nail plate.

A healthy nail will grow approximately 3–4mm per month and will grow faster in the summer, and in children and pregnant women. Children and pregnant women have higher levels of nutrients in the blood. In summer, due to the increase in temperature, blood circulation is faster. Toenails grow more slowly than fingernails (about 2 mm per month) and are often thicker and harder.

To produce healthy nails the vitamins A, B complex and D are needed together with the minerals calcium and iron.

The effects of nail care treatment

Nail treatments such as buffing and massage benefit nail growth by increasing the blood supply to the nail bed. In doing so, more nutrients and oxygen are available for the cells to grow and divide. This means that the nails will grow more quickly and will be stronger.

The effects of illness

Systemic illness, in other words disease or illness affecting a system of the body, can influence the rate of growth and appearance of the nails, as well as the skin and hair. Poor health or poor diet can cause the nails to be brittle or very soft, flexible, pale, discoloured or blue in colour and the cuticles to be dry, split and hardened.

Activity

1. Look closely at your hands. Write down what you see. Follow the look, touch, question routine. Now repeat the exercise on a colleague.

2. Observe as many different nail shapes as you can by looking at friends and family, and magazine photographs.

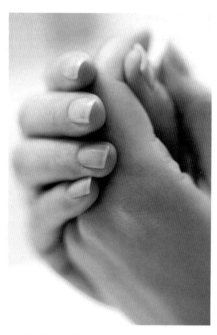

△ Healthy nails

Physical damage

Nail bed – a knock or blow that is hard enough to damage the nail bed will appear as a bruise under the nail. The blood vessels in the nail bed break, allowing blood to flow out under the nail plate. After a short time the blood vessels mend, leaving some under the nail plate. This dries, sticks to the underside and grows up with the nail plate until it reaches the free edge, where it can be removed.

Matrix – damage to the matrix can result in temporary loss of the nail or permanent damage to the nail plate. When the matrix is damaged by a severe knock or blow, some of the cells die. This results in a temporary halt in the production of the nail plate and nail bed. This can appear as a ridge in the nail or, if a lot of the matrix is damaged, the loss of the nail plate.

The dead cells need to be replaced and are made by the matrix itself. When fully healed, the matrix will begin to make the nail plate and nail bed again. If, however, the damage is severe enough, the matrix may not heal completely, leaving scar tissue. This will appear as a permanent condition in the nail, such as a vertical ridge or split.

Chemical damage

Strong chemicals such as detergents or even nail polish remover, with continuous use, will cause the nail and cuticle to dry out. The nail may appear brittle, discoloured (usually yellow), flaky and ridged. The cuticle will be dry, white in colour and inflexible.

Inflammation and infection

The signs of infection and inflammation are:

- redness
- swelling
- pain
- pus (which will be present where there is a bacterial infection).

Contraindications and restrictions to manicure

The presence of some conditions may contraindicate manicure services. A therapist must be able to recognise conditions in order to make the decision as to whether a nail care treatment can be performed or not but must not diagnose the condition. For more details regarding the correct course of action when the client presents with a contraindication that prevents treatment refer to Chapter 1.

Conditions that prevent treatment

Ringworm (tinea)

Not a 'worm', as the name implies, but a fungal infection that can affect the nails and the skin. The disease is highly contagious and is often passed on by pets. Do not touch the area but tell the client to see a doctor as soon as possible for suitable treatment.

Ringworm of the nail appears as yellow or white streaks in the nail plate that invade from the free-edge towards the cuticle, and subsequent thickening of the nail plate. Sometimes the top layers of the nail will peel off. This is also known as onychomycosis.

Ringworm of the skin appears as red, slightly raised patches of skin in the shape of a ring.

On the feet, ringworm appears as white, moist flaking or peeling between and around the bottom of the toes. Commonly called 'athlete's foot', it often spreads to the toenails.

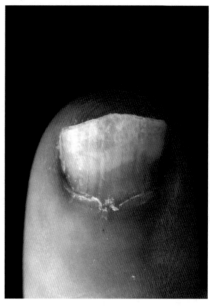

△ Ringworm of the nail

Whitlow (paronychia/onychia)

Whitlow is a contagious infection of the skin, cuticle or nail bed, caused by bacteria entering through an opening in the skin or cuticle. It can be caused by poor nail-care techniques, but is usually associated with nail biting. Severe cases may need lancing or a course of antibiotics, so advise the client to see a doctor. Look out for red, painful swelling of the skin surrounding the nail plate and the formation of pus.

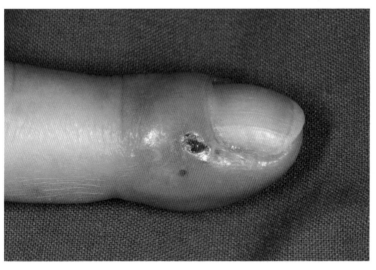

△ Whitlow

Warts

These are contagious conditions caused by a virus affecting the skin of the hands or feet. If minor, they can be covered with a dressing and the treatment can be performed. If severe, the client should see a doctor. Look out for raised, horny lumps with black dots on the hands. Horny lumps in an uneven shape, which grow into the skin on the soles of the feet, are characteristic of verrucae.

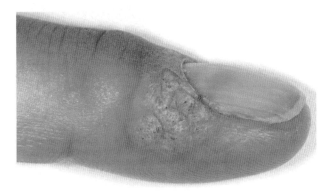

△ Warts

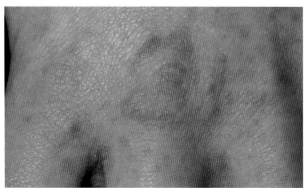

△ Scabies

Scabies or itch mite

Scabies is caused by an animal parasite that burrows under the epidermis and invades the hair follicles. Greyish lines appear on the skin where the mite burrows. Secondary infection may be present due to scratching, which may break the skin.

Eczema

An inflamed, red skin condition that is not contagious. It can be stress-related or the result of an allergy, for example to metals, chemicals, drugs, clothing or products such as nail enamels. If severe or with open sores, treatment would be contraindicated. When mild, however, treatment can go ahead, avoiding the area affected. Look out for redness, swelling, blisters, flaking, weeping and cracking of the skin. Eczema can give rise to changes in the nail, such as ridging and pitting.

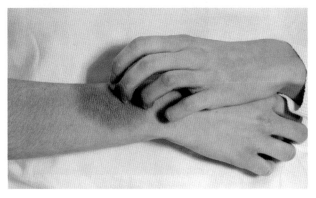

△ Severe eczema

Psoriasis

An inherited condition aggravated by stress, drugs or infection. Commonly found on knees and elbows, it is not infectious so treatment can go ahead but with restrictions. Some nail care treatments such as massage are thought to benefit the condition. However, if severe or open, cracked or infected, it is wise to refer the client to a doctor. Look out for:

- severe ridging or pitting of the nail plate
- raised, red, silvery, scaly skin patches, circular or oval in shape and with a definite outline.

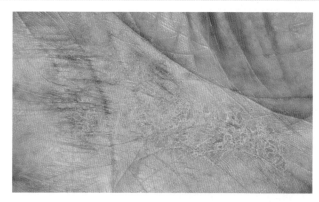

△ Psoriasis

Dermatitis

This is a term used to describe any inflammation of the skin caused by an external irritant, such as detergent. Care should be taken not to expose the skin to known allergens such as chemicals, metals and perfumed products.

Onycholysis (nail separation)

This term means the separation of the nail plate from the nail bed and is caused by systemic illness, injury, nail disease or infection, circulatory problems or as a reaction to drugs. It appears as a white area of the nail plate, due to loss of blood supply. In severe cases, the nail plate may be shed completely or discoloration can be caused by the invasion of fungi or bacteria. If severe and of systemic or disease origin, the client should be referred to a doctor. Mild cases restrict treatment, in that the affected finger should be omitted.

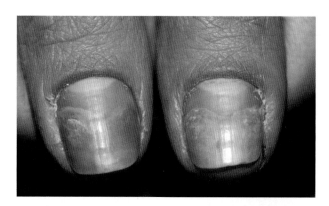

△ Nail separation

Conditions restricting treatment

Bruised nail

Bruised nails are caused by injury to the nail bed with bleeding under the nail plate. There is dark purple, blue or black discoloration. Perform nail treatments with care, avoiding pressure. If severe, involving the loss of the nail plate, refer the client to a doctor. If mild, miss out the finger from the treatment. Cover with a dark-coloured enamel if appropriate.

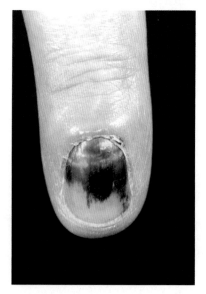

△ Bruised nail

Bitten nails

A nervous or stress-induced habit where the free edge, nail plate and cuticle are bitten to leave the hyponychium exposed and the cuticle and surrounding skin ragged. Nail biting is the most common cause of deformed nails, due to the increased risk of infection. Regular manicures help to overcome the habit. File the nails smooth to remove ragged edges, remove ragged cuticle, skin and hangnails with nippers to avoid temptation to bite. Give attention to the cuticles, massaging with oil or cream.

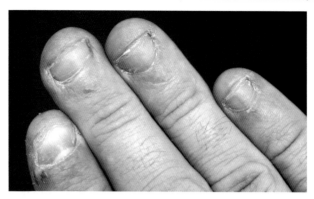

△ Bitten nails (onychophagy)

Arthritis

There are two types of arthritis. Osteoarthritis is the wear and tear of the joints and is more common in elderly clients. Rheumatoid arthritis is a disease that can affect a person at any age. Both involve painful joints, especially with movement or weight bearing. The conditions are usually treated with drugs and physiotherapy but, when under control, gentle massage can mobilise joints and eliminate fluid, reducing swelling. Such treatment should only be performed by a therapist who has medical permission to do so. The heat associated with paraffin wax treatments can give relief to painful joints.

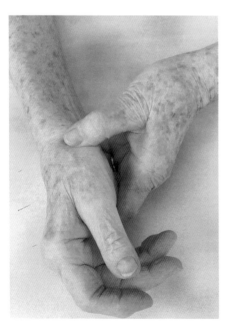

△ Arthritis

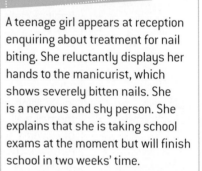

Activity

A teenage girl appears at reception enquiring about treatment for nail biting. She reluctantly displays her hands to the manicurist, which shows severely bitten nails. She is a nervous and shy person. She explains that she is taking school exams at the moment but will finish school in two weeks' time.

1. Write a short paragraph on how you think this client is feeling as she discusses her hands and nails with the manicurist, how the manicurist should handle the client and what advice should be given.

2. Write out a treatment plan for this client to include both salon and home care.

Open cuts/wounds

Where they can be avoided, open wounds can easily be covered with a waterproof dressing and the manicure carried out with special care in the affected areas.

The following table details common nail conditions, their causes and the relevant treatment required.

▽ Common nail conditions

Condition	Cause	Appearance	Treatment
Corrugations	Vertical ridging can be hereditary or caused by damage of the matrix with age, indicating dryness. Horizontal ridging, if present on all nails, indicates a temporary pause in growth due to illness such as measles. If present on only one nail, the ridge may be caused by damage to the matrix	Vertical or horizontal ridges or furrows within the nail plate	If the ridging is mild, use a buffer with paste polish to buff the nails. Horizontal ridges grow out with the nail but avoid the use of coloured enamel as it is difficult to remove from the ridge. If ridging is severe treat the nails as fragile
Hangnails (agnail)	Dryness, cutting off too much cuticle during manicure or the habit of chewing the cuticle	Hard, dry pieces of nail or cuticle found in the nail groove or wall. If pulled, can result in torn tissue and subsequent infection	Remove with cuticle nippers and suggest regular oil manicures, which will prevent dryness
Split nails (onychorrhexis)	Injury, filing too deeply into the nail wall, excessive use of solvents such as polish remover, chemicals and alkalines, pressure on very long nails	Horizontal or vertical splits in the free edge, often at flesh level or below. When associated with dry hair and skin, this suggests a glandular disorder	Perform oil manicures, use only the fine side of an emery board when filing, regular application of cuticle cream
Brittle nails (fragilitas unguium)	Dehydration of the nail plate due to overexposure to alkaline, solvents or immersion in water. Can also indicate an iron deficiency or anaemia	Yellow, thick nails that break easily	Avoid contact with chemicals and solvents, wear rubber gloves and use barrier creams. Regular use of cuticle cream, especially at night
Flaky nails	Dryness caused by exposure to solvents and chemicals	The layers of the nail plate separate at the free edge	Protect with gloves and barrier creams, regular use of nail strengtheners and cuticle cream, especially at night. File with the fine side of an emery board only and use polish remover containing oil
Blue nails	Poor circulation due to cold, hereditary defect or heart disorder	Nail plate appears blue instead of pink. May cause ridging of the nail plate	Increase the circulation by exercise, massage and buffing
White spots (leuconychia)	Mild injury to the base of the nail	White spots within the nail plate. The injury causes the layers of the nail to separate	They grow out with the nail plate. Avoid pressure on the cuticle during nail care treatment. Use the fine side of an emery board when present in the free edge

Pterygium	It is either hereditary or can be caused by infrequent attention to the cuticle	The cuticle is often dry, split and grows in excess. Grows forward and sticks to the nail plate	Careful use of the cuticle knife and nippers to remove the excess cuticle. Oil manicures help prevent the regrowth from sticking back down to the nail and keeps the cuticle soft and supple
Excess perspiration (hyperhydrosis)	Can be hereditary or caused by a stressful situation	Hands or feet are damp and clammy. Feet can suffer from odour as they are confined within shoes	Sweaty hands are difficult to treat, but a light dusting of talc can help. Feet should be washed daily and antiperspirant sprays or powders can be used. Socks or tights should always be worn and synthetic shoes should be avoided. Leather allows air to circulate around the feet. Special odour-absorbing inner soles can also be used in footwear
Hard skin (callous)	Thickening of the stratum corneum due to pressure and/or overuse, formed to protect the affected area	Dry, hard, inflexible overgrowth over a bony prominence such as knuckles or joints	Mild calluses may be removed by softening in warm water before the use of a corn plane or chemical hard skin remover. Severe calluses need referral to a chiropodist

Outcome 3: Carry out manicure services

Quick guide

The following is a quick reference guide to the work method for manicure service with polish. More detail for each stage is explained later in this chapter.

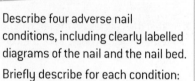

Activity

Describe four adverse nail conditions, including clearly labelled diagrams of the nail and the nail bed.

Briefly describe for each condition:

1. Salon treatment.
2. Home care advice.

Procedure for a manicure

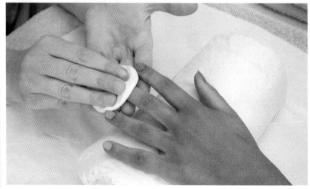

1. Remove nail polish from the nails of both hands (if you have not already done so).

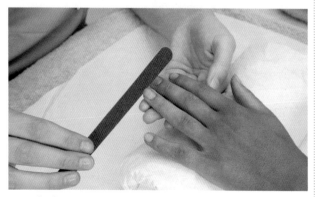

2. File the nails of the left hand (buffing can be done at this stage without buffing paste).

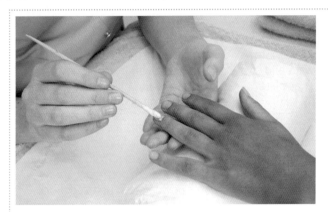

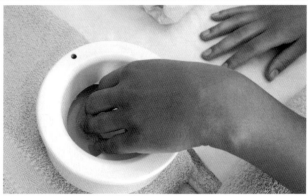

3. Apply cuticle massage cream.

5. Repeat steps 2, 3 and 4 on the right hand.

4. Soak left hand in the bowl of warm soapy water.

6. Dry left hand thoroughly.

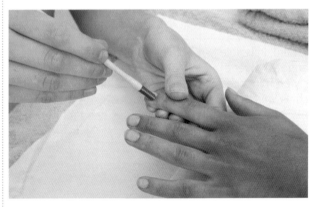

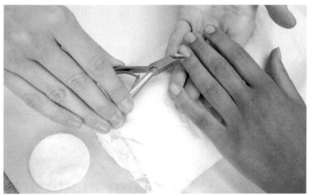

7. Treat the cuticles on the left hand by applying cuticle remover and pushing back the cuticle using a cotton wool-tipped orange stick and a hoof stick.

8. Remove excess cuticle using the cuticle knife and cuticle nippers.

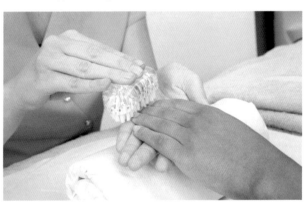

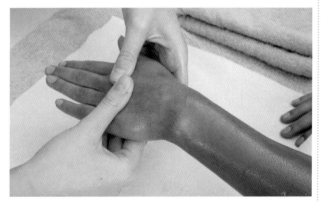

9. Use a nail brush to rinse off cuticle remover and any loose cuticle. Dry thoroughly.

10. Repeat steps 6 and 8–10 on the right hand.

11. Massage both hands.

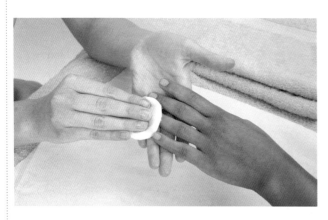

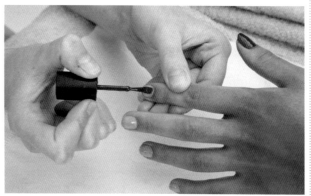

12. Remove grease from the nail plate on each hand using cotton wool and polish remover.

13. Apply nail polish. Base coat (once), coloured nail polish (twice) and top coat (once). If the client does not want nail polish, buff to a shine.

14. Allow polish to dry completely. The use of a light dryer speeds up the drying process.

15. Offer the client home care advice.

Shaping the nails

This is an important stage in the manicure.

You must discuss the shaping of the nails with the client. They may have very strong views. A number of factors must be taken into consideration at this stage:

- Natural shape and length of the nails – are they equal in length and shape?
- Condition and strength of the nails – are the nails brittle, dry, thin?
- Client's occupation – for example, a nurse cannot have long, pointed nails.
- Shape of the hands and fingers.

Natural nail shapes vary in individuals. Men tend to have square nails, due to them being kept short. Women tend to have varying shapes, from oval to fan shape.

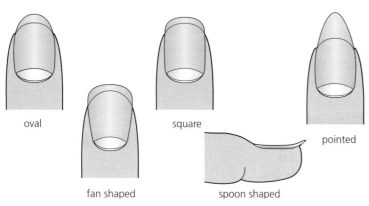

oval

fan shaped

square

spoon shaped

pointed

△ Nail shapes

- **Oval** – the ideal shape as it provides strength to the free edge.
- **Square** – a square shape is popular, particularly for long nails and nail extensions.
- **Pointed** – pointed nails require shaping down the nail wall, which causes weakness to the free edge. Splits low down in the nail plate can result.

Shortening the nails

It may be necessary to shorten excessively long nails. This is best carried out using sharp, curved nail scissors, followed by filing. The nail should be supported while cutting the free edge. Very hard brittle nails may require soaking first. The nail should be cut straight across, leaving it slightly longer than the finished shape to allow for filing.

Filing

Good quality emery boards should always be used. They should be flexible and 12–15 cm in length to allow long sweeping movements when filing. The emery board will have different degrees of coarseness on either side, indicated by the colour. The dark side is coarse and used for reducing the length of strong nails. The finer side is light in colour and used for shaping and smoothing the nails. The emery board should be held with the thumb on the side not being used, and four fingers on the other side.

Nails must be filed in one direction, from the side to the centre of the nail tip, making an oval-shaped movement. Long, swift, rhythmical strokes should be used. Sawing movements backwards and forwards can damage the nail, particularly if soft and delicate. Filing into the corners of the nail by pulling back the nail wall will weaken the nails and reduce the support to the free edge. This can lead to splits and breaking of the nail.

Bevelling is used after shaping to remove any fragments left after filing and to smooth the edge of the nail. The fine side is used to file under the free edge at 45 degrees.

Cuticle treatment

The aim of treatment is to reduce dryness and overgrown, torn or thick cuticles, leaving the skin around the nail neat, soft and pliable.

Cuticle work is an important stage in the manicure. The treatment required will depend on the condition of the client's hands and nails. It may take several manicures to treat poor cuticles. This should be indicated in the treatment plan.

1. Cuticle massage cream is applied first. A small amount is dispensed from the pot using an orange stick and applied to each nail. The cream is massaged into the nail and surrounding skin. The emollient makes the cuticles pliable and the massage increases circulation to the tips of the fingers.

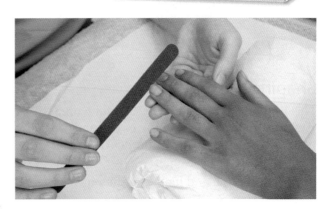

△ Filing the nails

2. Soaking the fingers in hot soapy water will soften the skin and clean the nails.

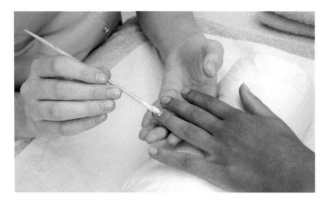

△ Applying cuticle cream to cuticles

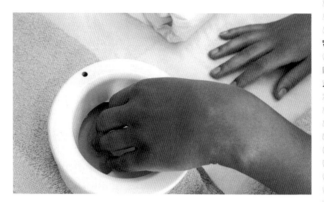

△ Soaking the cuticles

3. Cuticle remover and using implements is the next stage of cuticle treatment. One of the major problems with untreated cuticles is that the skin adheres to the nail plate and becomes torn, causing **hangnails**. Cuticle remover and the use of special implements to remove cuticle from the nail plate and trim excess cuticle from around the nail is advised.

    After soaking, the hands are dried and cuticle remover applied all around the cuticle and under the free edge. Cuticle remover is slightly caustic and breaks down the keratin in the skin, allowing the cuticle to be loosened. It may also remove stains from the nail plate.

4. A cotton wool-tipped orange stick is used to push back the cuticle. A rolling movement is used, starting halfway up the nail plate and rolling down to the base of the nail, gently pushing back the cuticle.

The **hoof stick**, with its flexible rubber hoof-shaped end, is designed to continue the lifting of cuticle from the nail plate. Use flat circular movements, working downwards to the base of the nail plate.

The **cuticle knife** should be held flat in the palm of the hand, not upright between the thumb and first finger, like a pencil. The flat position ensures that the length of the blade is used to gently 'scrape' any cuticle sticking to the nail plate, rather than using the point of the blade, which could damage the matrix.

> **Key term**
>
> **Hangnail** – torn cuticles which may become infected.

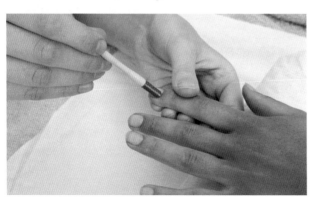

△ Pushing back the cuticles

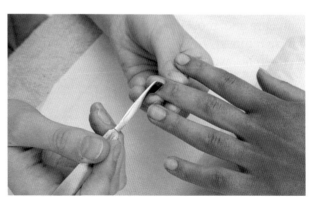

△ Using the cuticle knife

The blade is stroked in one direction and must be moistened throughout by dipping into the manicure bowl. This prevents scratching the nail plate.

Cleansing under the free edge to remove dirt and dead skin is carried out using a cotton wool-tipped orange stick, taking care not to dig into the nail bed.

The **cuticle nippers** are used to cut away excess cuticle that has been lifted from the nail plate during treatment or to cut off torn cuticle. Some clients require careful cuticle work at this stage, due to overgrown or damaged cuticles, often caused by the client biting the nails and surrounding skin or lack of care to hands and nails, resulting in dryness and damage.

Hangnail may be treated but special care must be taken not to pull at the skin, causing discomfort to the client.

Excessive forward-growing cuticle (**pterygium**) can be improved with very careful use of cuticle nippers. Cuticle nippers must be handled very carefully to avoid tearing the cuticle and causing bleeding, which could lead to infection.

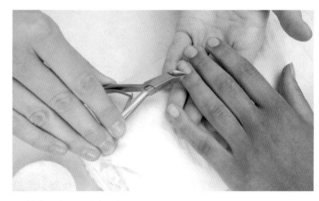

△ Using the cuticle nippers

The aim is to remove the cuticle in one piece so that there are no rough edges. This requires the correct holding of the nippers. They should be held in the palm of the hand with the spring between the handles moving smoothly. The nipper blades are then used in a 'nibbling' action in a curved movement around the base of the nail.

The pulling of the cuticle as a result of poor technique or blunt blades will cause tearing and possibly bleeding. Trimming the cuticles too closely will weaken the protection they give to the nail and increase the risk of infection.

It is not always necessary to use the cuticle nippers. For example, clients who have regular manicures and a good home-care routine may not accumulate a great deal of cuticle.

The nail brush is used next. Dipping the treated nails into the water in the manicure bowl, the brush is used from the cuticle to the free edge. This gets rid of the dead skin removed during this stage of the manicure and, most importantly, flushes away the cuticle remover, which is slightly caustic and, if left on the nails, would be very drying.

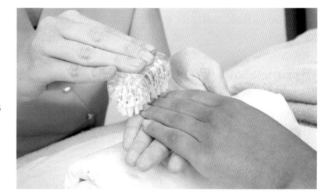

△ Using a nail brush

Inspect the nails and cuticles

When cuticle work is completed on both hands it is important to evaluate the treatment so far. Visual checks should include:

- Are the nails an even shape?
- Does the free edge of the nails need bevelling to remove any layers or snags left after filing?

- Do the nails require any repair?
- Are the cuticles pushed back exposing as much **lunula** as possible?

Any minor shaping or correcting rough or torn cuticle should be done at this stage.

You should gain the client's approval and refer to the treatment plan. Any future treatment to improve the nails and surrounding skin should be discussed and recorded in the treatment plan.

Key term

Lunula – the visible portion of the matrix commonly known as the 'half moon'; it is not present on all nails.

Hand massage

Hand massage can be the most enjoyable part of the manicure for the client. Allow sufficient time to ensure that the massage is not rushed and that the full benefits are experienced.

The benefits of hand massage are to:

- relax the client
- increase the blood and lymphatic flow to the hands and fingers
- improve mobility in the joints
- spread the hand cream or lotion
- nourish and smooth the surface of the skin by helping the skin to absorb the hand cream
- remove loose skin cells.

Massage of the hand uses:

- **Effleurage** – stroking movements using the palm of the hand or the tips of the fingers. These are flowing movements using very little pressure to spread the hand cream. Effleurage is applied in an upward movement, towards the heart and should start and end the routine.
- **Petrissage** – kneading movements, which are deeper and more stimulating. Petrissage increases lymphatic and blood flow and can aid the removal of loose skin cells.
- **Rotations** – circular movements applied to the joints to aid mobility.

Where possible, the client should remove long-sleeved items of clothing or roll sleeves up to the elbow to prevent hand cream from soiling clothing. The client may wish to have massage to the lower arm and hand, in which case short sleeves are essential. Otherwise the massage is applied to the wrist and hand only.

The massage routine

The area to be massaged can be divided into:

- the forearm and elbow
- the wrist
- the palm and back of the hand
- the digits (fingers).

If your routine follows a set pattern it will make it easier for you to remember and ensure a thorough massage.

Procedure for massage

This is a quick reference guide to help you while you are practising. The full procedure follows.

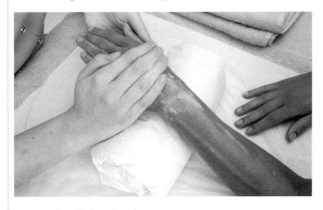

1. Apply sufficient hand cream.

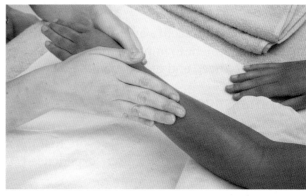

2. Effleurage from fingers to the elbow 3–4 times.

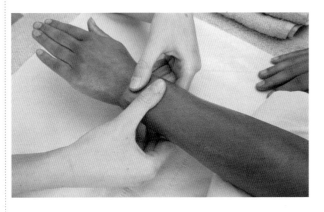

3. Petrissage (thumb-kneading) to the forearm (wrist to elbow) 3 times.

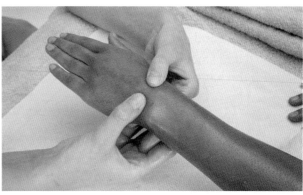

4. Thumb-knead the top of wrist (carpels).

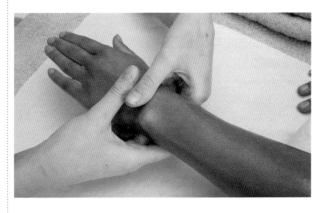

5. Criss-cross thumb movements (friction) to the underside of wrist.

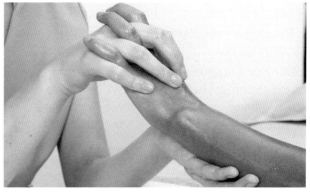

6. Rotate wrist 3 times in each direction.

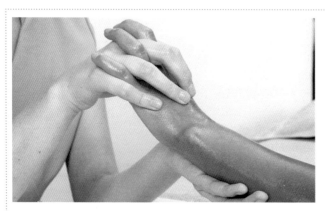

7. Flex wrist 2–3 times.

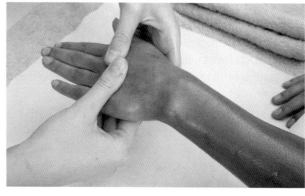

8. Thumb-knead the back of the hand.

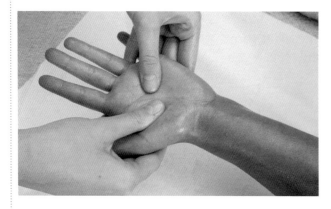

9. Thumb-knead the palm.

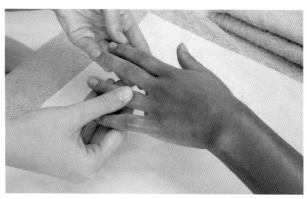

10. Thumb-knead the joints of the fingers.

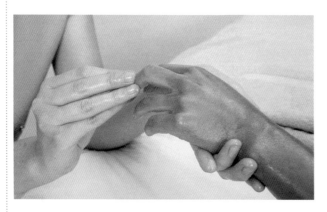

11. Rotate fingers 3 times in each direction.

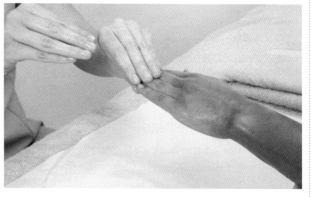

12. Finger 'snapping'.

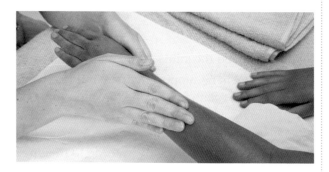

13. Effleurage to finish.

The forearm

1. Take sufficient hand cream from the container using a spatula or pour lotion directly into your hands. Take care not to apply too much lotion, as it becomes messy and your hands will not massage effectively if the skin is too slippery. It is also extravagant and wasteful.

2. Effleurage from the fingers to the elbow with a small amount of pressure to spread the cream evenly. Support the client's hand and mould your other hand around the upper surface of the arm as you move up to the elbow. Return, moving down the underside of the arm. It should not be necessary for you to alternate your hands. Use whichever is most natural and comfortable for you. Repeat 3–4 times.

3. Petrissage (thumb-kneading) to the forearm using the thumb of one hand in circular movements, while supporting the client's arm with the other hand. Slide back down to the wrist and repeat.

The wrist

1. Thumb-knead the wrist using small circular movements, as if you were feeling for all the intricate, small bones of the wrist.

2. Apply rapid thumb movements (friction) in a criss-cross action to the inside of the wrist. This stimulates the main artery (radial) leading to the hand.

3. Rotate the wrist by placing the client's elbow on the manicure cushion and, while supporting the forearm, grip the fingers and rotate in one direction and then the other. Repeat 6 times in each direction.

4. Flex the wrist by placing the client's elbow on the manicure cushion and, while supporting the forearm, interlock your fingers with the client's and push the hand back slowly and firmly. Repeat 2–3 times.

Palm and back of the hand

1. Thumb-knead the back of the hand from the knuckles to the wrist using both thumbs, in circular movements.

2. Thumb-knead the palm by turning the hand over and applying deep circular movements with both thumbs to the fleshy part of the palm.

The fingers

1. Thumb-knead the joints of the fingers and thumb.

2. Rotate fingers by supporting the hand and holding each finger individually, rotate first in one direction three times and then in the other.

3. Finger 'snapping' – use the first two fingers of your hand to twist and pull the finger from the knuckle to the fingertip, as if pulling blood through the vessels to the very tip of the finger.

To complete the massage

The final movement in the massage routine is to effleurage the hand and forearm 5–6 times, finishing with your hand slowly working to the tips of the client's fingers, placing them on the manicure cushion. The client's hand can be wrapped in a towel to keep it warm while repeating the massage routine on the other hand.

Effleurage can be used to link movements together or to warm up an area that has not been worked on for some time and may be getting cold.

Any excess massage cream/lotion left on the hands can be wiped off with a tissue. The client's hands should not be left oily or sticky.

Buffing

Buffing may be incorporated in the manicure at one of two stages in the routine:

1. After filing, without using buffing paste to increase the circulation to the nail, or with buffing paste to begin smoothing the surface of the nail plate. Nails with small ridges may benefit from buffing with paste as it is slightly abrasive. Buffing will not reduce deep ridges or damage to the nail plate.

2. After hand massage, as an alternative to nail polish:
    - for male clients
    - clients who want a natural shine to their nails
    - for those in occupations where polish would not be appropriate for hygiene reasons, for example nurses and those working with food.

Buffing method

1. A very small amount of buffing paste is taken from the container using an orange stick. Care should be taken not to use too much paste or to spread it onto the cuticle, as it is difficult to remove.

2. Place a small dot of paste on the centre of each nail plate of the hand being treated.

3. Spread the paste towards the free edge with the ball of the thumb before using the buffer.

4. Hold the buffer between the first two fingers, although this may depend on the style of the buffer. Holding the buffer correctly ensures that a light movement can be used, therefore avoiding thumping the nail.

5. Stroke the buffer fairly quickly *in one direction only*, from the cuticle to the free edge 15–20 times for each nail or until you have created a shine. Ensure that buffing paste is not spread onto the surrounding skin.

Choosing nail polish

You would normally discuss the colour and type of nail polish with the client during the consultation. The client may have definite views or rely on you to advise. The choice of colour should be recorded on the record card.

Points to be considered when choosing polish include:

- the age and colour of the skin – older hands that are uneven in colour and have red and blue tones do not suit orange and peach colours
- bright colours – these draw attention to the hands and require the nails to be an even length and shape
- dark nail polish – this draws attention to the nails and make small nails look even smaller
- pearlised polish – this shows up any imperfections in the nail plate
- special occasion – the client may require matching of the polish to an outfit or other make-up colouring.

Nail polish application

The final stage of the manicure is the application of nail polish. Ensure that you have allowed sufficient time when planning the treatment for careful application.

1. Place a tissue over the manicure cushion to avoid spoiling the towels.
2. Ask the client to replace jewellery to avoid smudging the nail polish at the end of the treatment. Ensure that the nails are free from grease and manicure preparations by wiping over with nail polish remover on cotton wool. Make sure there are no cotton wool fibres left on the nails.
3. It may be appropriate to ask the client to pay for the treatment at this stage so there is no risk of damaging the finished application.
4. Apply a base coat first, followed by two coats of coloured polish and then a top coat. Pearlised crystalline and frosted polish do not require top coat, so a third coat of colour may be applied.
5. To avoid risk of smudging the polish during application it is a good idea for the right-handed manicurist to start with the little finger of the client's left hand and work towards the thumb, repeating on the right hand. (The left-handed manicurist should reverse the procedure.)
6. The way in which the client's finger is supported is important to prevent catching the nails during application.

The colours and style of application of polish will depend on fashion and to some extent the length and shape of the nails:

- the whole of the nail plate can be polished
- the lunula can be left unpolished
- the nail plate can be polished, leaving a gap at the sides, to give an illusion of length, which is particularly useful on broad thumb nails
- the nail plate can be polished natural pink, with the free edge polished white (**French manicure**).

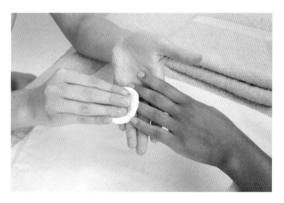

△ Removing grease

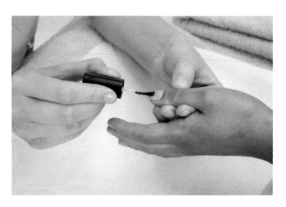

△ Applying base coat

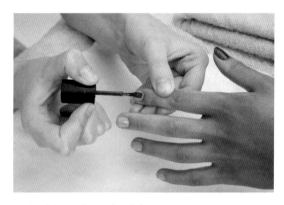

△ Applying coloured polish

> ### Key term
>
> A **French manicure** is where the nail plate is polished a natural pink and the free edge polished white.

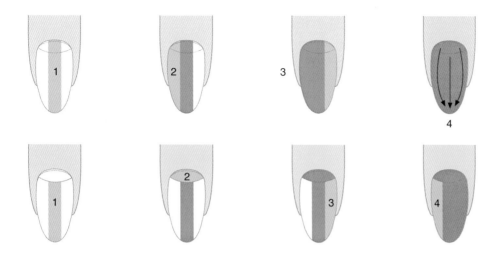

◁ Different polish applications

Allergic reaction to nail polish

Formaldehyde resin is thought to be the cause of allergy to nail polish. Itchiness and inflammation, followed by dry flaking skin, is likely to occur around the eyes or areas where the nails come into contact with the skin, such as the face and neck.

Removing excess polish

Polishing the nails is very skilled work and requires a great deal of practice. The most experienced manicurists sometimes make mistakes and too much polish on the brush can lead to flooding of the cuticle. This can be rectified by using a cotton wool-tipped orange stick dipped in polish remover to carefully work around the cuticle, taking off any polish. This method should only be used when occasional mistakes are made during application. Aim to apply polish without catching the surrounding skin.

Drying

It is essential that the polish is completely dry before the client leaves the salon. If possible, each coat should be allowed to dry before the next one is applied. Thick and poor quality polishes or over-thinned polish may not dry in the time available, so should be avoided. The client may request re-polishing if the polish smudges before a reasonable amount of time.

Dryers that use ultraviolet light are most effective, hardening the cellulose ingredient of the polish. The nails need to be in the unit for between three and six minutes. Quick-drying aerosols can speed up drying time by the rapid evaporation of the spray on the nails. A fine film of oil is left behind, which reduces the tackiness of newly polished nails.

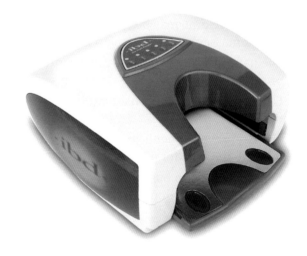

△ Light unit

Repairing a smudge

It can be annoying if the client or the manicurist catches the nails before the polish is dry. If the nail is badly smudged, then it is advisable to remove the polish from the nail and reapply, starting with base coat. Sometimes a minor smudge can be dealt with by applying polish remover to the nail. This must be done carefully by applying polish remover to the tip of your finger and smoothing over the smudged nail in one direction towards the free edge.

This may be repeated, taking care not to flood the nail with remover.

If successful, the nail should be left to dry and a further coat of coloured polish applied if necessary.

French manicure

The French manicure is very popular and enhances the free edge of the nail, giving the nails a natural look, and is designed to show off and enhance the natural appearance of healthy nails. A healthy nail has a pink nail bed, white lunula and free edge.

The manicure or pedicure follows the normal routine, with careful attention to cuticle work to expose the lanula and filing to provide a good shape to the free edge. The free edge is whitened by:

- using a white pencil under the free edge
- applying white tape to highlight the free edge
- applying white nail polish to the free edge. A stencil can be used to achieve a perfect line following the hyponychium (flesh line) or a flat brush dipped in polish remover can be used to form a clean flesh line.

The whole of the nail plate is then polished with a pink translucent polish to complete the look.

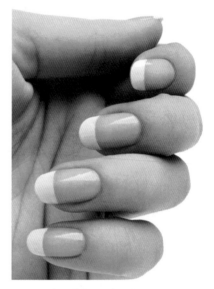
△ French polish application

Hints and tips

Remember to wipe the top of the polish bottle with polish remover immediately after use.

Adapting a manicure for a male client

It is necessary to adapt the routine of the manicure to meet the needs of male clients. Less time is required for varnish application and shaping the nails and more time may be spent on cuticle work and hand massage.

1. File nails to a shorter length and a gentle round or square shape.

2. Use unperfumed hand cream for the hand massage.

3. Use deeper movements in the massage and increase the time for massage.

4. Buff the nails with buffing paste to create a natural shine, rather than using polish. Some clients may wish to have a coat of clear polish.

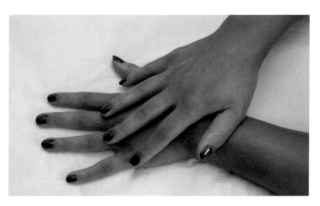
△ Dark polish application

Select a dark-coloured varnish and ask three friends or colleagues with different nail shapes and lengths to act as models. For example:

✤ short, square-shaped nails

✤ long, oval-shaped nails

✤ mis-shaped nails.

Begin by wiping over the nails with polish remover and apply a base coat. Do not choose old, thick polishes just because you are practising. Apply two coats. Do not use an orange stick to remove polish from the cuticle.

Evaluate your polish application in each case using the following checklist and add a comment on the suitability of the dark colour for each of the models.

Polish application checklist	Yes	No
Was the polish a good consistency?	☐	☐
Did you start with the finger and work towards the thumb?	☐	☐
Did you use the minimum number of strokes to apply the polish?	☐	☐
Was the polish smooth on the nail?	☐	☐
Did the polish cover the nail plate evenly?	☐	☐
Was there any polish on the cuticle or surrounding skin?	☐	☐
Were any of the nails smudged?	☐	☐

Contra-actions to manicure

Allergic reactions can occur to many of the products used in manicure, for example lanolin in hand cream, colour pigment, perfume or the solvents used in nail polish. The reaction may occur on the hands or around the nails, but it is quite common for allergies to occur around the eyes, or where the allergen has come into contact with the skin by touching, for example the face or neck.

A serious allergic reaction can be seen initially as:

✦ redness

✦ irritation

✦ swelling.

After a time the skin may become:

✦ dry and scaly

✦ blistered

✦ infected with weeping sores.

The product should be removed immediately and the reaction noted clearly on the record card.

After a manicure a client could complain of soreness around the cuticle of one or more of their nails. This may be due to infection around the nail where the cuticle has been over-trimmed or torn.

Reasons for polish not lasting

Sometimes a client will complain that the polish application did not last – either it chipped or it peeled off the nail. There are a number of possible causes:

- The nail plate was not cleaned with nail polish to remove oil or hand cream.
- No base coat was applied.
- Poor quality nail polish was used.
- The polish was not stored correctly. (Polish should be kept out of direct sunshine, stored in a dark cool place, and tops screwed tightly.)
- Successive coats were not allowed to dry sufficiently.
- The polish was too thick due to evaporation of the solvent. (This may be due to the top not being tightened sufficiently. Often, the bottle tops are left sticky with drips of polish.)
- Top coat was not applied.

Special hand and nail treatments

Treatments used by the therapist on other parts of the body can be adapted for use on the hands and feet. Special treatments can enhance the beneficial effects of a manicure. Treatments such as hand or foot massage have a number of beneficial effects, including:

- stimulating blood flow, bringing about erythema
- removing dry dead skin from the hands (desquamation)
- moisturising and softening the skin
- cleansing the skin
- lightening the skin, helping to removing sun spots
- relaxing the client.

Treatments include:

- paraffin wax
- hand masks, including lightening agents
- exfoliators
- warm oil.

The use of heat in conjunction with nourishing cream, oils or waxes can also be very beneficial.

Applying heat to the hands:

- Hot towels are placed over the hands or feet.
- Electrical equipment such as infra red lamp or electrically heated mitts are used.
- Wax or oil is heated before placing on the skin.

Paraffin wax treatment

Paraffin wax is a solid and cloudy white in colour. It comes in pellets or blocks, which are placed in a specially designed heater. The heater is thermostatically controlled to a working temperature of 29°C.

The wax is painted on to the skin and the hands wrapped in tin foil to retain the heat.

Benefits include:

- easing of stiffness in joints. Clients with rheumatism may find this treatment helps to relieve pain.
- improves texture, colour and condition of the skin.

> **Health and safety**
>
> - Ensure wax does not overheat.
> - Do not move the wax bath while it is hot.
> - Protect the client's clothing. It is extremely difficult to get wax out of fabric.
> - Dispose of used wax immediately after use.

Procedure for paraffin wax treatment

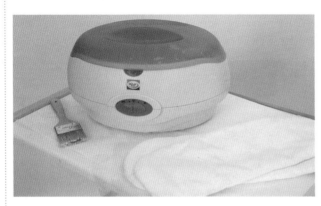

1. The wax must be heated in the wax bath at least 30 minutes before you need to use it. You will have to plan ahead to ensure the wax is properly melted and ready for use.

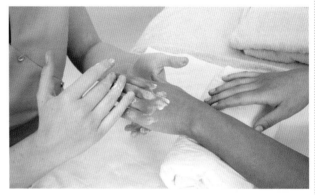

2. The manicure or pedicure is completed up to and including a brief hand/foot massage. A rich massage cream is applied and gently massaged into the area.

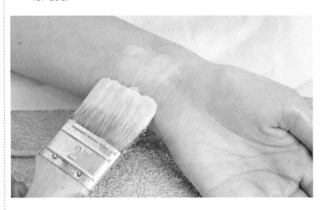

3. Test the temperature of the wax by first looking at its consistency. Then check the thermostat on the heater and apply wax to the inside of your wrist with a spatula.

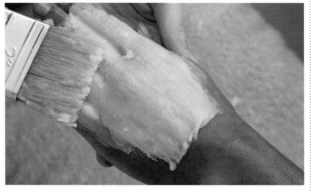

4. Dispense the heated wax into a small bowl and quickly brush the wax onto the client's hands or feet (a small paintbrush is ideal).

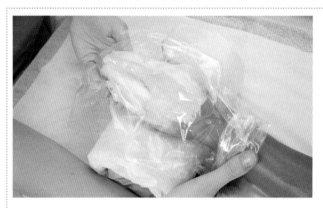

5. Wrap the hand or foot in tin foil or a plastic bag.

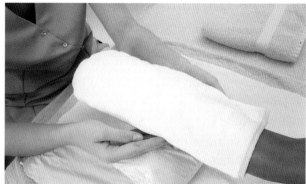

6. Cover with a towel or use thermal mitts or bootees. This process is repeated on the other hand or foot. The wax can be left on for up to 20 minutes, depending on how much time has been allowed for the manicure. Ten minutes is adequate. Make sure the client is seated comfortably and relaxed.

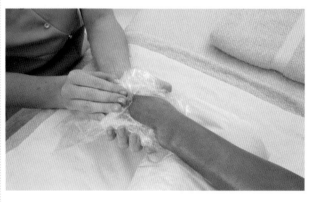

7. Remove the wax from the first hand or foot. The wax should peel off in one piece and be disposed of.

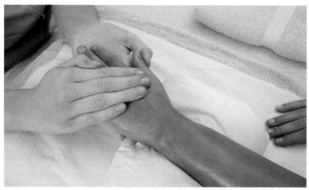

8. The hand or foot is now in an ideal condition for massage. A full massage of 10 minutes should be given to ensure that the client receives the full benefit of the treatment. Repeat on the other hand or foot.

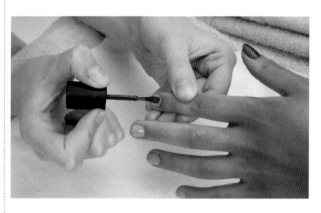

9. Continue with the application of polish, taking extra care when wiping over the nails with polish remover to ensure that there are no traces of wax left on the nails, which will prevent the polish adhering to the nail.

Safety precautions

1. Safety checks should be made on the electrical wax bath. The thermostat must be in good working order to ensure that the wax does not overheat.
2. Protect the client's clothing and the area around the wax bath during treatment. The process can be very messy.
3. Do not move the wax bath while it is hot.
4. Dispose of used wax immediately after use.

Oil treatment

The application of good quality warm vegetable oil to the hands and feet can be very beneficial in treating dry cuticles and nails. Almond oil is ideal, but because of the quantities required it can prove expensive for use in manicure and pedicure. Olive oil is most commonly used, although it tends to have a distinctive smell.

△ Oil treatment

Procedure for oil treatment

1. Place sufficient oil to cover the fingers of one hand up to the first joint in a small bowl. Place this in a larger bowl of hot water on the manicure table.
2. Ensure that the client's clothing is protected, particularly the cuffs of blouses and sweaters.
3. When the cuticle work is completed on the left hand, the fingers are placed in the bowl of warm oil while the right hand is being treated.
4. The left hand is removed and placed on a tissue. It will be necessary to replenish the hot water to warm up the oil for the right hand.
5. The left hand can now be massaged using the oil. Pay particular attention to the cuticles and dry areas of skin. Massage would normally be confined to the hands and wrists.
6. As this is a remedial treatment, the client should be discouraged from having polish applied. This allows the nails and cuticles to benefit from the oil soaking in. Any excess can be removed with tissues. If the client prefers, the hands can be wiped over with witch hazel on a pad of cotton wool. The oil treatment can also be used in an oil manicure as a substitute for soaking in soapy water.

Masks

The colour and condition of the hands can be improved by proprietary brand masks that hydrate the skin or remove unsightly sun spots by gentle bleaching. Pigmentation in the skin of the hands becomes patchy and large brown spots appear – common in fair skin. It is caused by the sun and as the skin ages. The masks are applied in the normal way, using a masking brush. If heat is required the hands can be wrapped in foil and a hot towel applied or thermal mitts may be used. The mask is removed after 10–15 minutes with warm water.

Exfoliating

Exfoliation is the removal of dead skin using mildly abrasive substances such as ground fruit kernels, oatmeal or salt. Exfoliation treatment for the hands removes dry dead skin scales, ingrained dirt and the stains that tend to build up on hard-working hands.

Chemical exfoliants are more often used on the feet to treat the build-up of hard skin. An alkali breaks down the keratin in the skin, softening it. The product also contains grains that loosen the softened skin. The product must be rinsed off thoroughly to remove any traces of the alkali, which would irritate the skin. (Cuticle remover is a similar product. It softens the cuticle to aid removal.)

Salt or oatmeal rub

Salt is mixed to a paste with water or oil and rubbed on the hands with the pads of the fingers, using gentle friction movements. Oatmeal that is mixed and applied in the same way has a similar effect, but is a little gentler. The salt or oatmeal rub would come before hand massage in the manicure routine.

Evaluation of the manicure

Always check the client's satisfaction in line with the treatment plan:

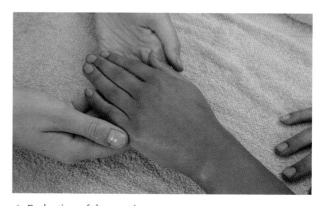
△ Evaluation of the manicure

- Have you completed the treatment as agreed?
- Is the client pleased with the manicure? (Always ask the client before they leave the salon.)
- Do you have any recommendations for further treatment to maintain or improve the client's hands and nails?
- Was the treatment completed in a commercially acceptable time of 45 minutes?
- If extra treatment such as paraffin wax was included, was this completed in 15 minutes?

Outcome 4: Provide aftercare advice

Offering the client aftercare advice is an important part of salon service.

You can use the opportunity to:

- advise on home care
- recommend further treatment
- retail nail products.

Advise the client to:

- wear protective gloves when doing gardening, housework and washing-up as detergents and chemicals will dry the skin and nails
- dry the hands thoroughly after washing and apply hand cream
- protect the hands in cold weather by wearing warm gloves
- use hand cream and cuticle cream just before going to bed
- not to use fingernails to open lids
- protect weak and brittle nails with nail strengthener
- always use an emery board for filing the nails, not a metal file as they create heat by friction and dry out the nail plate

- buff the nails as this will improve circulation to the nail bed and give the nails a natural shine
- ensure a good diet – calcium, iron and vitamin A are necessary for nail health.

 Remember...

Offer the client the opportunity to buy hand cream, nail polish and cuticle preparations.

Manicure is a treatment that shows instant results, helping the client to feel good about her hands and nails. It is therefore possible to recommend regular manicures and to follow a home regime that will care for her hands.

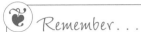 **Want to know more?**

Access HABIA Code of Practice for Nail Services at www.habia.org.uk

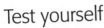

Test yourself

Test yourself on manicure services by answering the following questions:

1. What is the main reason for using buffing paste when buffing?
   a) to stimulate nail growth
   b) to condition the nails
   c) to improve the colour of the nails
   d) to give the nails shine.

2. Nitrocellulose is an ingredient found in:
   a) cuticle remover
   b) buffing paste
   c) nail varnish
   d) hand cream.

3. When shaping the nail the emery board should be used:
   a) with a sawing action across the top of the free edge
   b) in one direction towards the centre of the free edge
   c) across the surface of the nail plate
   d) by pulling back the nail wall and filing the free edge to a point.

4. Which product contains a solvent?
   a) hand cream
   b) buffing paste
   c) cuticle remover
   d) varnish remover.

5. Which is the correct way to hold a cuticle knife, to ensure that the blade and not the point is used?
   a) in an upright position between the thumb and first finger
   b) like a pen
   c) flat in the palm of the hand with the thumb and first finger guiding the implement
   d) between the thumb and middle finger.

6. Hot water is essential during the manicure:
   a) to soak the client's nails and cuticles
   b) to wash the towels
   c) to clean the manicure implements
   d) to wipe up any spillages.

7. Give two contraindications to manicure.

Are you ready for assessment?

> *Remember...*
>
> Practice makes perfect! The more opportunities you have to complete a manicure the more confident you will be when it comes to being observed by your assessor.

> *Remember...*
>
> Always keep your logbook handy.

The following checklist will help you to be fully prepared for your assessment

1. Practical observation

> *Remember...*
>
> Your assessor will observe your performance on at least three occasions each involving a different hand and nail treatment from the range.

Your assessor will look at how you:

- prepare the treatment area
- consult with the client and prepare a record card
- carry out a manicure on a client (not a fellow student or colleague) using a range of tools and products, carry out a special treatment from the range, carry out a hand and arm massage using suitable medium, apply nail polish covering each colour from the range
- carry out the manicure in a commercially acceptable time
- check with the client that the manicure meets her expectations
- provide aftercare advice
- demonstrate professional practice throughout the service
- carry out all treatments with regard to health and safety.

2. Knowledge and understanding

What you must know:

- Organisational and legal requirements.
- How to work safely and effectively when providing manicure services.
- Consult, plan and prepare for treatment with clients.
- Contraindications and contra-actions.
- Anatomy and physiology.
- Manicure treatments.
- Aftercare advice.

To ensure that you have the necessary knowledge and understanding of manicure services your assessor will:

- ask you questions before, during and after carrying out the treatment
- ensure that you have completed project work and written exercises relating to the unit

- check that you have recorded in a log/diary treatments you have carried out with signed record cards showing that you have completed three manicures competently

- that you have covered the range in your candidate logbook

- require you to take a written test.

Sources of evidence

Remember...

Simulation is not a valid means of assessment for manicure service.

- Photographs of completed manicures and nail polish application

- Client record cards

- Witness statements

- Feedback

- Video.

Remember...

The maximum commercially viable service time for a basic manicure is 45 minutes.

Chapter 12
Unit N3: Provide pedicure services

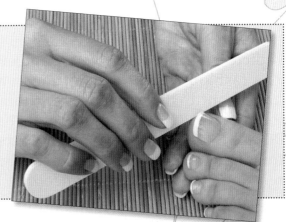

Learning objectives

This chapter covers the skills and knowledge required for Unit N3 'Provide pedicure services'.

There are four learning outcomes for Unit N3 and they are:
1 Maintain safe and effective methods of working when providing pedicure services.
2 Consult, plan and prepare for the pedicure service.
3 Carry out pedicure services.
4 Provide aftercare advice.

You will need to be competent in all of these outcomes in pedicure services, qualify for insurance and perform the treatment on members of the public.

Evidence requirements

Your assessor will need to observe you perform this service successfully on at least three occasions on three different clients. On each occasion you must perform a different foot and nail treatment from the range. You must:

1 Demonstrate the use of consultation techniques:
- questioning
- visual
- manual
- reference to client records.

2 Take at least one of the following necessary actions:
- encourage the client to seek medical advice
- explain why the treatment cannot be carried out
- modify the treatment.

3 Demonstrate the use of these feet and nail treatments:
- paraffin wax
- foot masks
- thermal boots
- exfoliators.

4 Demonstrate the application of both types of nail finish:
- dark colour
- French.

5 Provide treatment advice:
- suitable aftercare tools and products and their use
- avoidance of activities which may cause damage (contra-actions)
- recommended time intervals in between nail services.

Introduction

Pedicure has become a very popular salon treatment. The fashion trend for open toed shoes and sandals has meant that the need to care for the feet and the toe nails has become important. In general, people do not look after their feet. Pedicure is a therapeutic treatment for the feet and toenails but it is also a very relaxing treatment for most people.

Unit N3 appears as a mandatory unit in the Level 2 Beauty Therapy General and Nail services routes.

The purpose of pedicure is to:

- improve the appearance of the feet and nails
- relax tired and aching feet
- reduce hard skin on the feet
- offer advice on care of the feet and referral as necessary to a chiropodist.

The pedicure will include:

- reducing the length of the nails
- cuticle treatment
- removal of hard skin
- foot massage
- nail polish application as required.

Meet the professional

"Add-on treatments go well with a pedicure, such as glycolic peel on the feet. Be up to date with the newest colours and treatments. It is an ideal opportunity to inform your clients about other treatments you could provide, e.g. Minx, Shellac, 'Hollywood toes' and 'Glitter toes'."

Jacqui Bostock

Outcome 1: Maintain safe and effective methods of working when providing pedicure services

In general, people do not look after their feet. Women in particular will follow fashion trends in footwear at the expense of comfort and correctly fitting shoes. This can lead to long-term foot disorders such as bunions and calluses, as well as poor posture.

Choosing the correct shoes for everyday wear, particularly for work, is important. For example, the beauty therapist, who stands for long hours in a warm environment, should choose shoes that support the foot. A good fit is necessary so that the toes are not cramped and the heels are not chafed, causing blisters and hard skin.

A low heel rather than a flat shoe gives support to the arch of the foot. Equally, very high heels are extremely tiring if worn for long periods of time. They tend to change the natural posture by throwing the weight forward.

You will find further details about correct personal appearance and footwear for the therapist in Chapter 1 and about health and safety in Chapter 3.

 Remember . . .

The feet have to withstand pressure from the weight of the body and are essential for walking and balance. The therapist can help the client through advice and regular pedicures to appreciate the importance of caring for the feet.

The pedicure will include:

- reducing the length of the nails
- cuticle treatment
- removal of hard skin
- foot massage
- nail polish application as required
- specialist treatments.

Health and safety is of the utmost importance in the salon and must be a priority when preparing and carrying out any treatment on clients in the salon

Much of the routine for manicure applies to pedicure. The major differences are:

- the positioning of the client and therapist for treatment
- the treatment of hard skin and the implements and products used
- foot massage routine.

When assessing possible hazards, consideration must be given to:

- the salon environment/work area
- hygiene procedures
- equipment and pedicure products
- the necessary competence to carry out the pedicure safely.

 Health and safety

Access HABIA Code of practice for Manicure Services which will provide information relevant to pedicure treatment. (www.habia.org.uk)

Preparing the work area for a pedicure services

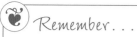 The increase in demand for nail treatment has led to the development of nail salons with specialist equipment. Banks of pedicure chairs with integral spa foot baths are now common. The client sits high in the chair (which may have a massage facility), allowing the pedicurist to work in a comfortable position at the feet of the client.

However, most beauty salons may only have a small space for manicures and pedicures.

Wherever you work, it is essential that:

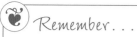 the pedicure table and stool are at the right height. Pedicure chairs with an integral spa foot bath provide a very comfortable work station for both client and therapist.

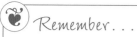 seating for the client and pedicurist is comfortable. You should not be in a slouching position as this can cause back problems over a period of time and will certainly cause fatigue.

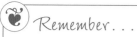 there is good lighting – it may be necessary to have a magnifying lamp or an angle-poise lamp to hand.

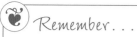 there is adequate ventilation – when working with solvents it is essential that fresh air circulates freely (this applies particularly when using artificial nail systems)

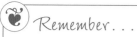 pedicure implements are clean, sterilised and arranged in a neat and organised manner with everything to hand

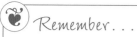 hot and cold water with liquid soap is available for washing your hands before and after treatment, for soaking the client's nails to soften the cuticle and to remove preparations from the nails during treatment

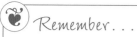 there are plenty of clean towels available

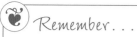 you have on hand disposable materials such as paper towels, tissues and cotton wool.

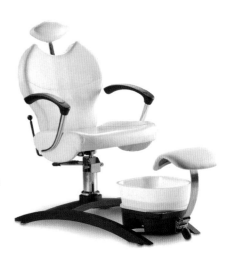

△ Pedicure spa chair

 Health and safety

Refer to safe working practice with regards to posture and repetitive strain injury

 Health and safety

Refer to Chapter 3 for information on heating and ventilation.

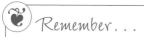 Remember...

Poor hygiene procedures in the salon can cause cross-infection. Fungal infection is particularly problematic when dealing with the feet.

Client care and preparation

Before examining your client's feet ensure that you have washed your hands thoroughly using a medicated hand wash to minimise the risk of cross-infection.

Ensure that your client is seated comfortably. Ask them to remove socks or tights and if they are wearing jeans or trousers they can roll them up or be offered a gown and remove them in a changing room.

Remember...

Before carrying out a pedicure treatment the client must be consulted to establish contraindications to the treatment (see Chapter 1).

Preparation and hygiene procedures

Preparation and hygiene procedures are an essential part of all salon treatments. Pedicure implements are small items that can be cleaned and sterilised quite easily and some are disposable.

The trolley must be wiped over with disinfectant. Sterilised and clean tools need to be set out in an orderly way that allows the pedicurist to have them close at hand while working. A mobile therapist may use a basket with sterilised tools. A covered bin should be available for waste. This bin must be emptied into the main bin after every treatment.

Refer to Chapter 3 for details on general health, safety and hygiene procedures.

Products, tools and equipment

Tools used in pedicure

Refer to Chapter 11 for further details on tools and equipment.

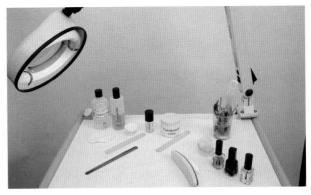

- **Nail scissors** – small, curved blades for reducing the length of the nails.
- **Nail clippers** – because the toe nails grow hard and thicken with age, it may be necessary to use nail clippers to shorten the nails.
- **Cuticle knife** – small, flat blade used to remove cuticle attached to the nail plate.

△ A range of implements set out on a trolley

- **Cuticle nippers** – small, scissor-like implement with a spring action to allow small movements, used to remove excessive, torn or damaged cuticle. Metal tools can be washed in hot soapy water and sterilised using an autoclave. They can be stored in an ultraviolet cabinet after sterilising. During the pedicure small implements should be placed in disinfectant on the trolley.
- **Callous file or rasp** – an essential tool for gently removing hard skin which can build up on the heels, toes and pads of the feet.

After use these items of small equipment can be washed in hot soapy water and placed in the ultraviolet cabinet for storage. Emery boards are made of fibrous board and therefore cannot be washed.

The orange stick, spatula and hoof stick should be placed in disinfectant during the pedicure and disposed of after each client.

- **Hoof stick** – orange-wood or plastic handle with a rubber end shaped like a hoof, used to gently push back the cuticle from the nail plate.
- **Nail brush** – used to remove all products before the application of nail polish; may also be required to clean dirty nails.
- **Orange stick** – disposable wooden implement with one end slanted and the other pointed, which should be tipped with cotton wool before use. The orange stick has a number of uses: pushing back softened cuticle with the cotton wool-tipped end soaked in cuticle remover, to clean under the nails with pointed end tipped with cotton wool and to remove small amounts of preparations from their pots.

> ☆ **Hints and tips**
> A small pack of disposable implements, such as emery board and orange stick can be costed into the pedicure and given to the client for home use.

- **Spatula** – used to dispense products from pots (may be made from plastic material that can be washed easily or wood that can be disposed of after use).

- **Emery board** – has a dark side which is coarse and used when nails are to be shortened in length or for filing very strong nails. The light side is fine and used for shaping and smoothing the nails. The emery board should be flexible and 12–15 cm long to allow for good technique during filing of the nails. If reusable files are used they must be washed and sterilised.

> *Remember...*
>
> Disposable emery boards used on the client can be costed into the pedicure and given to her to take home. Ensure that you explain to the client how to file correctly.

Products used in pedicure

- **Polish remover** – a solvent that removes nail polish. Amyl acetate (acetone) is the main ingredient in polish remover, with a small amount of oil added to help counteract the drying effect of the solvent on the nail plate.

- **Cuticle massage cream** – an emollient used to soften and nourish the cuticles. Lanolin or mineral oils are the main ingredients. Cuticle oil may be used in the same way.

- **Cuticle remover** – an alkaline substance that softens the keratin in the skin, allowing the cuticle to be lifted from the nail plate and the excess to be removed using cuticle nippers. Potassium hydroxide is the main ingredient, which is caustic and very drying if not removed thoroughly after use. Cuticle remover also has a mild bleaching effect and can help to remove stains from the nails.

- **Buffing paste** – a mild abrasive substance which, when combined with the friction action of the buffer, gives the surface of the nail plate a shine. Pumice, silica or stannic oxide (jeweller's paste) is the main ingredient. Buffing may help increase the circulation to the nail bed and smooth ridges in the nail.

- **Hand cream/lotion** – an emollient that softens and nourishes the skin and assists in the application of massage. **Lanolin**, **glycerol** or **vegetable oils** are used to make an oil-in-water emulsion. Other ingredients include perfume, colour and some natural products such as aloe vera.

- **Nail polish: base coat, top coat and coloured varnish** – a plastic film that is applied to the nail plate. Nitro cellulose and a solvent such as amyl acetate are the main ingredients of all nail polish, with various pigments added to give colour, or guanine from fish scales to give a pearlised effect. Good quality nail polish lasts longer, has a good range of colours, has a good consistency for smooth application and dries quickly and evenly.

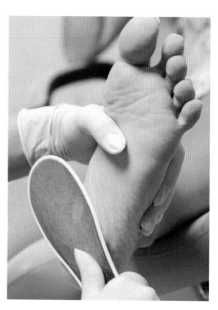

△ Hard skin removal products

- **Base coat** – provides a smooth base for the application of coloured varnish, protects the nails from staining (which can be caused by colour pigment), minimises ridges or irregularities in the nail plate and prolongs the life of polish by helping to prevent chipping and peeling.

- **Ridge filler** – provides a more even surface for polish when nails have ridges.

- **Top coat** – is used to give extra gloss to cream polish and to help the polish last longer by providing a hard surface, protecting the polish from chipping. Top coat is not required for crystalline polish as it can dull the finish.

- **Nail polish thinners** – a solvent used to thin down nail polish that has become thick. Ethyl acetate is the active ingredient. Thinner should be used very sparingly or the polish will not harden. Nail polish remover should not be used for thinning polish, as the oil it contains will prevent the polish from drying.

- **Nail strengtheners** – a product that hardens the keratin in the nail plate. Formaldehyde is the active ingredient in these products. Nail strengtheners may also be an acrylic substance that provides a hard plastic coating to reinforce the nail.

- **Nail white pencil** – a pencil that is dipped in water before applying to the underside of the free edge. This whitens stained nails. Titanium dioxide is the main ingredient.

- **Quick-dry spray** – the cooling effect can speed up the drying process. A solvent aerosol spray that evaporates quickly is the basis of this product, although polish that is allowed to dry naturally is longer lasting.

- **Exfoliants** – a product containing abrasive ingredients that remove dead skin and help to smooth calluses and rough skin.

- **Masks** – can be adapted from facial products to draw impurities from the skin, soften and improve the texture of the skin.

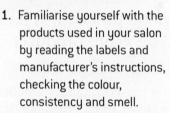

Activity

1. Familiarise yourself with the products used in your salon by reading the labels and manufacturer's instructions, checking the colour, consistency and smell.

2. Make a list of the products needed for a pedicure.

3. Visit a department store or chemist shop and look at the range and cost of products and tools available to your clients.

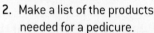

General items of equipment and materials for pedicure

As well as specialist items of equipment and products, you will need some more general equipment and materials that include:

- **Foot bath** – many salons provide a foot spa with the beneficial effects of pulsating water, which gently massages the feet. Soaking the feet before starting the pedicure is essential to soften the skin, nails and cuticle and to ensure the feet are clean.

- **Surgical spirit** – for cleansing the client's feet prior to examination and for disinfecting implements and surfaces.

- **Jar of sanitising fluid** – to hold pedicure implements during treatment. This may be disinfectant or sterilising fluid.

- **Cotton wool** – for wiping over the feet when soaked in surgical spirit, for removing nail polish when soaked in polish remover and for tipping the orange stick before use.

- **Tissues** – for wrapping sterilised implements before use, for covering the towelling cushion during polish application to protect the towel.
- **Disposable towels** – to dry the feet after soaking prior to inspecting and carrying out the consultation.
- **Towels** – for drying client's feet during the pedicure. A towel should be placed on your lap during the pedicure for drying your hands.
- **Hot towels** – for keeping feet warm during mask or paraffin wax application.
- **Waste bin** – for immediate disposal of waste materials. A small pedal bin is ideal.
- **Disposable toe separators** – required during polish application to avoid the toe nails touching and causing a smudge.
- **Disposable flip flops/footwear** – after polish application it is essential to wear these to avoid smudging.
- **Thermal bootees** – used to keep feet warm during paraffin wax or mask treatments.

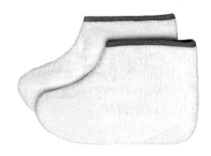

△ Thermal bootees

Hygiene procedures and care of small implements and pedicure products

Small tools

Always buy good quality, stainless steel tools such as cuticle knife and nippers, so that they can be sterilised without damaging them. Make sure blades are sharp, particularly the cuticle nippers, to avoid tearing the cuticle. Ensure that the hinge moves easily on the nippers to allow for the correct technique to be used.

All small tools must be sterilised after use, whether by autoclave or chemical sterilising fluid, as appropriate. (Refer to Chapter 1 for sterilising methods.) The items should be dried and stored either in an ultraviolet cabinet or placed in a tool roll.

Pedicure products

Many products used in pedicure and manicure services contain solvents and must, therefore, be handled and stored carefully. The COSHH risk assessment for your salon will identify hazards when using these products.

It is important that tops are secure on bottles to avoid evaporation of polish remover and solvent in polish.

Particular attention is needed when caring for nail polish. Your clients will want to choose from a wide range of polish colours. Polish should be of excellent quality to ensure a long-lasting finish and good colours.

The necks of the bottles should be wiped after use to ensure that the top fits securely. When the solvent is allowed to evaporate from the polish, it becomes thick and impossible to apply to the nails. Polish will require thorough shaking before use to ensure a smooth, well-mixed colour. Small beads are placed in some bottles to ensure thorough mixing. Slight separation may occur in cream polishes, leaving a white deposit or sometimes, dark layers form at the top of the bottle.

Coloured polish needs to be stored upright, away from direct sunlight to avoid fading of colour pigments and thickening of the polish due to changes in temperature.

Health and safety

COSHH regulations are outlined in Chapter 3.

Outcome 2: Consult, plan and prepare for the pedicure service

Client consultation is a very important part of the service offered to a client. A client's health and circumstances can change between visits to the salon so it is important to go through the consultation process every time, whether the client comes for treatment regularly or for a one-off visit. You may also need to check progress against the treatment plan.

Remember . . .

The therapist should ask the age of the client, as you are required by law to gain parental or legal guardian's consent in writing before treating a minor (someone under the age of 18 in England and under 17 in Scotland). The parent or legal guardian should also accompany the minor for the duration of the service if they are 16 or under. Treating a child of pre-school age is legal with parental or guardian consent, though some salons refuse to do this as part of their own salon policy.

Full details of client consultation and treatment planning can be found in Chapter 1.

Assessing the client for pedicure services

It is essential that the feet have been soaked prior to inspecting and carrying out a consultation. The feet should be dried with disposable paper in case there is infection present. The paper should then immediately be disposed of in a bin.

Assessing the client for treatment involves:

- visual – looking at the feet
- manual – touching the skin and checking in between the toes and the soles of the feet
- question – questioning the client
- reference to the client's record card.

Look and touch (visual and manual assessment)

To carry out this stage, go through the following steps.

1. **Check under the foot and between the toes**. Check immediately for any signs of infection, for example between the toes for signs of athlete's foot, and the nails for signs of fungus. Check the soles of the feet and toes for build up of hard skin and rough, dry patches of skin, any cuts or broken skin. The age of the client will affect the texture of the skin, and conditions such as arthritis may be apparent.

2. **The cuticles**. The condition of the cuticle of the nails will immediately indicate whether the client cares for their feet and has regular pedicures. Overgrown, torn and dry cuticles will require extra work during the pedicure and home care advice to the client. The cuticle becomes attached to the nail plate and hardens in areas of pressure, so cuticle removal in pedicure is an important part of the treatment.

3. **The nails**. Inspect each nail for:

   - **shape** – toe nails should be square or slightly rounded. It is important that the nails are not filed into the corners where pressure can cause in growing toe nails

   - **colour** – a slightly pink colour is an indication of healthy nails. Discoloured nails may be an indication of infection, particularly from a fungus.

Nails will vary in thickness, flexibility and strength. This is normally a hereditary factor although illness, disease and certain drugs can severely affect the condition of the nails. Nails of the feet become thicker with age and especially where there is pressure from footwear. Flaking and splits in the nail should be noted.

Question

Discussion with the client at this stage is a very important part of the consultation. If there are any conditions of the feet or nails that are contraindications and prevent you continuing with treatment, this must be handled in a very sensitive manner. You must explain to the client about the condition and why it prevents you from continuing. This will usually be because there is infection present that could be passed on to other clients or therapists. It may be appropriate to explain to the client how the condition could spread and infect others in the home or workplace. For example, clients are often not aware of athlete's foot (fungal infection).

Gentle questioning will enable you to establish the lifestyle, habits and occupation of the client, all of which will have an effect on the condition of the client's feet and nails. You may be able to establish the cause of any condition by asking an open question:

- What type of shoes do you wear regularly? This can help to establish the reason for corns or excessive hard skin being present.

By talking to the client you will be able to identify their needs and expectations. You will be required to advise them on what the treatment entails, what the end result will be, and whether you can meet their expectations. It is important that you discuss the cost of the pedicure, especially if you have agreed to include a special treatment that will take extra time.

The questioning phase of the client assessment will allow you to build a rapport with the client and help them to relax, making the treatment more enjoyable.

Reference to the record card

All the details that you discover through looking, touching and questioning should be included in the treatment plan or record card.

Remember . . .
All the information you gain from your client that is written on a record card is confidential.

The client's record card is an important source of information, providing the therapist with details on previous treatments and any contraindications.

Treatment times for pedicure

The table below provides the commercially accepted treatment times for pedicure services.

▽ Pedicure treatment times

Service description	Service time
Pedicure with polish, including French	50 mins
Pedicure without polish (buffed)	35 mins
File and re-polish	15 mins
Specialist hand and nail treatment	(add 15–20 mins to treatment)

Activity

Look closely at your feet. Write down what you see. Follow the look, touch, question, routine. Observe: areas of hard skin, the shape of the nails and the condition of the cuticles. Now repeat the exercise on a colleague.

Healthy nails

- Healthy nails appear firm but flexible, smooth and slightly pink in colour. The surrounding cuticle should be unbroken, flexible and should not be stuck to the nail plate.
- Toenails grow more slowly than fingernails (about 2 mm per month) and are often thicker and harder. They will grow faster in the summer, and in children and pregnant women. Children and pregnant women have higher levels of nutrients in the blood. In summer, due to the increase in temperature blood circulation is faster.
- To produce healthy nails the vitamins A, B complex and D are needed together with the minerals calcium and iron.

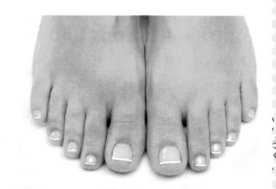

△ Healthy feet

The effects of nail care treatment

Nail treatments such as a paraffin wax treatment and massage benefit nail growth by increasing the blood supply to the nail bed. In doing so, more nutrients and oxygen are available for the cells to grow and divide. This means that the nails will grow more quickly and will be stronger.

The effects of illness

Systemic illness, in other words disease or illness affecting a system of the body, can influence the rate of growth and appearance of the nails, as well as the skin and hair. Poor health or poor diet can cause the nails to be brittle or very soft, flexible, pale, discoloured or blue in colour and the cuticles to be dry, split and hardened.

Physical damage

Nail bed – a knock or blow that is hard enough to damage the nail bed will appear as a bruise under the nail. The blood vessels in the nail bed break, allowing blood to flow out under the nail plate. After a short time the blood vessels mend, leaving some under the nail plate. This dries, sticks to the underside and grows up with the nail plate until it reaches the free edge, where it can be removed.

Matrix – damage to the matrix can result in temporary loss of the nail or permanent damage to the nail plate. When the matrix is damaged by a severe knock or blow, some of the cells die. This results in a temporary halt in the production of the nail plate and nail bed. This can appear as a ridge in the nail or, if a lot of the matrix is damaged, the loss of the nail plate.

The dead cells need to be replaced and are made by the matrix itself. When fully healed, the matrix will begin to make the nail plate and nail bed again. If, however, the damage is severe enough, the matrix may not heal completely, leaving scar tissue. This will appear as a permanent condition in the nail, such as a vertical ridge or split.

Chemical damage

Strong chemicals such as nail polish remover, or continuous use of nail polish, will cause the nail and cuticle to dry out. The nail may appear brittle, discoloured (usually yellow), flaky and ridged. The cuticle will be dry, white in colour and inflexible.

Contraindications and restrictions to pedicure

The presence of some conditions may contraindicate pedicure services. A therapist must be able to recognise conditions in order to make the decision as to whether a nail care treatment can be performed or not but must not diagnose the condition. For more details regarding the correct course of action when the client presents with a contraindication that prevents treatment refer to Chapter 1.

Conditions can be divided into two types:

- those that prevent treatment being carried out and may need medical referral, for example open cuts and abrasions
- those that restrict treatment, for example bruising, arthritis in an area that can be avoided during the treatment, or in the case of painful joints where treatments such as paraffin wax are very beneficial.

The presence of some conditions may contraindicate pedicure treatment for example:

- infectious conditions – clients may be unaware of conditions of the feet that require referral to a doctor or chiropodist (e.g. verrucae, athlete's foot)
- open wounds such as burst blisters, cuts or abrasions.

A therapist must be able to recognise conditions in order to make the decision as to whether a treatment can be performed or not.

Other conditions that would contraindicate treatement include:

- infection in the area of the feet, which can be recognised by the presence of **redness, swelling, pain** and **pus**
- infectious nail disease
- allergic reaction to products, the symptoms being **itching, swelling, redness** or **raised blisters**.

Conditions that prevent treatment

Common diseases caused by micro-organisms may require treatment by a medical practitioner. When referring a client to their GP, it is important to do so without causing alarm or embarrassment.

Verruca plantaris

These are contagious conditions caused by a virus affecting the skin of the hands or feet. Do not touch. If minor, they can be covered with a dressing and the treatment can be performed. If severe, the client should see a doctor. Look out for raised, horny lumps with black dots on the feet and horny lumps in an uneven shape which grow into the skin on the soles of the feet, characteristic of verrucae.

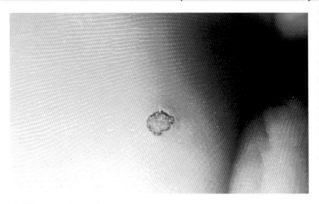

△ Verruca plantaris

Ringworm (tinea)

Not a 'worm' as the name implies, but a fungal infection which can affect the nails and the skin. The disease is highly contagious and is often passed on by pets. Do not touch the area but tell the client to see a doctor as soon as possible for suitable treatment.

Look out for:

- Yellow or white streaks and thickening of the nail plate. Sometimes the top layers of the nail will peel off. This is known as onychomycosis.
- Red, slightly raised patches of skin in the shape of a ring.
- On the feet, it appears as white, moist flaking or peeling between and around the bottom of the toes. Commonly called 'athlete's foot', it often spreads to the toenails.

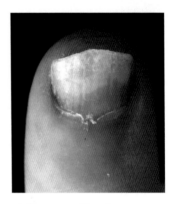

△ Ringworm (tinea)

Conditions restricting treatment

Ingrowing toenails (onychocryptosis)

Can affect the fingers, but most common on the toes. The edges of the nail cut into the nail wall, which then can become infected by bacteria. The problem is caused by restrictive footwear, by clipping the corners of the nail too low at the nail wall or it can be a congenital defect. If inflammation or infection is present, the client should be referred to a doctor; if not, the condition should be referred to a chiropodist and the nail omitted from the nail care treatment.

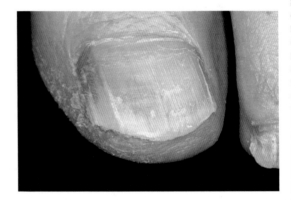

△ Ingrowing toe nails

Chilblains

Caused by poor blood circulation and, therefore, common on feet and toes. The condition appears in cold weather. When severe, refer the client or delay treatment until the condition has improved. If mild, avoid the affected area. Look out for red, itchy swellings that become painful in the cold.

Corns

These are similar to calluses in that they are formed by an increase in pressure or overuse. A corn, however, develops a root-like structure that penetrates into the skin and when it presses on a nerve it causes pain. A client with a deep, developed corn needs referral to a chiropodist. Soft, new corns can be treated in the same way as calluses.

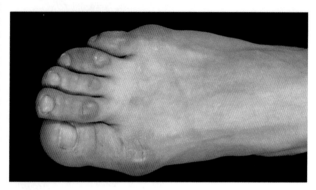

△ Corns

Bunions (hallus vulgus)

This is a condition where the big toe is forced towards and under the other toes due to pressure and friction from tight or pointed footwear. This causes the joint to swell and become inflamed, causing pain. Another cause may be an inherited weakness in the arches of the foot. The therapist can assist with massage when the bunion is newly formed but in most cases the condition needs to be treated by a chiropodist or by referral to a doctor for surgery. During pedicure, take care with the area as pressure may be painful. Filing and cuticle work can be performed with care although enamelling may be difficult if the toe is severely affected.

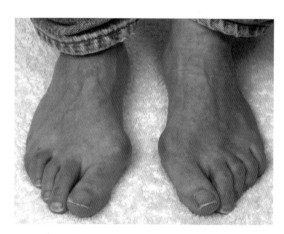

△ Bunions

Diabetes

A client who suffers from diabetes will have reduced skin healing so therefore it is necessary to take very great care when applying the cuticle nippers that may, if handled incorrectly, cut the skin. This is particularly a problem with the feet as poor circulation may be a result of diabetes.

Outcome 3: Carry out pedicure services

Hygiene procedures for pedicure

All general hygiene procedures for salon treatments apply, as do the routine hygiene procedures for pedicure relating to implements, equipment and the work area. Refer to Chapter 3 for details.

Client preparation

Soaking the client's feet prior to thorough examination and treatment is essential. A quick visual check of both feet is required and you should question the client regarding any foot problems.

1. Prepare a foot bowl with warm water and antiseptic liquid soap.

2. Place both feet in the water for 3–5 minutes. This will help relax the client, as well as freshen the feet prior to treatment.

3. It is a good idea at this stage to dry the feet with disposable paper towels in case, after closer examination, infectious foot disease is present.

Clients are often unaware of conditions such as athlete's foot and you may not be able to see it without close examination between the toes. This can be carried out discreetly while drying the feet. The client can be advised and referred to a chiropodist or doctor. The treatment should be cancelled until the condition has cleared. The foot bowl will need to be disinfected, paper towels disposed of immediately and you must wash your hands very thoroughly.

Products, implements and equipment

Pedicure treatment will require the same products and implements as for manicure, with the following additions:

- foot bowl/foot spa
- nail clippers or curved scissors
- cuticle trimmer
- callous file or corn rasp for removing hard skin
- exfoliating cream or hard-skin remover.

(A buffer is not required.)

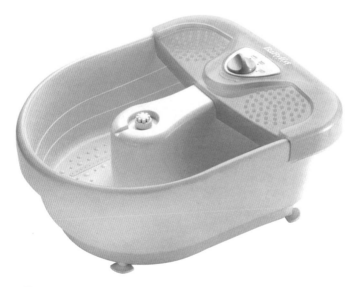

△ Foot spa

The basic manicure routine is followed throughout, except where extra treatment is required to deal with foot-specific conditions such as hard and dry skin, overgrown cuticle and thickened nails. These are discussed later in this chapter.

Procedure for pedicure

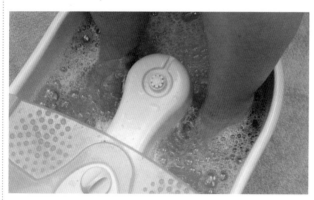

1. Soak both feet in warm soapy water.

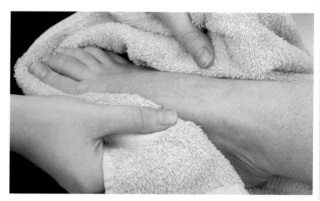

2. Dry both feet with disposable paper and inspect the feet closely.

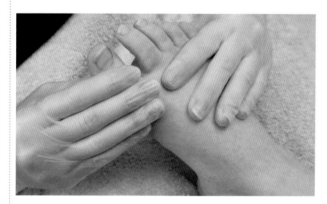

3. If there are no contraindications present continue with treatment.

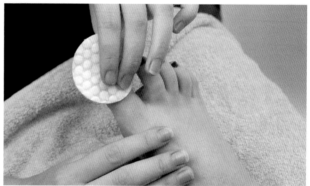

4. Remove nail polish.

5. Replenish the water in the foot bath to ensure that it is warm.

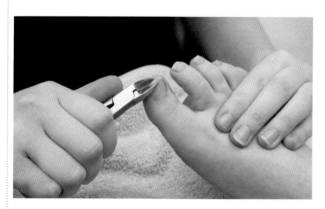

6. Cut nails on the left foot with curved scissors or nail **clippers as required.**

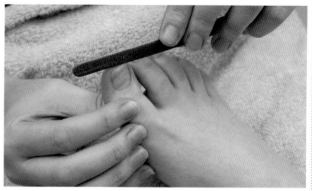
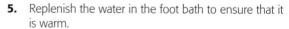

7. File.

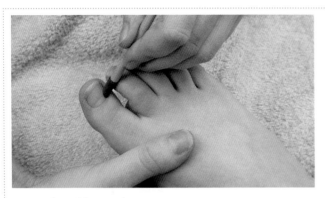

8. Apply cuticle massage cream.
9. Soak.
10. Repeat steps 6–9 on the other foot.
11. Dry the left foot thoroughly.
12. Soak the right foot (check with the client that the water is still warm).

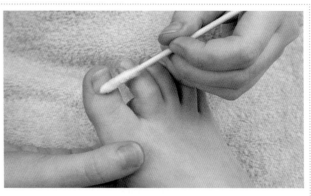

13. Treat the cuticles on the left foot by applying cuticle remover and pushing back the cuticle using the cotton wool-tipped orange stick.

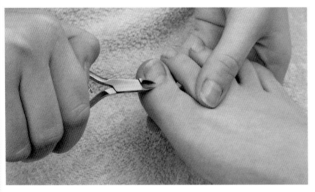

14. Remove excess cuticle with the cuticle knife and cuticle nippers.
16. Apply hard-skin remover to the sole of the foot, heels and tops of the toes, as required. Using the heel of the hand apply with vigorous rubbing to help exfoliate the hard skin.
18. Dry the left foot and wrap in a dry towel to keep warm.

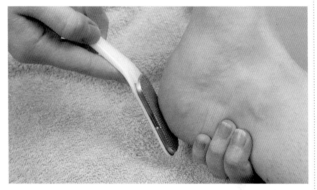

15. Use a callous file or rasp, if required, to remove the build-up of hard skin, usually on the pads of the foot, heel and little toes.
17. Rinse off the cuticle remover, hard-skin remover and exfoliated skin in the foot bath using a wad of cotton wool.
19. Repeat stages 13–18 on the right foot.

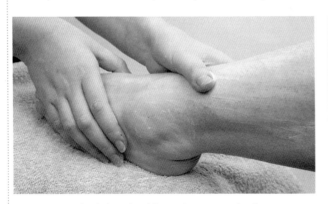

20. Massage both feet (and lower leg as required).

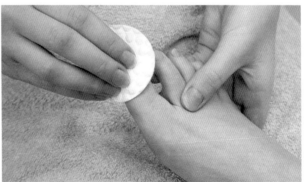

21. Remove any remaining massage cream from the nail plate on each foot with polish remover on a pad of cotton wool.

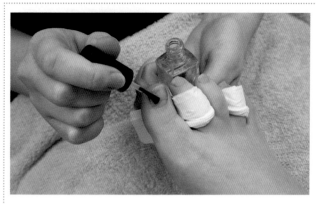

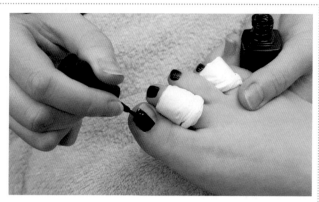

22. Use toe separators or tissues twisted between the toes to separate the toes and prevent the polish smudging.

23. Apply polish. Base coat (once), coloured polish (twice) and top coat (once).

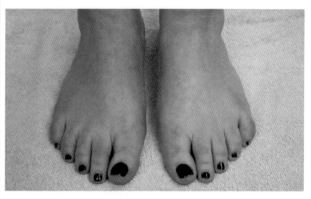

24. Allow polish to dry completely. This is absolutely essential before replacing tights/stockings and shoes. The use of a light dryer will harden the cellulose in the polish.

25. Give home care advice to the client.

Cutting the toenails

Toenails should be cut straight across to avoid ingrowing nails. After soaking the feet to soften the nails, the nail clippers or sharp scissors can be used, followed by filing with the coarse side of an emery board.

 Remember...

Nail clippers are most effective in cutting hard thick nails. Toe nails can become thick and hard due to pressure from footwear or age.

Pressure from wearing shoes can cause the nails to thicken, particularly the big toenails. Thickened toenails are particularly common in older clients. It may be necessary to refer the client to a chiropodist for nails to be cut.

The nails protect the ends of the toes and should not be cut too short, as this will cause discomfort and pressure on the ends of the toes.

Cuticle work

The cuticles on the toes are often quite thick and overgrown unless the client cares for their feet and has regular pedicures. The cuticles can be treated in the same way as in a manicure, but extra time will be needed for using the cuticle nippers or cuticle trimmer to cut excess cuticle from around the nails. The cuticle trimmer should only be used on hard raised cuticle. It is a small V-shaped implement. The 'V' has a sharp cutting edge that trims excess cuticle as the trimmer is passed around the base of the nail.

Removing hard skin

Hard skin develops on the feet as a form of protection in those areas that receive the greatest pressure and rubbing. The balls of the feet and heels are commonly affected. Only unsightly dry skin should be removed or smoothed to improve the appearance of the feet.

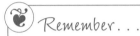 *Remember . . .*

It is the job of the chiropodist to deal with excessive hard skin including calluses and corns.

A range of implements and products can be used for treating hard skin. The callus file and corn rasp are metal files used to lift dead hard skin from the foot using a quick filing movement. Hard-skin removers or exfoliants use chemicals (alkali) or abrasive ingredients to remove hard skin.

Activity

Research how an alkaline solution helps to remove hard skin.

Foot massage

Foot massage is very relaxing for the client. It is important that the client is positioned comfortably to avoid strain as pressure is applied during the massage.

It is usual to massage the feet and lower leg, but if the client is wearing trousers they may wish to have just the feet and ankles treated. Remember to protect clothing from the lotion by using tissues.

Follow a sequence, as for hand massage. Divide the area to be massaged as follows:

- lower leg
- ankle
- top and sole of the foot
- toes.

Health and safety

It is important to take account of positioning the client to avoid unnecessary strain which could cause injury to the therapist or the client. Refer to Chapter 3.

Procedure for foot massage

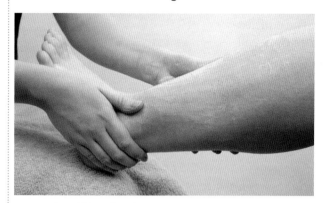

1. Apply sufficient hand cream.

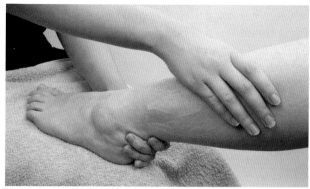

2. Effleurage from foot to the knee six times.

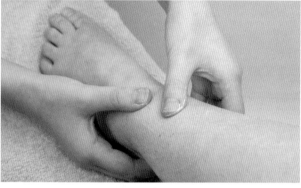

3. Petrissage (thumb-kneading) the front of the leg.

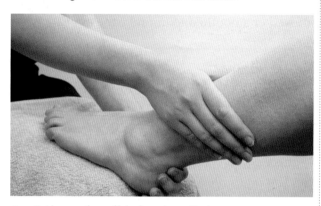

4. Petrissage the calf (palmar kneading).

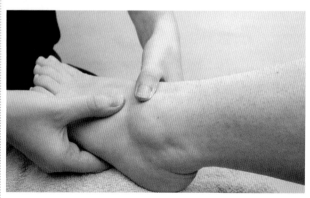

5. Thumb-kneading round the ankle bone.

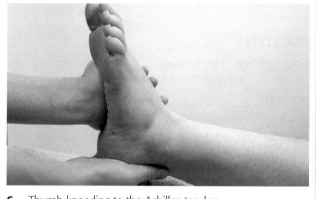

6. Thumb-kneading to the Achilles tendon.

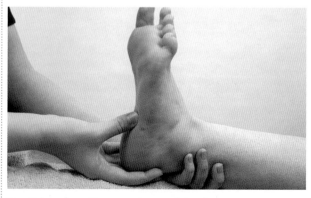

7. Palmar kneading over the medial arch.

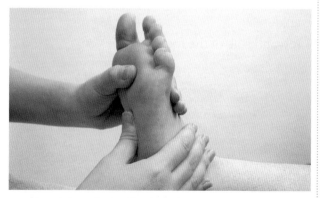

8. Thumb-kneading underneath the foot and toes.

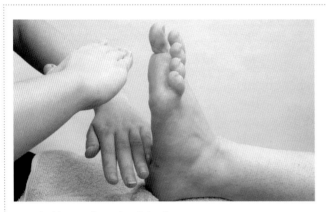

9. Hacking to the sole of the foot.

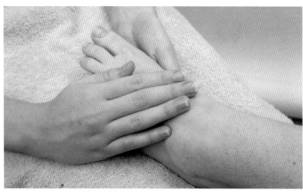

10. Deep stroking of the foot.

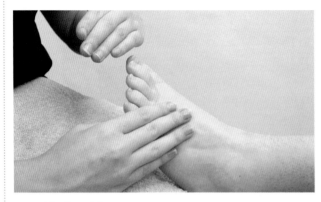

11. Whipping of the toes.

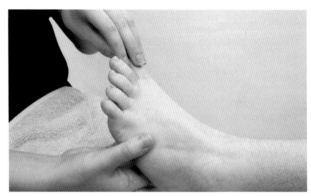

12. Toe snatching.

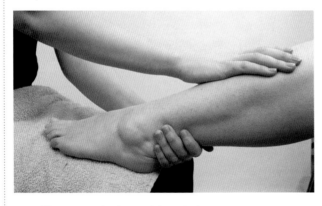

13. Effleurage to the leg and foot six times.

Nail polish application

The procedure for applying polish is very similar to manicure (as set out in Chapter 11), except that the nails, apart from the big toenail, are often small, making application more difficult.

Toes do not span naturally like fingers, so toe separators are required to keep them apart while the polish is drying. Toe separators made from foam can be obtained from beauty suppliers. However, as they cannot be sterilised easily, it is more appropriate to use folded tissues that can be disposed of after treatment. Disposable toe separators are also available.

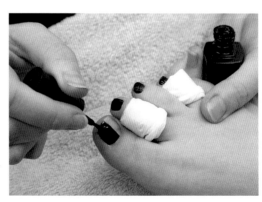

Special treatments

Re-polish

Regular pedicure clients may on occasions request that their nails are polished without a full pedicure. It may be that the client needs to change the nail colour to match an outfit or that they dislike the colour applied. Whatever the reason, a re-polish must only be carried out on perfectly pedicured nails to ensure that a professional finish can be achieved.

Re-polish routine

1. Cleanse the client's feet with surgical spirit. Soaking is not necessary unless the client requests it or you feel it is beneficial.

2. Briefly check the shape of the nails and file if necessary.

3. Remove polish from the nails of one foot and place in the pedicure bowl to soak. This will remove all traces of polish remover and cleanse the nails.

4. Remove the polish from the other foot and place it in the pedicure bowl, having removed the first foot.

5. Thoroughly dry the foot and check the cuticles. Remove any obvious bits of cuticle.

6. Apply hand cream and do a short massage routine to the feet.

7. Repeat on the other foot.

8. Wipe over the nails with polish remover soaked in cotton wool.

9. Apply nail polish in the usual way.

Heat treatments and skin conditioners for the feet and nails

A number of treatments can add to the enjoyment of a pedicure and also help to improve the condition of the client's feet and nails.

Treatments used by the beauty therapist on other parts of the body, for example moisturising masks and exfoliating treatments, can be adapted for use on the feet. The use of heat in conjunction with nourishing creams, oils or waxes can also be very beneficial. The heat required to increase the effectiveness and pleasure for the client can be supplied by:

- heating the material before application, as for paraffin wax or warm oil treatment

- applying hot towels that have been warmed either by soaking in hot water or by warming on a radiator or drying cabinet

- using electrical equipment such as an infrared lamp or thermastatically controlled electrically heated bootees.

Paraffin wax

Paraffin wax is solid and cloudy white in colour when cold. It is heated in a thermostatically controlled wax bath to a working temperature of around 49°C. Paraffin wax treatment is used to ease stiffness in the joints and to improve the texture, colour and condition of the skin. It heats the tissues by enclosing the area with warm wax.

This encourages:

- the skin to perspire
- erythema to develop
- increased activity in the sebaceous glands
- the pores to open, helping the nourishing cream, which has been applied to the hands or feet as part of the treatment, to be absorbed.

Some clients who suffer from rheumatism find this treatment helps to relieve pain and stiffness in the joints. The application of heat to the feet is very relaxing.

Procedure for paraffin wax treatment

The treatment is similar to that used in manicure. Refer to Chapter 11 for more details.

1. The wax must be heated in the wax bath at least 30 minutes before you need to use it. You will have to plan ahead to ensure the wax is properly melted and ready for use.
2. The manicure or pedicure is completed up to and including a brief hand/foot massage. A rich massage cream is applied and gently massaged into the area.
3. Test the temperature of the wax by first looking at its consistency. Then check the thermostat on the heater and apply wax to the inside of your wrist with a spatula.
4. Dispense the heated wax into a small bowl and quickly brush the wax onto the client's hands or feet (a small paintbrush is ideal).
5. Wrap the hand or foot in tin foil or a plastic bag and cover with a towel or use thermal bootees.
6. This process is repeated on the other foot.
7. The wax can be left on for up to 20 minutes, depending on how much time has been allowed for the pedicure. Ten minutes is adequate. Make sure the client is seated comfortably and relaxed.
8. Remove the wax from the first foot. The wax should peel off in one piece and be disposed of.
9. The foot is now in an ideal condition for massage. A full massage of 10 minutes should be given to ensure that the client receives the full benefit of the treatment. Repeat on the other foot.
10. Continue with the application of polish, taking extra care when wiping over the nails with polish remover to ensure that there are no traces of wax left on the nails which will prevent the polish adhering to the nail.

Safety precautions

1. Safety checks should be made on the electrical wax bath. The thermostat must be in good working order to ensure that the wax does not overheat.
2. Protect the client's clothing and the area around the wax bath during treatment. The process can be very messy.
3. Do not move the wax bath while it is hot.
4. Dispose of used wax immediately after use.

Oil treatment

The application of good quality warm vegetable oil to the feet can be very beneficial in treating dry cuticles and nails. Almond oil is ideal, but because of the quantities required it can prove expensive for use in pedicure. Olive oil is most commonly used, although it tends to have a distinctive smell.

Procedure for oil treatment

1. Apply warm oil liberally to the nails and feet.
2. Pay particular attention to the cuticles and dry areas of skin.
3. Wrap the feet in foil or cling film and apply hot towels or bootees.
4. Massage one foot at a time paying particular attention to the cuticles and hard skin.

As this is a remedial treatment, the client should be encouraged not to have polish applied.

This allows the nails and cuticles to benefit from the oil soaking in. Any excess can be removed with tissues. If the client prefers, the feet can be wiped over with witch hazel on a pad of cotton wool.

Masks

The condition of the feet can be also improved by proprietary brand masks that hydrate the skin. The masks are applied in the normal way, using a masking brush, and are removed after 10–15 minutes with warm water.

Exfoliating

Exfoliation is the removal of dead skin using mildly abrasive substances such as ground fruit kernels, oatmeal or salt. Exfoliation treatment for the feet is an important part of the pedicure and is used after applying the foot rasp. Exfoliants remove dry dead skin scale and smooth rough areas of skin.

Chemical exfoliants

These are more often used on the feet to treat the build-up of hard skin. An alkali breaks down the keratin in the skin, softening it. The product also contains grains that loosen the softened skin. The product must be rinsed off thoroughly to remove any traces of the alkali, which would irritate the skin. (Cuticle remover is a similar product that softens the cuticle to aid removal.)

Salt or oatmeal scrub

Salt is mixed to a paste with water or oil and rubbed on the feet with the pads of the fingers, using gentle friction movements. Oatmeal mixed and applied in the same way has a similar effect, but is a little gentler. The salt or oatmeal rub would come before foot massage in the pedicure routine.

Outcome 4: Provide aftercare advice

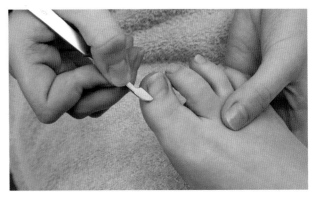

△ Therapist working on a client's feet

Aftercare advice

Offering advice to your clients after the pedicure will help them look after their feet between visits. It is also an opportunity to recommend retail products such as foot powders, sprays, foot baths and hard-skin remover.

Aftercare advice will differ for each client, depending on the condition of their feet. It may include the following:

- ❧ wash feet daily (more often if suffering from excessively sweaty feet and in hot weather)
- ❧ make sure feet are thoroughly dry after washing, especially between the toes
- ❧ change socks or tights daily
- ❧ allow the air to circulate around the feet by going barefoot whenever it is comfortable and safe to do so
- ❧ buy good quality shoes that fit properly (changing to shoes with different heels can help with tired feet)
- ❧ wearing very high heels over long periods of time should be avoided as they cause tired sore feet and poor posture
- ❧ avoid wearing synthetic shoes such as trainers over long periods of time as they cause the feet to sweat
- ❧ any infection or serious condition of the feet must be referred to a doctor or chiropodist (regular visits to a chiropodist may be necessary for some clients with ongoing foot problems).

Evaluation of treatment

It is essential at the end of any treatment to evaluate the treatment against the treatment plan.

- ❧ Have you met the client's expectations? Are they satisfied with the pedicure? Have you done what you set out to do in your treatment plan? This could be special attention to the cuticle or hard-skin removal, for example.
- ❧ Was the pedicure carried out in a commercially acceptable time? A pedicure will take longer than a manicure because of the time needed to treat the cuticles and hard skin. A client who cares for their feet and has regular pedicures will require 30–35 minutes for treatment. If the feet require extra attention, 50 minutes will be needed. The time you expect to take should be discussed with the client as part of the treatment plan.

Activity

Evaluate your pedicure treatment.

Evidence of your performance can be judged by:

- ✤ the client's comments – enter verbal or written comments in your diary or log
- ✤ colleagues in the workplace, who work with you and observe you – ask them to provide a written witness testimony
- ✤ your teacher or assessor, who will mark your assessment book.

≥• Was the pedicure of professional quality? You must aim to provide careful and accurate treatment in the best possible time to be commercially viable. Following your evaluation of the pedicure, was it the best you could do or are there things that require improvement and more practice?

Test yourself

1. Give two reasons why it is essential to soak the feet before starting a pedicure.

2. Name two professional practitioners to whom you might refer a client during the consultation for a pedicure treatment.

3. It is necessary to take extra care when using cuticle clippers on a client who has diabetes, to avoid cutting the cuticle too closely and causing bleeding. Why? (There are two possible answers.)
   a) It is unprofessional
   b) It can lead to infection
   c) It will stain clothing
   d) It will take a long time to heal

4. Name two conditions of the feet caused by wearing tight-fitting shoes

5. Toe nails should be cut and filed straight across
   a) because it is fashionable
   b) to avoid ingrowing toe nails
   c) to make it easier to apply nail polish
   d) so the nails do not press on the shoes.

6. Give one example of each of the following which may be found on the feet
   a) Fungal infection
   b) Viral infection
   c) Bacterial infection

Are you ready for assessment?

Remember . . .

Practice makes perfect! The more opportunities you have to complete a pedicure the more confident you will be when it comes to being observed by your assessor.

Remember . . .

Always keep your logbook handy.

The following checklist will help you to be fully prepared for your practical assessment.

The range of clients/treatments you must cover:

1. **Practical observation**
   Your assessor will look at how you:
   ≥• prepare the treatment area
   ≥• consult with the client and prepare a record card

Remember . . .

Your assessor will observe your performance on at least three occasions each involving a different foot and nail treatment from the range.

- carry out a pedicure on a client (not a fellow student or colleague) using a range of tools and products, carry out a special treatment from the range, carry out a foot and leg massage using suitable medium, apply nail polish covering each colour from the range
- carry out the pedicure in a commercially acceptable time
- check with the client that the pedicure meets her expectations
- provide aftercare advice
- demonstrate professional practice throughout the service
- carry out all treatments with regard to health and safety.

2. **Knowledge and understanding**

What you must know:

- Organisational and legal requirements.
- How to work safely and effectively when providing pedicure services.
- Consult, plan and prepare for treatment with clients.
- Contraindications and contra-actions.
- Anatomy and physiology.
- Pedicure treatments.
- Aftercare advice.

To ensure that you have the necessary knowledge and understanding of pedicure services your assessor will:

- ask you questions before, during and after carrying out the treatment
- ensure that you have completed project work and written exercises relating to the unit
- check that you have recorded in a log/diary treatments you have carried out with signed record cards showing that you have completed three pedicures competently
- check that you have covered the range in your candidate logbook
- require you to take a written test.

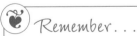
Remember . . .
Simulation is not a valid means of assessment for pedicure service.

Sources of evidence

- Record cards
- Treatment plans
- Video
- Witness statements
- Client feedback.

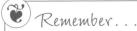
Remember . . .
The maximum commercially viable service time for a basic pedicure is 45 minutes.

Chapter 13

Unit N4: Carry out nail art services

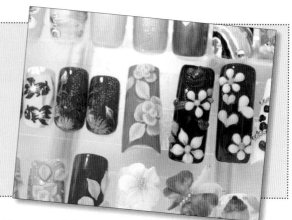

Learning objectives

This chapter is about creating designs for nail art and their application to the nails of the hands and feet.

> There are four learning outcomes for Unit N4 and they are:
> 1. Maintain safe and effective methods of working when providing nail art services.
> 2. Consult, plan and prepare for the nail art service.
> 3. Carry out nail art services.
> 4. Provide aftercare advice.
>
> You will need to be competent in all of these outcomes in nail art services.

Evidence requirements

Your assessor will need to observe you perform this treatment successfully on at least four occasions, each involving a different client. On one of these occasions nail art should be carried out on the feet. You must:

1. Demonstrate the use of consultation techniques:
   - questioning
   - visual
   - manual
   - reference to client records.

2. Take one of these necessary actions:
   - encourage the client to seek medical advice
   - explain why the treatment cannot be carried out
   - modify the treatment.

3. Apply these nail art techniques:
   - coloured polishes
   - transfers
   - glitters
   - foiling
   - flatstones
   - rhinestones
   - marbling
   - striping
   - dotting
   - freehand.

4. Provide this advice:
   - suitable aftercare products and their use
   - avoidance of activities which may cause contra-actions
   - recommended time intervals between nail services.

Introduction

Colour has been applied to the nails to improve their appearance and attract attention for many years. In China, thousands of years ago, coloured nails represented social class: colours such as gold and silver, black and red were reserved for use by royalty only and there were fatal consequences if this rule was not abided by.

Modern nail art involves the use of colour, transfers, glitter, stones and foils to take nail adornment to a new level. Nail art can complement an outfit and add that extra something for a special event or add a unique flair to the appearance of the nails every day.

Unit N4 'Carry out nail services' is for Level 2 NVQ Diploma in Nail Services only, and is worth four credits.

Meet the professional

"If you've got a creative flare use it. Experiment wherever possible. The possibilities are endless and you need to keep your clients interested. Your clients want the best and newest trends so keep up to date. This is a very fast-moving area so go to seminars, workshops and enter competitions. Learn more than one system – acrylics, gels, fibreglass and sculpting should all be considered. The more background information you have, the better.

Subscribe to professional nail magazines. These offer a wealth of latest ideas and courses. Advertise your skills to promote interest. Ask your clients if you can photograph the finished result to display in a reception booklet. This is a great way of building a portfolio to promote your work. Listen to what your clients are saying: they may have read an article in a magazine or seen a promotional event on daytime TV. If they've mentioned it to you they're more than likely to want to try it! Research it! The internet is excellent for finding out which star has had the latest new nail treatment.

Be a perfectionist! Clients can pick up the tiniest of details."

Jody Camplin

Remember . . .

Information on the structure and function of the skin, structure of the nail unit and the process of nail growth can be found in Chapter 19.

Outcome 1: Maintain safe and effective methods of working when providing nail art services

Preparing the work area for nail art services

A professionally set up area and a wide range of materials, tools and equipment are an essential part of a nail art service. Make sure you have a clean and steady desk to work at and a height-adjustable stool to maintain your posture. The client will also require a comfortable chair in which to relax.

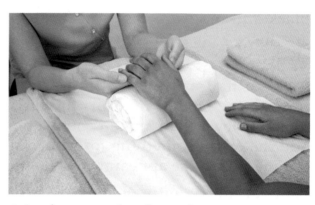

△ A work area set up for nail art services

- Tools and equipment should be readily available as designs can sometimes require a whole range of techniques.

- Have your polishes and a range of accessories to hand as this can sometimes catch the eye of potential new nail art clients.

- Lighting and ventilation are an important part of the service. Magnifying lamps or angle-poise lamps may be necessary to ensure you can see clearly. As you are working with solvents, adequate ventilation is also important.

- Hand-washing facilities need to be available, with a nail brush to clean the client's hands if you are not undertaking a full manicure service prior to a nail art service.

> ★ *Hints and tips*
> *Always have a portfolio of examples of your work to help your clients to understand the techniques involved in the designs. This can also advertise your skills to potential new nail art clients.*

 Remember . . .

All health and safety rules apply, as does a full client consultation, in which you can gain an understanding of the client's nail shape, condition and type, along with their requirements for the service. (Refer to Chapters 1 and 3.)

Personal appearance

If nail art services are being performed by a beauty therapist, the guidelines for personal appearance laid down in Chapter 1 apply. However, with the advent of nail salons and bars, a variation of the acceptable professional appearance for a nail technician can be described as follows:

- Clean comfortable clothing and footwear that meets the individual salon's or nail bar's requirements.

- Long hair should be tied back.

- Any jewellery that could come in contact with the client such as rings, bracelets or necklaces should be removed when performing nail services.

- Long nails and the wearing of nail enamel and nail art is acceptable and can act as promotion for the salon.

- A high level of personal hygiene is still expected.

Sterilisation, disinfection and hygiene procedures

To maintain levels of hygiene to avoid cross-infection the following procedures should be applied when carrying out nail art services:

- Clean towels and linens should be provided for each client.

- Towels and linens should be washed at a minimum of 60°C.

- Client's and nail technician's hands should be thoroughly washed using liquid soap and hot water before the commencement of the treatment.

- Disposable towels should be used to dry the hands.

- Work surfaces should be washed with detergent before wiping down with a disinfectant between services.

- Creams, lotions and sprays should be dispensed from pump-action bottles if possible, or a spatula should be used to dispense products from containers.

- Metal tools and equipment that could become contaminated with body fluids such as blood should be sterilised by a suitable method such as an autoclave.

- Use of single-use items is advised, so they can be disposed of after use

Chapter 1 gives more detail on suitable sterilising procedures.

Equipment, materials and products for nail art techniques

Tools required for a nail art service:

- Dotting/marbling tools – to create designs incorporating dots and marbling colours.

- Nail art brushes (fan, striping, shading, sable) – a variety of sizes for striping, freehand designs, rolling glitter, swirls and mixing colours.

- Foils – to create instant nail art.

- A variety of polishes – to provide a base for nail art, to blend colours, marble and create freehand pictures and designs.

- Rhinestones and flat stones – using a variety of sizes and colours to complement a design.

- Glitters – to complement all nail art designs.

- Transfers and stickers – a variety of sizes and designs to create fast and effective nail art designs.

- Polish securers and top coats – to fix the design in place and maintain the look.

- Adhesives and base coat – to adhere the designs, rhinestones and polishes to the nail.

- Orange wood stick – used for picking up small objects such as rhinestones.

> **Key term**
>
> **Sterilisation** – the process of making something free from germs.
>
> **Disinfection** – the process of cleansing something of infection; to destroy disease or germs.

 Remember . . .

Keep your nail art kit clean and tidy. Look after your products and clean your tools. This gives a good impression of your services.

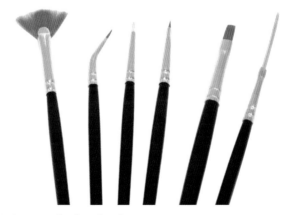

△ A range of nail art brushes

As a professional nail artist, a full range of tools, equipment and materials is required. A kit can never be complete – collecting materials, transfers, colours, gems, etc., can be an ongoing task. Remember to invest in a range, not just to your own taste – some clients may want all sorts of colours so do not presume the colours you like will suit everyone.

Nail art service times

Service times for nail art are dependent on the design and skill level of the student and the artwork required. As a general guide a 30-minute appointment is an acceptable time for a Level 2 student completing:

- basic freehand design
- opalescent paint effect
- marbling designs
- designs incorporating rhinestone and flatstone application, glitters, foils or transfers.

Outcome 2: Consult, plan and prepare for nail art services

Consultation techniques

As a professional nail artist you require good communication skills to obtain the correct information from a client and make them feel comfortable. There is a certain amount of personal information required, so a polite and friendly manner is vital in making a client feel at ease.

The consultation process is a very important part of any treatment. Gaining an understanding of a client's lifestyle and personality is key to understanding the client's choice of nail art design.

The medical history, personal details and hand and nail analysis should be recorded on the consultation card, along with signed consent or permission for the service to take place.

Every time a client has an appointment, the details of the service should be recorded as this shows the client a professional record of the previous design plans, which can be looked back on by the nail artist for future designs.

Treating minors

Nail art can be very exiting for young children as it is bright, colourful and often sparkling. It is becoming increasingly popular for children's parties and special occasions.

When treating minors you must ensure parental or guardian consent is obtained prior to any service. The parent or guardian must also be present during the service of minors under the age of 16.

 Hints and tips
There are so many easy ways of creating quick and effective nail art, so if you aren't as creative invest in some special-effects polishes or transfers that do the work for you.

Remember . . .
Always have a supply of disposable equipment and materials to hand, such as nail wipes, cotton wool and manicure roll.

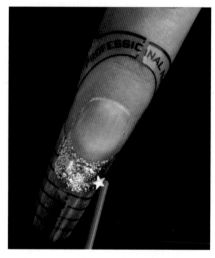
△ Some materials used in nail art: stones, glitters, foils and transfers

Hints and tips
Encourage clients who want a particular design to draw out or find a picture of the design they want as misinterpreting a design can be very easy.

 Remember . . .
Data Protection Act 1998 – the regulations governing the recording of individuals' personal details.

Contraindications

There are many conditions that can prevent a nail art service taking place. As a professional you must be able to recognise whether you can treat a client or not and give professional recommendations if you have to turn a client away.

Skin and nail diseases and disorders have already been described in Chapters 4 'B4 Provide facial skin care treatment' and 11 'N2 Provide manicure services' respectively.

Analysis of the hands and nails

During the consultation process an analysis of the hands and nails must be carried out. This process is usually carried out if a client is having a manicure prior to the nail art service as part of the manicure consultation. If the client is only having the nail art then the same process must be carried out. Wipe over the hands and nails with surgical spirit or an antibacterial product before you begin the visual and manual analysis, checking the skin, cuticles and nails.

For more detail about how to assess your client's hands and nails please refer to the 'Assessing the client's hands and nails for manicure' section in Chapter 11.

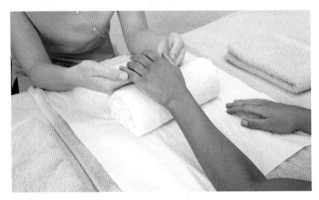

△ It is important to carry out an analysis of your client's hands and nails

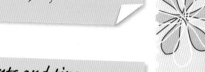

☆ **Hints and tips**
Never diagnose a condition as you could cause undue alarm to the client. Always refer them to a doctor.

☆ **Hints and tips**
Refer to the manicure unit for a detailed description and pictures of the most common contraindications

Recommendations for nail art design

As a professional nail artist it is important to choose designs to suit a client's lifestyle, occasion and personality. Gaining an understanding of the client's needs and expectations is vital to creating a suitable design for your client.

An up-to-date portfolio of your skills and previous designs can help a client identify what look and design they desire.

The nail shape, nail bed length, nail plate condition and the length of the free edge need to be considered when choosing a design with a client. A short nail bed and free edge will not suit an elaborate design as it can look too much; a simpler design can look classy and professional. If the nail plate is uneven or ridged then some careful buffing or ridge filler may be required prior to treatment.

Colour theory

A very important part of creating a nail art design for a client is to understand colour theory. Colour choices can be the making of a design or can just as easily ruin it. What looks good on one client may not suit another because of their skin tone. Some colours can make skin look radiant, while others can make a skin look dull.

Invest in a colour wheel to work with your client to see which shades of which colours suit their skin tone.

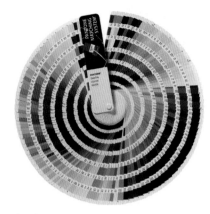

△ Colour wheels are useful when assessing what colours will suit a client's skin tone

Contra-actions

As with the use of all chemicals, the client may be allergic to the products used. An allergic reaction would appear as swelling and irritation around the nails and on the hands, but also – as with any allergic reaction – the eyes may become red and watery or, in the worst cases, breathing difficulties may occur.

Because nail art is invariably applied to nail extensions, the health and safety measures for nail extensions must be taken into account (see Chapter 14 for more information on this).

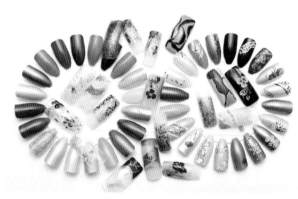

△ Nail art designs

If the allergic reaction occurs when the client is having nail extensions or nail art applied the process should be stopped immediately and the products removed. If the reaction occurs some time later (the curing of nail extension chemicals continues for up to 48 hours after the nail application) the nails must be removed with acetone. It may be the solvents used in nail extensions that are causing the reaction. In severe cases medical advice is required before attempting removal.

Outcome 3: Carry out nail art services

Preparation of the nail for nail art

After the consultation process and the nail art design have been planned, the preparation of the nail is vital. Not all clients will wish to have a manicure; it is, however, very important to prepare your canvas before applying your art. The skin and cuticles must be tidied and moisturised prior to treatment and the nail filed and buffed to a smooth finish. If the design requires a base coat of enamel this is the time to apply it. A base coat and two coats of colour will provide a good base to create the design. The application of the enamel has to be perfect to enhance the look.

If no base enamel colour is required, apply a base coat to give extra adhesion to the design.

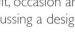 **Hints and tips**

Nail art is becoming increasingly popular on the toes, so don't miss an opportunity to increase business. Some clients don't think about their feet so advertise designs for the toes as well as the finger nails.

Remember...

Always consider the client outfit, occasion and style when discussing a design plan.

Activity

Practise some designs on nail tips – this can help to perfect your techniques and colour blending skills.

Applying nail art

There are no set rules in applying nail art. The way to achieve the best results is to play around with ideas and have fun with the products.

By using a selection of techniques, gems and glitter, etc., the therapist can produce original designs or work from templates and pictures.

French manicure (see Chapter 11 'N2 Provide manicure services') is the most basic type of nail art that a therapist will be asked to do for a client. This technique enhances the nail tip and the natural colour of the nail bed. The polish can be made to stand out even further by using different colours such as blue and white or red and yellow. The French manicure is a good base for nail art.

A basic technique for freehand decoration

1. Polish all ten nails, either with a coloured polish or a natural French manicure polish.
2. Select paint colours and a design.
3. Create a design by selecting from a range of freehand techniques: use a marbling tool to create dots of colour, a fan brush to create swirls, a liner brush for straight lines, or a shading brush to mix colours on the nail.
4. Always keep the design simple for a striking effect. The surface available does not allow for complicated designs.
5. Allow the paint to dry thoroughly. The nail paint tends to look dull when dry so a top coat is needed.
6. Apply a top coat – one coat to fix the paint and give shine and a second coat to give added protection to the artwork.

Opalescent paint effects

1. A dark nail polish is used on each nail and a thin application of opalescent nail paint that complements the nail colour is applied.
2. The nail paint can be applied with a fan brush, sweeping from side to side on the nail plate, or a liner brush can be used following the same action.
3. The paint appears white during application but dries to give an iridescent effect.
4. Take care not to over-blend and lose the effect.
5. Allow the nail paint to dry and apply two layers of top coat.

 Hints and tips
Well-manicured nails will complement nail art designs. Always advise your clients to have a manicure before the nail art service or incorporate it into treatment.

Hints and tips
Practice makes perfect and the simplest art can look just as effective as complicated designs.

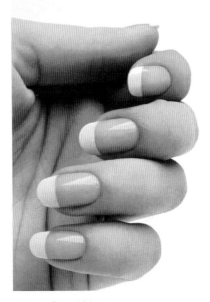
△ French manicure

Hints and tips
There are many special effects nail polishes available for creating fast and effective designs. Use these to enhance your designs or for an instant and easy design.

Marbling

This is a simple technique using the marbling tool.

1. Discuss the design and choice of colours with the client.
2. Apply the base coat and two coats of coloured nail polish, ensuring good coverage of the nail plate.
3. Place two different colours of nail paint on the artist's palette. Use only small amounts to avoid wastage.
4. Using the large end of the marbling tool, place one drop of each colour on one corner of the nail.
5. Make sure the marbling tool is clean before swirling one colour into another to create a marbling effect. Do not overwork or the effect will look messy.
6. Allow the paint to dry and apply two coats of top coat.

Water marbling

Another method of creating a marbling effect can be to use water. This is a little messy but can be very effective.

1. Prepare a medium-sized bowl of water (big enough to place your hand in) and fill half full with water.
2. Select two or three colours that will contrast well and try and select a black or white with your colours.
3. Add 2–3 drops of each colour into the water, one colour on top of another. Be careful not to drop the colours from too high or too fast as they will sink to the bottom of the bowl, they need to sit on the surface of the water.
4. Using your marbling tool, gently pull through the colours to marble them together. Less is more: do not mix up, just pull one colour into another.
5. Gently touch the nail plate on top of the water onto the polish design; do not push through the polish, just touch the surface.
6. To finish the look, clean around the cuticle and surrounding skin and apply a top coat.

Applying rhinestones and flat stones

Nail designs can be enhanced by the application of glitter, tiny stones and diamanté.

1. Flat stones and rhinestones come in a vast range of colours, sizes and shapes.
2. The stones are applied to wet polish early in the application of a design or at the end of the design by using a dot of top coat, or during the application of top coat.
3. A selection of stones can be placed on the artist's palette and when needed they are picked up individually using an orange stick dampened at the pointed end with water.

> ⭐ **Hints and tips**
> The choice of colours will depend on the client's preference, perhaps to match an outfit, or the therapist's creative skill.

> ⭐ **Hints and tips**
> Using acrylic paints instead of nail polish can give you more time to create your design. Nail polish can be used but with less time to perfect your design as it dries quicker.

> ⭐ **Hints and tips**
> This can create a great design but can be messy so practise your technique to perfect the design and eventually you will find ways of working without too much mess.

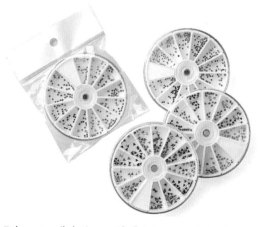

△ Enhance nail designs with flatstones or rhinestones

4. Flat stones have a flat edge and sit well on the nail.

5. The design and the stones are further secured and protected with two coats of top coat.

Applying glitter

Applying glitter involves rolling the glitter on the nail with a sable brush that has been dipped in glitter dust mixer.

1. Discuss the design and choice of colours with the client.

2. Apply the base coat and two coats of coloured nail polish, ensuring good coverage of the nail plate.

3. The glitter may be part of a design or complete the design.

4. Use the mixer product, allowing the glitter to stick to it and then apply by rolling the bead of glitter over the nail.

5. Circular movements are used to distribute the glitter rather than drag the product over the nails, which tends to separate the glitter particles.

6. Leaving some parts of the nail free from glitter allows the polish colour to shine through, giving a good effect.

7. Apply two coats of top coat.

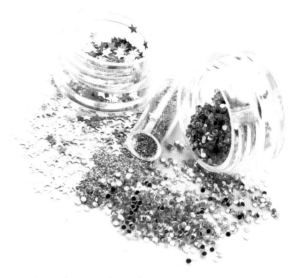

△ Applying glitter on the nail

> **Remember . . .**
> Taking care of the tools and materials used in nail art ensures they will last for a long time.

Foils

Foiling produces a unique effect. There is no other technique that quite matches the effect achieved with foil.

The foil comes in rolls or sheets and is bonded on to a clear backing. The foil adhesive that is placed on the nail releases the foil from the backing, leaving the design made by the adhesive on the nail.

1. Base coat and nail polish is applied to each nail. A clear nail can be achieved by using two coats of good quality base coat.

2. Ensure the polish is dry and apply foil adhesive sparingly in the area where the foil is to be placed. The adhesive is white, making it easy to see the design made, especially on dark polish.

3. Once the adhesive becomes clear it is ready for the foil to be applied.

4. Place the foil over the adhesive and rub the foil with a cotton bud to ensure it is firmly stuck to the adhesive.

5. Lift the backing away from the nails.

6. Apply two coats of top coat to seal and protect the design.

> ☆ **Hints and tips**
> Allow enough time for the adhesive to go clear. Do not rush this process as it can spoil your design if the adhesive has not dried completely clear, as the foil will not stick and you can end up with a gap in your design.

Transfers

Applying designs to the nails using transfers is less time-consuming than freehand designs and does not require so much skill and creative ability. Transfers may be self-adhesive or released by moistening the back of the transfer with a wet cotton-wool bud. The transfer is applied to the polished nails and covered with two coats of top coat.

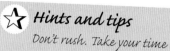
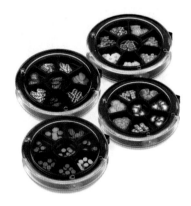

△ Transfers

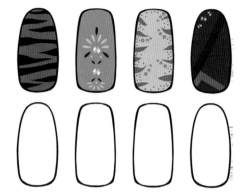

△ Try out your own ideas

The art of nail design

The range of nail designs is endless. It is the creativity of the therapist or nail technician that comes to the fore when designing and applying nail art. By using the vast range of products, colour combinations and techniques available, the therapist can be as creative as their imagination and skill allow.

Finishing the nail art design

On completion of your design apply a nail art sealer to hold your design in place, allow drying for a few minutes before applying a top coat to give the design a high-gloss finish.

You can advise your clients to apply a top coat every 2–3 days to keep the design looking shiny and maintain the polish.

Allow the whole completed design to dry for up to 10 minutes (which we call touch dry) and apply a cuticle oil all over the surface of the nail and cuticle. Allow time for the oil to be absorbed into the cuticle. This will cut off the oxygen supply to the polish and allow for faster drying; it will also rehydrate the cuticles and make the skin look moisturised and healthy.

Disposal of waste and completion of the treatment

To complete the treatment ask your client's permission to photograph the design. This will build your portfolio and show your clients you are proud of what you have created. Ensure you retail the necessary products to your client to maintain the design and to profit your business, as this is added income for your salon.

Waste disposal is a very important part of the service. Non-contaminated waste, for example cotton wool and paper towel should be placed in a lined metal bin with a lid. This will keep any

Activity

Create some of your own nail design ideas.

Don't forget when designing to take account of:

❖ the colours of nail paint and polishes you have available

❖ the material you have available

❖ the client's preferences

❖ the degree of skill you have. Do not attempt something too difficult and complicated. Simple designs often look the most effective.

⭐ *Hints and tips*
Know your own limits. Don't try a new design on a client – practise on a nail tip first and don't agree to it if you're not confident. An unpractised design can be very unprofessional and ruin the service.

vapours from solvents such as enamel remover and polishes inside. This waste should be removed every day, sealed and placed into a normal rubbish bin.

Any spillages or unused solvents that require disposal must be soaked up into paper tissue while wearing gloves and disposed of in the metal bin.

Client record cards

To comply with the Data Protection Act accurate client records are to be made on completion of each service and stored securely for future reference. Whether records are stored electronically with a password or paper-based and stored in a locked filing cabinet, the records must be updated on every visit to the salon.

The salon's insurance will require the records to be updated with the history of the client's visits, the service they had and updated medical history, with dates they attended for treatment.

This can also help a nail artist to gain an understanding of the client's history of nail art, what they have had before and the type of designs they like.

Outcome 4: Provide aftercare advice

Advice and recommendations

As a professional nail artist offering aftercare advice is part of the service. Advice on how to maintain the nail art and future treatments is essential to complete the treatment.

For future treatments it really depends on your client. A manicure would be advised every 2–4 weeks, therefore if the client requires a painted finish then that could be applied following the regular manicure. Some clients will only have a nail art design for special occasions and some will want a different design every week.

Retail advice is expected to increase the profit of the business as well as ensuring your clients leave the salon with the correct products to apply to their nails. A top coat and cuticle oil are key to the longevity of the design, while a nail enamel remover can be recommended to remove the design.

As well as retail advice, recommend to your client how to look after the design and their nails:

- Always wear gloves when washing up or gardening.
- Do not use your nails as tools.
- Always dry your hands thoroughly when washing and apply a hand cream to moisturise.
- Use a nail strengthener or protein to maintain the health of your nails.
- Apply a top coat every 2–3 days to prevent the design chipping and to keep the shine.
- Apply cuticle oil or cream at night to nourish and condition the cuticles.

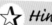

☆ *Hints and tips*

Home care for your nail art clients is essential to allow the designs to last longer. Applying a top coat to maintain the design and a cuticle oil to moisturise the cuticle are also a great way to retail products to your client.

Want to know more?

A copy of the Code of Practice for Nail Services can be downloaded from the Habia website at www.habia.org.

Test yourself

1. How do you dispose of solvent waste?
   a) place it in a plastic bin with no lid
   b) soak the solvent up in paper tissue and place it in a metal bin with a lid
   c) make sure the lid is on tight and throw the whole bottle in the bin
   d) dispose of the solvent down the sink.

2. Which of the following contraindications would prevent the nail art service taking place?
   a) viral, bacterial and fungal infections
   b) minor eczema and psoriasis
   c) brittle nails
   d) overgrown cuticles.

3. What age is a client considered a minor?
   a) under 21
   b) under 12
   c) under 16
   d) under 14.

4. From the following list what do you consider are important questions on a consultation card?
   a) medical history
   b) client signature
   c) contraindications
   d) all of the above.

5. Following a nail art service which product would you recommend for aftercare advice?
   a) a nail file
   b) top coat
   c) exfoliate
   d) a buffer.

6. List three nail art techniques.

7. What is the legal act that protects clients' personal information?

8. When setting up your work area for a nail art service, what do you consider to be essential?

9. What information do you require from your client when choosing a nail art design?

10. Name three pieces of aftercare advice you would give to a client following a nail art service.

Are you ready for assessment?

 Remember...

Practice makes perfect! The more opportunities you have to complete a nail art service the more confident you will be when it comes to being observed by your assessor.

The following checklist will help you to be fully prepared for your practical assessment.

The range of clients/treatments you must cover:

1. **Practical observation**

 Remember...

Your assessor will observe your performance on at least four occasions, each involving a different client. You must include and use all of the techniques from the range, all consultation techniques and at least one necessary action and provide all of the service advice.

Your assessor will look at how you:

- prepare the treatment area
- consult with the client and prepare a record card
- carry out a nail art service on a client (not a fellow student or colleague) using a range of tools and products
- carry out nail art services using a range of techniques
- carry out the nail art service in a commercially acceptable time
- check with the client that the nail art service meets her expectations
- provide aftercare advice
- demonstrate professional practice throughout the service
- carry out all services with regard to health and safety.

2. **Knowledge and understanding**

What you must know:

- Organisational and legal requirements.
- How to work safely and effectively when providing nail art services.
- How to consult, plan and prepare for nail art services with clients.
- Contraindications and contra-actions.
- Anatomy and physiology.
- Nail art services.
- Aftercare advice.

 Remember...

Simulation is not a valid means of assessment for nail art service.

To ensure that you have the necessary knowledge and understanding of nail art services your assessor will:

- ask you questions before, during and after carrying out the treatment
- ensure that you have completed project work and written exercises relating to the unit
- check that you have recorded in a log/diary treatments you have carried out with signed record cards showing that you have completed four nail art services competently
- that you have covered the range in your candidate logbook.

 Remember...

The maximum commercially viable service time for a nail art service is 30 minutes.

Chapter 14

Unit N5: Apply and maintain nail enhancements to create a natural finish

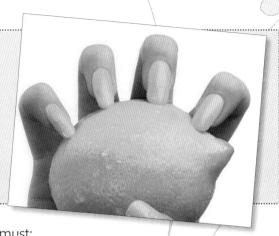

Learning objectives

This chapter is about the application of nail enhancements to create a natural finish on the nails of the hands and feet, and the maintenance and removal of nail enhancements.

There are seven learning outcomes for Unit N5 and they are:
1 Maintain safe and effective methods of working when enhancing, maintaining and removing nail enhancements.
2 Consult, plan and prepare for nail enhancement services.
3 Apply natural overlays.
4 Apply tip and overlays.
5 Maintain nail enhancements.
6 Remove nail enhancements.
7 Provide aftercare advice.

You will need to be competent in all of these outcomes in the application and maintenance of nail enhancements to create a natural finish, qualify for insurance and perform the treatment on members of the public.

Evidence requirements

Your assessor will need to observe you using one of: gel, liquid and powder, or wrap, on at least six occasions, which must include:
- one application of a full set of natural nail overlays
- one full set of tips and overlays
- two maintenance and repair of a full set of nail enhancements
- one removal of a full set of tips and overlays.

You must:

1 Demonstrate the use of consultation techniques:
- questioning
- visual
- manual
- reference to client records.

2 Take one of the following necessary actions:
- encourage the client to seek medical advice
- explain why the treatment cannot be carried out
- modify the treatment.

3 Apply these types of service:
- full set of natural nail overlays
- full set of natural tips and overlays.

4 Carry out these types of nail maintenance:
- infill
- rebalance.

5 Provide advice on:
- suitable aftercare products and their use
- avoidance of activities which may cause contra-actions
- recommended time intervals between nail services.

Introduction

Nail enhancements have been used for many years. The UK industry has grown and to support this increase in demand, many more salons and nail bars have opened to provide up-to-date services in nailcare, nail enhancement and nail art. The nail industry is changing constantly so it is important for the therapist or nail technician to keep up to date through training courses and by reading manufacturers' literature.

When a therapist is qualified in different nail enhancement systems there are a number of career opportunities: specialising as a nail technician, working in a nail salon or adding nail enhancement services as an extra dimension to treatments offered as a beauty therapist.

Unit N5 'Apply and maintain nail enhancements to create a natural finish' is a mandatory unit for Level 2 NVQ Diploma in Nail Services and is worth eight credits.

Meet the professional

"Practise! Practise! Practise! Don't leave rough edges. Buff to a very high shine so etching on the surface can't be seen. Get the nail shape right and the balance. Most systems have a different application and ratio (liquid/powder) technique. Perfect this before you work on clients. If you don't, clients will complain about lifting and breaking and they won't come back. Always check the length and shape with the client and advise accordingly."

Outcome 1: Maintain safe and effective methods of working when enhancing, maintaining and removing nail enhancements

Preparing the salon environment for nail enhancement

During nail enhancement services, strong chemicals are used and hazardous dust is created. Without protection and with continued exposure, the nail technician or therapist will be at risk from work-related disease or disorders. Under the Control of Substances Hazardous to Health Regulations 1988 (COSHH), the employer has a duty of care to put control measures into place for their employees' protection.

By carrying out a risk assessment, the employer can determine the main sources of fumes and dust and the types of exposure (inhalation, digestion and absorption). Appropriate control measures must be put in place.

Health and safety

COSHH regulations are about the use, storage and disposal of potentially harmful substances used during everyday activity while at work.

Preventing inhalation

Natural ventilation such as an open window allows fresh air to circulate through the work area, reducing exposure to fumes. The installation of artificial ventilation such as extractor fans is expensive but may be necessary and should 'extract' to the outside environment and not into another room in the building. The immediate work position or nail station should have an extraction facility that contains within it a filter mechanism. This will greatly reduce the amount of dust by drawing it into the filter and away from the lungs. Additionally, portable extractor fans, which work in a similar way, can be placed on the station during the 'dust creating' procedures of the service. The filters in such units and stations must be changed frequently to be effective.

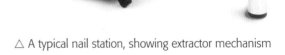

△ A typical nail station, showing extractor mechanism

The technician or therapist should follow some general rules in order to reduce the risks of exposure even further. They are:

1. Do not dispense chemicals for use until needed.

2. Dispense only small quantities of chemicals for use at the nail station.

3. Wipe brushes and spills. Soak excess chemicals into a tissue and dispose of into a lined metal pedal bin.

4. Use only lined metal pedal bins with lids that close automatically for the exposure of such chemicals, so that the fumes are contained. Do not use an open bin.

5. Empty the waste bin frequently. Tie the liner tightly, then place into an external bin. Do not allow the full bin liner to sit in a storage area within the building.

Preventing ingestion

Measures to prevent ingestion require the technician or therapist to wash their hands thoroughly after performing each nail enhancement service and before eating food. No food or drink should be consumed at the nail station but water contained within a sealed plastic bottle can be made available. Clients should also be made aware of such risks and be told not to place the nails or fingers in their mouths.

Preventing absorption

The technician or therapist can greatly reduce absorption of the chemicals through their skin by covering open wounds on their hands and by washing the hands thoroughly should any chemical accidentally get onto them. Non-latex, powder-free gloves can be worn by the technician or therapist throughout the treatment if exposure cannot be avoided.

The technician or therapist should regulate the amount of exposure to the chemicals that clients receive by avoiding the skin surrounding the nail as much as possible. Clients must be given good aftercare advice so that they are made aware of the potential risks to themselves while wearing a set of nail enhancements.

Care must also be taken when dispensing chemicals to avoid spillages as well as absorption, ingestion or inhalation.

Providing personal protective equipment

Personal protective equipment (PPE) such as non-latex, powder-free gloves should be worn for the dispensing of chemicals used in nail enhancement from large containers to smaller ones. They should also be worn by the technician or therapist when using such chemicals if it is recommended on the manufacturers" Material Safety Data Sheet (MSDS). Safety glasses should be made available and worn where there is a risk of 'splash' from such chemicals or flying debris when clipping nails. These should be made from a solvent-resistant material and have side protection panels in addition to the front panels to provide adequate protection. Safety glasses can be offered to clients for use during the nail enhancement service.

A dust mask offers the technician or therapist some protection from the dust created during a nail enhancement service. However, most are generally ineffective against the fumes created by the chemicals in use. Natural and artificial ventilation are more effective control measures to protect against the harmful effects of fumes from hazardous chemicals.

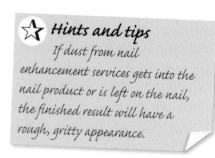

☆ *Hints and tips*
If dust from nail enhancement services gets into the nail product or is left on the nail, the finished result will have a rough, gritty appearance.

Lighting, mood and atmosphere

There should be sufficient light to enable the therapist or nail technician to carry out close and detailed work. A lamp over the nail station can provide more intense light when needed during the service.

A nail bar can be a lively work environment with music playing that is upbeat and popular (for example, a favourite radio station). Nail technicians and clients sit in close proximity and the atmosphere may be similar to that of a hairdressing salon.

A nail treatment station within a spa area or traditional beauty salon may be very different to that of a nail bar, with music and decor that creates peace and tranquillity and an atmosphere where clients can relax away from the stresses of everyday life.

Preparing the technician or therapist for nail enhancement

The importance of professional personal hygiene and appearance and good communication skills is dealt with in Chapter 1.

The technician or therapist must wash their hands thoroughly before and after each client but the hands can be sterilised during the service with an appropriate hand-steriliser spray containing alcohol. The wearing of polish, nail art and enhancements by the nail technician is acceptable work place practice as this acts as a promotional tool for the services offered.

It is advised that contact lenses should not be worn when handling nail enhancement products and chemicals as any accidental 'splashes' into the eye will cause the lens to melt and adhere to the eye. In addition, the dust produced during nail enhancement services can be absorbed by contact lenses and scratch the surface of the eye. Protective safety glasses should be worn when dispensing products and by clients who wear contact lenses.

Preparing the work station for nail enhancement

Both the client and the technician or therapist must be sitting comfortably to avoid repetitive strain and musculo-skeletal disorders (RSD and MSD), which may be caused by over-stretching and bending when sitting at the nail station for a long time.

1. Ensure the nail station is at the correct height for working. It should be a standard desk height but narrower to prevent the need for over-stretching.

2. Chairs with a supportive back pad that can be adjusted to the correct height should be used.

3. Foot rests should be used if the technician or therapist cannot place their feet flat on the floor with their chair at the correct height for work.

4. Store items for use between knee and shoulder height.

5. Do not twist or turn the body to access products and equipment. Instead, move the feet, taking them in the same direction as the body.

6. An elbow- or wrist-support pad should be provided for the technician or therapist and for the client to prevent RSD at the wrist.

7. Avoid gripping tools and equipment tightly. Use only sufficient grip to use and control the item.

8. Practise stretching exercises for the fingers, hands, wrists, arms, shoulders and neck regularly.

9. Take regular breaks from an activity. By managing the booking system, tasks can be varied, breaking up long and demanding tasks with smaller tasks that are less straining.

The nail station and trolley should contain all the tools, products, materials and equipment required for the service. This saves time and avoids unnecessary disturbance to the client. The trolley should be covered with disposable, absorbent paper to soak up any spillages and the clean tools and equipment laid out for ease of reach and application. For suitable sterilisation methods and procedures for tools and equipment, refer to Chapter 1.

Treatment times for nail enhancement services

The table below provides the commercially accepted treatment times for nail enhancement services.

▽ Nail enhancement treatment times

Service description	Service time
Nail enhancements – full set	2 hours
Nail wraps – full set	2 hours
Nail enhancements – infill	2 hours
Nail enhancement – maintenance	60–90 minutes
Overlays	90 minutes

Products, chemicals and equipment

Specialised products, tools and equipment are used in nail extensions. In particular, the chemicals used can be toxic if not handled with great care.

Nail sterilisers are alcohol-based sprays that are used before the nail enhancement system to prevent bacterial and fungal growth occurring between the natural nail and the nail extension.

Primers cleanse and dehydrate the nail plate. They draw moisture from the nail and remove surface oil and bacteria from the nail plate, and provide a surface for the acrylic to adhere to. Primers must not be allowed to come into contact with the surrounding skin as they are highly caustic They must be allowed to dry before continuing to the next stage of the procedure.

Nail tips are plastic or nylon nail shapes that are used to extend a short, natural nail.. They are available in different sizes, lengths and curvatures to suit and fit most natural nails with some customisation.

Acrylic powders are polymers; a long chain of chemical units such as polymethyl methacrylate.

Acrylic liquids are monomers such as ethyl methacrylate; chemical units that can form a polymer.

 Health and safety

Nail primers are corrosive and must therefore be used sparingly. Systems are being developed that do not require primer.

When mixed together, the liquid and powder create a chemical reaction that produces a substance that is a durable and strong nail enhancement. The powder comes in a range of colours, for example pink and white, to create a French manicure effect.

Gel products contain monomers, which, when exposed to ultraviolet light (UV), form polymers that harden to form the nail enhancement.

Wrap products include paper, fibreglass, silk and linen mesh, usually in strips that are cut to size. The strips may have adhesive backing to aid positioning on the nail.

Wrap adhesives are used if the fabric has no adhesive backing.

Adhesive sprays are used to set the wrap adhesive.

Fibreglass resin is a liquid used with the fibreglass system to provide overlays on tips.

Resin activator is a chemical that is sprayed onto the fibreglass and resin to speed up the setting/hardening process of the resin.

> **Health and safety**
>
> Methyl Methacrylate (MMA) has been banned for use in the USA and several local health authorities in the UK due to the extreme exothermic reaction and the effect of this heat on the nail and skin. It has been replaced by Ethyl Methacrylate (EMA).

Tools and equipment

Cuticle tools – a variety of tools can be used but the most popular are the cuticle pusher, which is used to push and lift the cuticle from the natural nail plate. This is important to ensure that the nail enhancement system adheres to the natural nail and the finished extension fits as closely as possible.

Stork scissors – a very fine bladed pair of scissors, used to cut and trim nail wrap fabric such as silk.

Nail forms – these are made of pliable metal, plastic or paper and enable a nail to be built up using a range of systems.

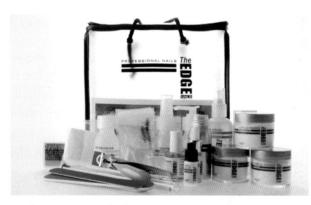

△ The variety of nail enhancement products

Brushes – these are usually made of sable and are available in different sizes. They are important tools for applying the products that form the nail. The brushes must be cared for by being cleaned immediately after use. A monomer liquid is effective for cleaning brushes, rather than soap and water. However, it dries out the sable hair.

Files and buffers – there are various shapes and sizes based on a grading according to their 'grit' size. The coarser the surface, the lower the grit number: 60–100 are coarse files used for shaping; 100–180 are used on acrylic and UV gel; while 240 grit is fine grade and is used for blending and smoothing.

Tip cutters – these are designed to give a clean cut when shortening and shaping nail tips.

Dappen dishes – these are small, glass screw-top containers that are used to hold small amounts of monomer liquid. The small neck of the dish reduces the surface area of the liquid exposed, limiting evaporation of the product.

A UV light box is used to cure UV gel nail enhancement systems. The product is placed under the light to cure or harden in the required shape. The light may 'flicker' when it is first turned on, so clients or therapists suffering from epilepsy should be advised to look away at this time. Viewing the light is not hazardous but looking directly at the UV bulb when illuminated should be avoided.

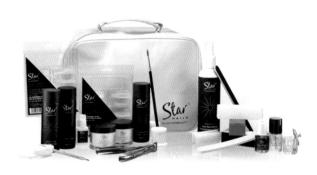

△ Tools and equipment used in nail enhancement services

Outcome 2: Consult, plan and prepare for nail enhancement services

The specific requirements of consultation for nail enhancement are to establish the client's needs, preferences and suitability for the service. It is particularly important to carry out a consultation, to prepare a treatment plan and agree the finished result.

Client suitability for nail enhancement services

As with all services of this kind it is important to check for contraindications to treatment. Details of appropriate questioning techniques to use during the consultation are given in Chapter 1. These techniques should be used to identify the presence of skin and nail diseases and disorders, as described in Chapters 11, 12 and 13.

Some conditions that will prevent or restrict nail enhancement services are:

- onycholysis (separation of the nail from the nail bed or other damage)
- severe eczema, psoriasis or dermatitis
- allergic reactions to the chemicals and products used.

Those that restrict treatment are:

- onychophagy (severely bitten nails)
- mild eczema, psoriasis or dermatitis
- minor nail separation
- bruising of the nail or finger
- cuts or torn cuticle around the nails
- swelling due to unknown cause
- erythema.

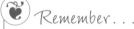

Remember...

The guidelines for treating minors – in England a client is considered a minor if they are under the age of 18 years of age; in Scotland it is 17 years of age and written parental/guardian permission is needed before treatment. The parent/guardian will need to also accompany the client if they are under 16 years of age.

Conducting a nail and skin analysis

A thorough analysis of the nail and skin condition will not only ensure the client's suitability and safety for treatment but also establish their needs and requirements. You should include a visual and manual assessment. Referral to the client's record card can reveal the details of any previous treatments.

A healthy nail has a pink nail body and a white free edge; is smooth and shiny, firm but flexible and is free from splits, flaking and damage. Thin, fragile and ridged nails do not provide a suitable surface on which to fix nail enhancements.

The cuticle and nail wall should be smooth, flexible and unbroken for safe and hygienic nail enhancement services to take place and there should be no cuticle adhering to the nail plate. Skin should appear smooth and unbroken and free from disease.

Assessing the client's needs and expectations

You will need to discuss the following with the client to enable you to make recommendations and prepare a treatment or service plan:

- the client's reasons for wanting nail enhancement applied
- the occupation/lifestyle of the client to establish whether nail extensions are suitable
- the suitability of each system
- nail shape and length required
- aftercare advice and maintenance.

There are many reasons why a client may seek nail enhancement services. For example:

- to enhance poor quality nails
- for a special occasion
- fashion trends
- for good personal grooming
- professional reasons (for example, model, actress)
- out of curiosity.

There are certain professions/occupations, hobbies and activities where nail extensions would be unsuitable, for example:

- occupations: nurses, those working with food, cleaners, dentists, those handling money
- activities: most sports, caring for young children, housework
- hobbies: using computers, playing cards, pottery, gardening.

Nail shape and length

Nail technicians have become more creative, designing the most dramatic looks through new products, new technology and nail art. These designs are always great for fashion photography, competitions and styling, but most clients need a design that is natural and durable. The client's lifestyle and occupation will therefore influence the length and shape of the artificial nails applied.

There are a number of factors that the technician or therapist must take into consideration when deciding the length and shape of the artificial nails.

Client's occupation:

- Do they work with their hands all day?
- What type of equipment or tools do they work with?
- Are their hands in water for much of the day?

Hobbies:

- Do they play sport, and if so, what type?
- Do they swim?

Lifestyle:

- Do they have young children?
- Do they do a lot of housework?
- Do they have the time to maintain the nail enhancements?

The occasion:

- Are the nails for a special occasion, for example a wedding?
- Are they for a holiday and will the client be swimming?
- Are the nails to help the natural nails grow?
- Does the client intend to keep the nail enhancements on for a long period of time?

Some clients have natural nail shapes that are not suitable for nail enhancements, or the condition of the nails is so poor the technician or therapist has to advise the client to have regular manicures to improve the condition of the nails and cuticles before embarking on nail enhancement services.

By obtaining the above information a technician or therapist can decide on:

- how best to meet the client's needs and preferences
- how long the nail extensions should be
- the best system to use
- the maintenance requirements.

A client who works with their hands, be it at home or at work, may be advised to keep nails a more natural length and shape due to the stress and strain that may be applied to them. There will be less need to repair breaks and replace nails.

A client who is having the enhancements for a special occasion, perhaps a wedding or a holiday, may prefer a more exotic design. Many clients request that nails are kept at the longest length possible. However, they must be advised that the nails may not be durable, are not as easy to maintain and are less practical.

A client who is having the enhancements to help support their natural nail, for example in the case of very brittle nails or if they bite their nails, is best advised to keep the extension to a shorter length. This will give the natural nail beneath support and help the client to get used to the feeling of a longer nail.

Remember . . .

Client consultation is essential to establish the length and shape of the artificial nails.

A client who is having the enhancements for a one-off occasion and does not intend to keep and maintain them can afford to have whatever length they desire. However, they should understand the restrictions that very long nail enhancements are subject to in terms of everyday activities, such as washing up. For example, long nails can easily be torn from the natural nail plate if they catch in clothing, causing damage to the natural nail and surrounding cuticle. The nail technician or therapist must ensure that they follow manufacturer's guidelines to ensure the nails are secure and stable.

> ★ *Hints and tips*
> The application has to be practical as well as flattering. Straight-sided nails with a slightly rounded tip have a strong shape and have the effect of making the fingers appear longer and more slender.

Nail enhancement systems

When you have analysed the client's nails and skin and determined their needs and expectations, you can choose the most appropriate nail enhancement system.

There are three main systems:

- acrylic liquid and powder
- UV gel
- wrap – fibreglass or silk.

Acrylic powder and liquid system

This system consists of two components: a monomer liquid and a polymer powder, which when brought together form a soft paste that can be moulded with a brush onto the nail or nail form to create the desired shape and length.

The brush is dipped into the liquid first, then into the powder to form a bead that is transferred to the nail and shaped with the brush. Keep the product away from the cuticle and nail wall. The brush used to apply the product is very important because it will affect how much liquid can be held and this can alter the bead size. The brush should be good quality sable and tapered, with no flared hairs to spoil the bead size.

Care of the brush is equally important. It should be cleaned with monomer after use and reshaped before storing. The brush should not be cleaned with soap and water as the detergent will dry out the sable hairs, making it difficult to use.

The process is repeated, shaping the paste until the desired effect is achieved and the product hardens on the nail. This hardening is achieved by a process called polymerisation and will result in the production of a mild heating sensation.

▽ Advantages and disadvantages of acrylic powder and liquid system

Advantages	Disadvantages
The nails are strong, flexible and hard-wearing	It is the most difficult system to master
A permanent French manicure can be achieved	The nails take time to remove
Maintenance is quick and easy	Very good ventilation is required as odours can be a problem
Irregular nail shapes can be corrected	
When nails are applied well they look very natural	

UV gel system

Gel systems are either derived from acrylic gel or the type of gel used to mould false teeth. Most gels are hardened by exposing the product to a source of UV light such as a specially designed lamp but some harden when sprayed with a special product called a 'gel activator'.

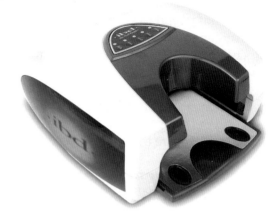

△ A typical UV lamp or light source

The gels come in containers already mixed and have a thick consistency with a low odour. They are available in different colours to give the appearance of wearing nail polish, including 'French'. Those used in gel overlay services have a 'self levelling' feature. The gel is taken from the container with a clean brush, placed onto the nail and shaped with the brush (keeping the product away from the cuticle and nail wall). When all the nails on one hand are ready they are placed under the UV lamp to 'cure' (harden).

This system is one of the easiest to use. It works very well for clients who have their hands in water a great deal because it cannot be soaked off. Removing the application can take some time: 30–45 minutes using buffing and files. Extreme care must be taken when removing the gel to avoid damage to the natural nail plate.

▽ Advantages and disadvantages of the UV gel system

Advantages	Disadvantages
It is easy to apply	Gels are not as strong and hard-wearing as liquids and powders
It cannot be soaked off	The nails are not easy to remove
The nails can be slightly more flexible than with other systems	Gels have a higher risk of allergic reaction
This system produces a permanent high gloss	Some gels produce heat during the curing process
When nails are applied well they look very natural	Very good ventilation is required

Wrap or fibreglass/silk system

This system is made up of three products: fabric mesh or wrap (which can be fibreglass mesh or a natural silk fibre providing a cross linked structure for strength), a resin of ethyl cyanoacrylate or a liquid adhesive and a resin activator used to dry or cure the resin.

Wraps and resins vary considerably, so it is essential that the manufacturer's information and instructions are read carefully.

The fabric is bought in strips, usually in a dispenser, to avoid dust or handling by uncovered hands, as oil from the skin will create a barrier to the resin. There are different weaves of fabric and some have a gentle adhesive backing to aid application.

Resins also vary in consistency and when they age they become yellow and brittle, which makes them unusable. Resins are hardened (cured) by an activator or accelerator, which speeds up the time needed to set. The activator may be spray or brush-on.

This system has always been known as the weakest of them all. However, there are positive aspects to choosing this system over the others.

▽ Advantages and disadvantages of the wrap or fibreglass/silk system

Advantages	Disadvantages
It is a very gentle system for the natural nail, as it requires very little buffing and there is no need for the use of primer	This system is recognised as being very fiddly and some therapists prefer not to use it unless requested by the client
It can be soaked off very easily and in the minimal time (10–15 minutes)	The spray activator can cause allergic reactions such as breathing problems or skin reaction
The overlay that is produced is not very thick and is flexible	The resin vapours can cause sore, watery eyes
This system is also useful for natural nail repairs as it is thin and will not look different to the other nails	

Preparation for nail enhancement services

To prepare to give a nail enhancement treatment, carry out the following steps.

1. Prepare the work area by ensuring that surfaces are wiped down with disinfectant and all tools are sterilised or disinfected as appropriate. Use disposable items wherever possible.

2. Begin by washing your hands thoroughly.

3. Ensure that the client has washed their hands and that they are clean and dry. The client's hands and nails must be wiped with isopropyl alcohol or a proprietary brand spray sanitiser. Surgical spirit should not be used for this purpose, as it leaves an oily film on the nail plate that will prevent proper adhesion of the artificial nails. It is important to ensure that the hands are completely dry, as water may be absorbed into the nail plate and it may lead to lifting of the nail extension at a later date.

4. A mini manicure should be carried out at this stage to ensure that the nails are fully prepared for the application of nail extensions:

   - Remove any nail polish on the nails.
   - Push back the cuticle from the nail plate, using either an orange-wood stick or hoof stick.
   - A cuticle knife or cuticle pusher may be necessary to loosen any cuticle adhering to the nail plate. A clean nail plate is essential. If the cuticle is not removed fully the overlay product will not bond to the nail plate and lifting may occur.
   - Remove excess cuticle with nippers if necessary.
   - File the nails so that they are even in length and all of the edges are smooth. Doing this will ensure the correct fit of a nail tip if it is to be applied.

The next step in preparing the natural nails is to remove the shine from the nail. Doing this gives optimum adhesion, as the nail's surface is naturally smooth and shiny. Two shiny surfaces do not adhere or bond together effectively. It is necessary to slightly roughen the nail plate both to aid adhesion and to remove any trapped bacteria. This is done by using either a white block or a 240-grit file, lightly buffing from the base of the nail to the free edge, making sure the side-wall area is buffed.

Dehydrating the nail plate is an important stage in the preparation. This is done to remove any traces of oil or moisture from the nail plate. Dehydrators that are used on the nail also act as sanitisers, removing oil and moisture as well as ensuring the nails are free from bacteria or fungal spores that could later cause problems. There are many dehydrators on the market and they must be applied following the manufacturer's instructions.

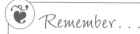
Remember...
For assessment purposes you only have to demonstrate competence in one nail enhancement system: acrylic liquid and powder, UV gel or wrap.

Remember...
Remember that the dehydration process is only effective for approximately 20–30 minutes and once this time has elapsed, the nail will naturally rehydrate and the process will have to be repeated.

The nails are now clean and prepared for the next stage of the treatment.

Outcome 3: Apply natural overlays

Natural nail overlays are when the nail enhancement system is placed directly onto the natural nail that has some natural length to give it strength. Natural nail overlays can be achieved using fibreglass and UV gel systems. This technique relies on a sound knowledge of the products and their application but also the suitability of the client's nails:

- A flat natural nail shape makes it difficult to create a good shape.
- Bitten nails with bulbous finger ends are unsuitable.
- Thin or poor nail plates do not provide a sufficiently good foundation for direct application of the product.
- Ski-jump nails (nails that curve upwards at the tip) are not suitable as it is impossible to achieve a good shape.
- The product won't last on the nails of clients who perform heavy work.

Application procedure for natural overlays using wrap system

1. Prepare the natural nails as described earlier:
   - remove polish
   - push back and remove excess cuticles
   - file the free-edge so smooth and even
   - remove the natural shine from the nail plate
   - dehydrate the nail.
2. Cut the fabric (fibreglass mesh or silk) the same width as the natural nail with the stork scissors. Take care not to handle

the fabric, as oil from your fingers will prevent the fabric from adhering to the natural nail.

3. If the fabric comes with a paper backing, carefully peel it away and adhere the fabric to the natural nail. Use the paper to press the fabric firmly onto the natural nail so that it is positioned as close as possible to the cuticle and nail wall without touching.

4. With the stork scissors trim the fabric so that it is slightly shorter than the free edge. This will allow the resin to seal the free edge when it is applied.

5. Repeat the procedure on all the nails of both hands so that all are covered in the fabric.

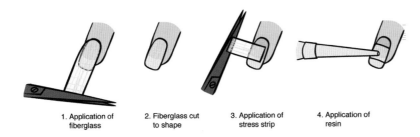

1. Application of fiberglass   2. Fiberglass cut to shape   3. Application of stress strip   4. Application of resin

◁ Applying fibreglass mesh

6. With the free-edge pointing downwards, apply the resin with a nozzle or a brush down the centre of the nail from cuticle to free-edge.

7. Work the resin into the fabric with the nozzle or brush using a side-to-side action. Ensure that all the fabric is covered; it should turn transparent. Carefully apply more resin if needed.

8. If a spray activator is being used, mist the activator over the whole of the nail. Hold the spray at least 30 centimetres (12 inches) from the nails and spray once, making sure that all nails have been covered.

9. If a brush-on activator is being used, apply only a small amount of the resin, as the activator will spread it. Spread the resin with the brush-on activator, making sure that you avoid the surrounding skin. Make sure that a brush cleaner is available to clean the brush between each application.

10. Repeat steps 6–8 or step 9 on all nails

11. Apply another layer of the resin to the nail; ensure that the resin is spread evenly and that there are no traces on the surrounding skin.

12. Repeat application of resin activator.

13. If more strength is needed, the application of resin and activator can be repeated.

14. The overlay should be smooth and require a minimal amount of buffing. To achieve a high shine use a soft file to buff and a white block to remove any scratches and to refine the surface.

15. Remove all file dust with a brush and apply oil to the nail and cuticle.

16. Apply polish if requested and ensure that aftercare advice is given.

The UV gel system can be used as a natural nail overlay by following the procedure set out in Outcome 4, omitting the techniques for applying the nail tips.

Outcome 4: Apply tip and overlays

The application of a nail tip before the nail enhancement system provides length and strength to short nails. The correct selection of the tip to be applied is very important and will affect the durability and look of the finished result. Time should be taken to get this vital stage of the procedure correct.

Nail tip application

The use of plastic nail tips developed from the traditional plastic false nail, which covered the whole of the nail. Huge improvements in the manufacture of materials have brought a durable plastic tip that covers only a small part of the nail plate. The tips come in a range of different shapes and sizes, ensuring that those selected meet the needs of the wide range of natural nail shapes. It is important to select the right tip to fit the client's nails to ensure a natural look and the longevity of the nails.

Tip selection

There are certain characteristics that ensure a well-fitting and natural-looking nail tip. They should:

- be made from good quality plastic (look for ABS plastic)
- be flexible
- be a good natural opaque colour
- bond well with the adhesive
- be a good range of shapes and sizes
- be easy to blend to the natural nail.

These qualities are reflected in the cost of the tips. Cheap tips can be difficult to fit, look unnatural and are more prone to breaking.

When selecting the tips, certain guidelines should be followed:

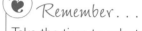

> **Remember...**
> Take the time to select the right tip as it will affect the final look, durability and the finished result.

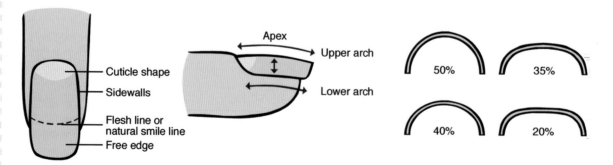

△ Parts of a nail tip

- Choose a tip that follows the same curve of the natural nail. Some clients may have a very flat nail, while others may have a curved nail. Look for the 'C' curve of the client's nails. Matching the curve incorrectly could cause a number of problems, such as air bubbles between the tip and nail plate. This will show through the overlay and will look very unnatural. The risk of infection is increased, as bacteria or fungus may grow in the spaces.

- Choose a tip with the correct 'stop point'. This is the area of the tip that fits into the free edge of the natural nail. The correct contact area or well area is very important and must be large enough to fit snugly. The contact area on tips will vary. Some will cover a larger area of the natural nail than others. Some may have a 'V' cut into the well area to make blending easier. The weakest bond on a nail extension is between the natural nail and the tip, so it is vital that the tip covers only a small portion of the nail plate. If the nail is very short or bitten it may be necessary to use a tip with a smaller contact area. It is also important as a larger contact area used on the wrong shape of nail will cause the tip to tilt upwards at an angle and this will look very unnatural.

- The side walls of the client's nails must be taken into account. If the tips do not fit perfectly into the natural nail grooves at the side walls, the nail could lift and result in infection or the nail coming off.

- The nail tips come in 10 different sizes, 1 being the largest and 10 the smallest. When choosing the size of tip for each finger it is important that it covers the nail plate from side wall to side wall. If needed, a plastic tip can be filed to shape to fit the nail prior to application, so if necessary opt for the larger size to ensure the best fit. There should be no gap at the side walls when the skin is pulled back. Although it is not very noticeable when a new set is applied, as the natural nail grows the gap will become evident.

Tip application

1. Select a suitable nail tip for each nail and place them in a logical sequence for application.

2. Carry out the nail preparation procedures as described earlier.

3. Apply a small amount of adhesive directly onto the well of the tip. In doing this, rather than applying it to the natural nail, you are ensuring that the adhesive does not run onto the skin around the nail.

4. There should be no more than 30 per cent of the tip on the natural nail plate.

5. Apply the tip to the nail at a 45-degree angle. Using a rocking movement, apply it to the natural nail, making sure that you release any air bubbles and it forms a perfect bond. Hold the nail in position for about 10 seconds ensuring that your pressure is not too heavy. If you need to apply a lot of pressure you might find that the tip is too small.

6. Ensure no excess adhesive is left under the free edge or around the side walls. It must be cleaned off before it dries.

> **Activity**
>
> Look at the 'C' curve of the nails of two of your colleagues and your own nails and discuss the differences. Find someone with a concave nail shape (ski jump) and a convex nail shape (claw) and discuss why it is difficult to apply nail extensions to these.

7. Once all 10 tips have been applied, the length and shape must be decided on. Consult the treatment plan and discuss once again. Always advise the client on the length that will suit their hands, occupation and lifestyle. Cutting the tip to size requires a sharp tip cutter.

8. The tips must now be filed to shape using a fine board of 240-grit or above. There are three different shapes that the client has to choose from, oval, squoval (rounded square) or square.

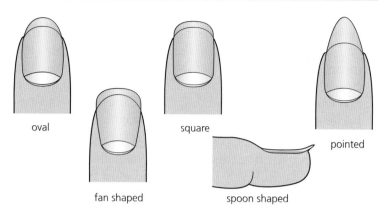

△ Different nail shapes

9. Check the side walls and taper if necessary.

10. The next step is to blend the tip to the natural nail. Use a grit file of 240 to thin the entire tip. Blend in one direction and use long sweeps with the file to avoid friction to the nail bed. Begin at the free edge of the tip (zone 1), working down towards the seam (zone 2). When blending the seam line, make sure that the line disappears. Using very light pressure, file over the base of the tip near the seam, avoiding the natural nail. The contact area on the tip will become thinner and the nail will be translucent.

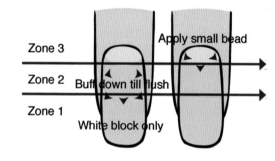

△ The zone areas

11. Use a white block to buff the area to ensure that there is no evidence of a visible seam line and the surface is smooth and free of scratches.

12. Check the tip application and remove any file dust from the free edge.

The tip application is follow by the application of a nail enhancement system such as UV gel, or the acrylic powder and liquid or wrap system described previously.

Application of gel system

1. Ensure the work area is well prepared and sterilisation and cleaning procedures have been completed.

2. Follow the nail preparation and the tip application procedure.

3. Ensure that all filing dust is removed by using a soft brush. If any dust gets into the gel it will cause a very bumpy overlay.

4. Take a small amount of gel and place at the tip of the nail using a clean brush. Apply a thin layer of the gel to the whole nail, leaving a small margin round the cuticle to ensure no gel touches the skin and cuticle. This is the base layer.

5. Turn on the ultraviolet lamp and ask the client to place their hand under it for the gel to cure for two minutes, or however long is required by the manufacturer's instructions.

6. While the first hand is under the lamp, repeat steps 3 and 4 on the second hand.

☆ **Hints and tips**

When using a wrap system for the tip and overlay technique, an additional strip of fabric should be cut and placed at the join of the nail tip with the natural nail, then sealed with resin to give extra strength to this weak 'stress area'.

7. Apply the second coat of gel to the first hand while the second hand is under the lamp. This second layer is the building layer. Place a large bead of gel in the centre of the nail. Spread the gel down the nail plate, leaving the bulk of it in the centre or stress area to give strength. Ensure that all sides of the free edge are sealed. As the second layer is thicker than the first it is important to make sure that no gel has come into contact with the surrounding skin. Cure for two minutes.

8. Repeat step 7 on the second hand.

9. Remove any residue from the nails with a nail wipe.

10. To get the perfect shape to the extension, the nail is buffed. Use a high-grit file.

11. Always check the shape of the nail by looking down the barrel of the nail to make sure it is even all over.

12. Use a white block to remove any scratches from the nail.

13. There are two ways of finishing the gel system. A three-way buffer can be used to produce a natural shine, or applying a very thin layer of finishing gel and curing for two minutes will produce a very high shine. Make sure that any residue is removed using a nail wipe if the nails are finished in this way.

14. Apply oil to the nail and cuticle area.

15. Apply polish if requested. Remember to remove traces of oil from the nail.

Safety points when applying gel

The safety points to remember when using the UV gel systems are:

- always read and follow the manufacturer's instructions
- use extraction ventilation
- check the ultraviolet lamp regularly and change bulbs every 6–12 months, depending on use
- apply thin layers of gel
- always use strict hygiene procedures.

Application of acrylic powder and liquid system

1. Prepare the nails in the usual way.

2. Apply tips, shape and blend.

3. Follow the procedure for acrylic nail application, as recommended by the manufacturer of the product to be used.

4. Apply a very small amount of primer at the base of the nails on one hand. The primer must be dry before applying the acrylic.

5. While the primer is drying, ensure that the brush is prepared to begin the overlay. Fill a Dappen dish with the monomer liquid. Clean the brush by submerging the bristles into the liquid to free it of air pockets and to prime it. Then wipe it on a paper towel.

6. Dip the brush back into the monomer and then press the sides of the brush against the Dappen dish to release any excess liquid.

7. Start on the little finger of one hand. Pick up a bead of powder and place it onto zone 1. Wait for five seconds for the bead to set, then, holding the brush at an angle, press the bead with the tip of the brush, using a combination of gentle patting and pressing motions to glide the product across zone 1. Check the shape by looking down the barrel of the nail to make sure the overlay is even.

8. Wipe the brush on a paper towel to remove any excess product.

9. Repeat stages 4, 5 and 6 for zone 2.

10. Then repeat stages 6, 7 and 8 for zone 3. Make sure that the bead is applied carefully to the cuticle area but leave a 1.5mm gap. Gently press the overlay to thin the zone and create a good bond with the nail plate.

11. Apply the overlays to the other nails by following the same procedure. This application requires practice to ensure a smooth, even coverage is achieved.

12. By the time the overlays have been applied to both hands, the first hand will be ready for the next stage.

13. Wipe any excess product from your brush and clean it by dipping it into the Dappen dish and brushing it on a paper towel.

14. Check that the acrylic has set by tapping the nail with the handle of the brush; if it is ready a clicking sound can be heard. If the acrylic has been applied carefully and not too thickly, finishing should not require excessive filing and buffing.

15. Using a 240-grit file, buff the surface of the overlay to help smooth out any bumps, ridges and unevenly distributed product. Check the overlay from all angles, not forgetting to look down the barrel, to ensure a perfect nail structure.

16. Use a white block to buff over the surface to refine and remove any surface scratches to the nail.

17. Use a three-way buffer, if required, to give a shine and seal the overlay.

18. Apply oil to the nail and cuticle to nourish the nail and surrounding skin.

19. Apply polish if desired.

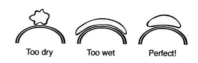

Too dry   Too wet   Perfect!

△ The correct consistency of acrylic liquid to powder

Outcome 5: Maintain nail enhancements

As the natural nail grows a gap will appear at the cuticle, which will require 'maintenance procedures' known as 'infills'. The procedure involves the filling in of this gap to maintain the appearance of the nail enhancement application.

Wrap system infills

The wrap system should be maintained every two–four weeks depending on the rate of growth of the client's natural nails. The system of infills is relatively easy and should take between 30 minutes and an hour, unless there are problems such as lifting or lost nails. If the client is returning for an infill for the first time they may not need fabric applying in the growth area, as the growth of the natural nail will be minimal.

Procedure

The same materials and equipment are required as for a new set of nails.

1. Ensure that all equipment is sanitised and available.
2. Sanitise both your own and your client's hands.
3. Use non-acetate polish remover to remove polish from the nails.
4. Using a cuticle tool, remove any new cuticle that has grown on the nail plate.
5. Replace any lost nails.
6. Using a 100-grit file, blend the edge of the overlay near the cuticle (zone 3) until it is flush with the natural nail, taking care that the natural nail is not buffed during this process. It is at this stage that any area of lifting on the overlay is removed and buffed down.
7. Use a 240-grit file to buff away the surface shine from the whole nail and buff over the area with a white block to remove any scratches.
8. Apply a thin strip of fabric in the growth area (zone 3).
9. Apply a small amount of resin to the growth area of the nail (zone 3) and blend it to the rest of the nail.
10. Apply the activator as before.
11. Another thin layer of resin may be needed, followed by activator.
12. Use a white block followed by the three-way buffer. Buff the nails to achieve a high gloss.
13. Apply polish if required.

UV gel infills

UV gel nails should be maintained every 2–4 weeks depending on the rate of growth of the client's natural nails. Gel infills should take about an hour to do, longer if some tips have been broken or your client has left it more than two weeks for their appointment.

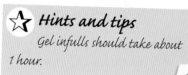

⭐ **Hints and tips**
Gel infills should take about 1 hour.

Procedure

The same materials and equipment are required as for a new set of nails.

1. Ensure that all equipment is sanitised and available.
2. Sanitise both your own and your client's hands.
3. Using cuticle tools, remove any new cuticle that has grown on the nail plate.
4. If there are any nails missing these must be replaced.
5. Check the shape of each nail and length and carry out any corrections needed.
6. Gently buff the surface with a 240-grit file.
7. Using a 100-grit file, working in zone 3, blend the edge of the overlay until it is flush with the natural nail. Take care to ensure that the natural nail is not buffed during this process. It is at this stage that any area of lifting on the overlay is removed and buffed.

8. Remove all the shine from the surface and buff over the area with a white block to remove any scratches.

9. Remove file dust from the nails and use a nail dehydrator to cleanse the new growth.

10. Apply a small amount of the gel to the infill area and blend it onto the rest of the nail. If it is the second or third infill you may need to apply two layers for added strength. Cure for two minutes.

11. Remove the residue from the nails and buff as for the first application.

12. Use a white block to remove any surface scratches to the nail.

13. End with either a three-way buffer or a layer of gel as necessary. Remember that it must be cured for two minutes.

14. Apply oil and polish if required. Remember to remove traces of oil from the nail before applying polish.

Acrylic infills

Clients should be recommended to return in two weeks. Acrylic infills should take about an hour to do; longer if some tips have been broken, if the client has left it more than two weeks for their appointment, or if the natural nails have grown quickly.

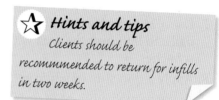

Hints and tips

Clients should be recommended to return for infills in two weeks.

Procedure

1. Ensure that all equipment is sanitised and available.

2. Sanitise both your own and your client's hands.

3. Using cuticle tools, remove any cuticle that has grown on the nail plate.

4. Look at the shape and length of the nails and adjust as necessary. Remember to check the treatment plan and discuss the length with the client. As the natural nail grows the nail extensions will get longer. This may not be what was agreed or recommended at the first treatment. If the client requests the nails to be left longer, remind them of the greater risk of breaking and lifting.

5. Use a 240-grit file to gently file down the side walls to straighten.

6. Continuing with the 240-grit file, blend the edge of the overlay until it is flush with the natural nail, making sure that care is taken and the natural nail is not buffed during this process. Remember the stress line has moved up the nail towards the free edge. Ensure that only the nail in zone 2 is buffed to avoid changing the shape of the rest of the nail. It is at this stage that any area of lifting on the overlay is removed and buffed down.

7. Remove all the shine from the surface and buff over the area with a white block to remove any scratches.

8. Ensure that filing dust is removed from the nails.

9. Apply a primer to the new growth area. Wait for this to dry before applying the overlay.

10. Apply a small bead of acrylic to zone 3 and press into shape, making sure that you blend it down to zones 1 and 2. Take care around the cuticle area and leave a gap of 1.5 mm.

11. Use a file to smooth the surface and buff around the cuticle area. Check the shape and look down the barrel to make sure that a perfect overlay is achieved.

12. Use a white block to smooth and remove any surface scratches.

13. Use a three-way buffer to seal and shine the nail.

14. Apply oil to the nail and cuticle area.

15. Apply polish if required.

Other maintenance

Other maintenance may also be required, such as repairing any damage or lifting that may have occurred during the wearing of the nail enhancements. The correct application of the nail enhancement system in the first instance will prevent most of these problems occurring. However, the client's misuse of her nails can lead to problems.

Lifting

The nail enhancement product lifting from the natural nail will be recognised by a cloudy appearance within the nail. This can occur around the edge of the nail, usually at the cuticle in zone 3 and at the side walls. This must be removed by filing before any further product is applied but do not clip away the lifted nail enhancement as this can lead to even more lifting.

Pocket lifting

This is where the product begins to lift in the middle of the nail plate but still has product bonded to the nail plate surrounding it. The lifted area will again appear cloudy in comparison with the rest of the nail. Little can be done to repair this and there is a risk that bacteria may grow underneath so the nail enhancement should be removed and reapplied.

Curling

This can occur at the free edge; the natural nail becomes dry and separates from the artificial nail causing it to start to curl. Again, the nail enhancement should be removed and reapplied, as there is a risk of bacteria growing underneath.

Cracks

Fine cracks or in more severe cases the crack can be deep, causing the artificial nail to bend slightly. The apex in zone 2 is more prone to this sort of problem. Remove the nail enhancement and reapply.

Broken nails

This occurs when the artificial nail has broken off, leaving some of the structure still attached to the nail bed. In some cases the natural nail plate can also split. The remaining nail product should be removed and reapplied.

Chipping

This usually occurs in zone 1. The free edge can become damaged and product chips away leaving a 'ragged' free edge. As long as the natural nail is not affected the nail enhancement can be repaired but if the natural nail is exposed there is a risk of bacterial growth and the nail should be removed and reapplied.

Outcome 6: Remove nail enhancements

Remember. . .

It is very important to remove nail enhancements carefully to avoid affecting the natural nail.

The safe removal of nail enhancements is important to avoid affecting the health of the natural nail. It should be carried out if the client no longer wishes to wear the nails or if sufficient damage has occurred to a nail before reapplication. Guidelines for safe removal include the following:

- Removal of nail enhancements should be performed by a professional nail technician or therapist. This service should be readily available in the salon.
- Products should be removed in a quick and safe way to avoid damage to the natural nail.
- Never sell or give clients professional products to remove their own nails at home.
- Constantly 'soaking off' nail extensions and reapplying will cause damage to the natural nail.

There are two methods of removing nail extensions:

1. the soak-off method
2. the buff-off method.

The soak-off method

Acetone is commonly used for the soak-off method, although it should be used with care as it is extremely drying and can affect the natural nail plate and surrounding cuticle. The solvent breaks down the polymer chains in the chemicals. The easiest system to remove is fibreglass as the resin used has the weakest chains. The liquid and powder system is the next easiest to remove, although it will take longer and requires some buffing. UV gel is substantially more difficult to remove. It has strong bonds and requires considerably more filing and buffing to remove the artificial nail.

Procedure

1. Place two glass or china bowls filled to a depth of about 3 cm with solvent. The bowls should be placed in hot water. The heat will accelerate the removal process.
2. Remove polish from the nails and cut back the length of the nails.
3. Submerge the nails into the solvent and cover with a towel to keep in the heat. It may be necessary to change the water to keep it hot. The process will take about 20 minutes.
4. Take one hand out of the bowl and gently remove the dissolved nails with an orange stick. Continue on the other hand.

5. The client will need to wash their hands to remove all traces of the solvent.

6. Check the cuticles and reshape the natural nails as necessary.

7. Reapply nail extensions or continue with hand massage and polish as required.

Another method of removal involves applying cotton wool soaked in solvent to each nail and then wrapping the hands in tinfoil to retain the heat. A plastic bag or heated mittens can be used to increase the heat and speed up removal.

Outcome 7: Provide aftercare advice

The client must be informed at the outset of what is involved in maintaining the nail enhancements. While some nails may be temporary, others remain on the nail as it grows and require infills to maintain a perfect shape.

Because of the pressure put on the tip of the nail they can come off or break. The longer the extended nail, the more likely this will happen. Replacing the nails will require a visit to the salon and a cost to replace the nail.

Advising clients on aftercare

Make sure that clients are fully informed of the 'dos and don'ts' of how to care for their nails at home. Stress to the client just how important it is that they follow a strict routine to maximise the life of the nail extensions.

An aftercare leaflet will ensure that clients have the information on how to care for the nail extensions. Clients who are offered an aftercare leaflet are less likely to blame the therapist if the nails do not last or meet their expectations. However, a leaflet does not replace clients' statutory rights.

You should discuss the following points with clients before they leave the salon:

- Contact the salon if any problems occur with the nails.
- If using polish remover, ensure that it is non-acetone.
- Always use a base coat before applying polish.
- Rebook for maintenance or infill treatments every two or three weeks.
- Apply oil or cuticle cream two or three times a day to the nail and cuticle.
- Use hand cream regularly to keep hands soft.
- Wear cotton-lined rubber gloves for daily housework jobs, especially if cleaning chemicals such as bleach and detergents are to be used.
- Take special care with fibreglass nails, as they are prone to damage from knocking.
- Take care not to catch the nails on clothing or grab at things, as this can cause breakage and damage to the natural nails.

Activity

Design an aftercare leaflet that gives the client clear information on the care of hands and nails. Include a section on the maintenance procedures required to keep nail extensions looking immaculate.

Contra-actions specific to nail extensions

These may occur during or after the nail enhancement service:

- allergies
- overexposure and exothermic reactions
- bacterial infection
- nail separation
- lifting of product
- premature loss of the enhancement.

Clients sometimes complain that their natural nails appear thinner after nail enhancement services have been removed. This is usually due to the fact that they have become used to a thicker nail plate produced by the overlay.

If the correct procedures are followed, the therapist is skilled at the system used and careful consideration is given to the client's needs, the nail enhancements should look natural and be long-lasting. However, poor practice when carrying out nail extensions can cause a number of problems. The table below shows the problems that may arise, the possible causes and suggested solutions.

▽ Solving problems

Problem	Possible cause	Solution to the problem
Thinning of the natural nail	Constant buffing and filing, over-priming, nail plate not dehydrated before applying products, product has lifted and moisture is trapped between the layers	Use correct grit files, use a light touch when filing, apply primer very sparingly and allow to dry, always carry out meticulous preparation of the natural nails, do not soak the nails if giving a manicure before nail extensions
Splitting and flaking of the natural nail	Over-blending of tips, nail extension too long or too thick, client picks or bites the extension off, maintenance not carried out on time	Light touch when filing, advise client on appropriate length, make sure client is aware of maintenance needs and the correct removal of the extensions
Premature loss of the nail extension	Poor preparation of the nail plate, nail extensions too long, nails do not fit client's lifestyle, incorrect selection of system	Ensure good preparation, carry out a full consultation into client's lifestyle, occupation and expectations, consider the appearance and shape of the natural nail before selecting a system
Discoloration of the natural nail plate	Poor preparation of the nails, overuse of primer	Ensure thorough preparation of the nail plate before applying products, use nail primer sparingly and allow to dry
Obvious infills	Poor blending, too much product, client not attending maintenance appointments	Use correct infill technique, follow manufacturer's instructions, blend correctly, emphasise to clients the importance of keeping appointments to maintain their nails
Lifting from the natural nail	Nails too long, improper preparation of the nail leaving the nail moist or oily, maintenance appointments not kept, nail extension unbalanced, poor home care	A thorough consultation to establish how the client will manage the nail extensions in relation to their job and lifestyle, correct preparation of the natural nails, the correct amount of product used

The finished nails pointing upwards or downwards	Incorrect placing of the tip or nail form	Check regularly throughout the application that the angles and curves are correct
The 'C' shape of the nail extension is irregular	Product applied unevenly or too much product applied, product too wet causing it to run	Practise to ensure high levels of skill, check throughout the application of the nails that the transverse arch and the 'C' shape are even
Infection of the nail	Bacterial or fungal infection due to cracks or spaces in the extension, infection caused by the client picking, tearing or biting the nail extension leaving the cuticle and nail bed exposed to infection, lifting of the product at the free edge, side walls or cuticle allowing moisture to become trapped between the layers	Careful preparation, regular maintenance, advice to client on home care, skilful application to ensure there are no spaces between the natural nail plate and the extension

Want to know more?

The 'Nails Code of Practice' can be downloaded from the Habia website at www.habia.org

Test yourself

Test yourself on nail enhancements with a natural finish by answering the following questions:

1. Nail primer contains a fungicide to:
   a) harden the nail
   b) help the artificial nail to stick
   c) prevent disease
   d) soften the nail plate.

2. The nail plate is buffed with an abrasive file to:
   a) smooth the nail plate
   b) reduce the length of the nail plate
   c) help the false nail stick to the nail plate
   d) clean the nail plate.

3. Fibreglass nail enhancements provide the most natural effect because:
   a) they are strong and flexible
   b) they are thick and heavy
   c) they are a natural colour
   d) they are easy to apply.

4. Give three contraindications to nail enhancement services.

5. What is a Dappen dish?

6. Why is a Dappen dish used in nail enhancement services?

Are you ready for assessment?

Remember...

Practice makes perfect! The more opportunities you have to complete a nail enhancement service, the more confident you will be when it comes to being observed by your assessor.

The following checklist will help you to be fully prepared for your practical assessment.

1. **Practical observation**

Remember...

Your assessor will observe your performance on at least six occasions, each involving a different client. You must use one of gel, liquid and powder, or wrap and this must include one application of a full set of natural nail overlays, one full set of tips and overlays, two maintenance and repair of a full set of nail enhancements and one removal of a full set of tips and overlays.

Your assessor will look at how you:

- prepare the treatment area
- consult with the client and prepare a record card
- carry out a nail enhancement service on a client (not a fellow student or colleague) using a range of tools and products
- carry out nail enhancement services using a range of techniques
- carry out the nail enhancement service in a commercially acceptable time
- check with the client that the nail enhancement service meets her expectations
- provide aftercare advice
- demonstrate professional practice throughout the service
- carry out all services with regard to health and safety.

2. **Knowledge and understanding**

   What you must know:

- Organisational and legal requirements.
- How to work safely and effectively when providing enhancements.
- How to consult, plan and prepare for nail treatment with clients.
- Contraindications and contra-actions.
- Anatomy and physiology.
- Nail enhancement services.

🍃 Maintenance and repair.

🍃 Aftercare advice.

To ensure that you have the necessary knowledge and understanding of nail enhancements your assessor will:

🍃 ask you questions before, during and after carrying out the treatment

🍃 ensure that you have completed project work and written exercises relating to the unit

🍃 check that you have recorded in a log/diary treatments you have carried out with signed record cards showing that you have completed six nail enhancements competently

🍃 that you have covered the range in your candidate logbook.

Chapter 15
Unit B7: Carry out ear-piercing

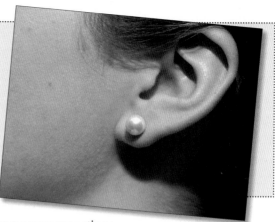

Learning objectives

This chapter covers Unit B7 'Carry out ear-piercing', that is, the piercing of the ear lobe and the skills and knowledge needed to perform the service.

> There are four learning outcomes for Unit B7 and they are:
> 1 Maintain safe and effective methods of working when piercing ears.
> 2 Consult, plan and prepare for ear lobe piercing with clients.
> 3 Pierce the ear lobes.
> 4 Provide aftercare advice.

You will need to be competent in all of these outcomes in ear-piercing, to qualify for insurance and to perform the treatment on members of the public.

Evidence requirements

Your assessor will need to observe on two different clients. You must:

1 Demonstrate the use of consultation techniques:
  - questioning
  - visual
  - manual
  - reference to client records.

2 Take necessary action:
  - encourage the client to seek medical advice
  - explain why the treatment cannot be carried out
  - modify the treatment.

3 Demonstrate the use of equipment, materials and products:
  - ear-piercing gun
  - sterile marker pen
  - sterile ear studs
  - mirror
  - consumables.

4 Provide relevant aftercare:
  - suitable home care products and their use
  - regular movement of the studs
  - possible contra-actions
  - removal of studs.

Introduction

Ear-piercing is a quick, inexpensive and profitable treatment to perform. Unit B7 is as optional and is worth two credits. It appears in both the general and make-up routes of the NVQ qualifications. As well as therapists and make-up consultants the unit could be offered to complement the training of receptionists, hairdressers, barbers, nail technicians and Afro-type hairdressers and those of other associated industries, such as jewellers.

Meet the professional

"As an Ear Piercing Technician, professionalism and procedure are key. Always ensure that your client is correctly informed about the process and that they are comfortable before carrying out the piercing. A Piercing Technician has a responsibility to remain attentive to their client and read any signs of nervous behaviour. By remaining relaxed, informative and chatty, you will help your client feel comfortable and confident, ensuring a stress-free piercing.

Educating clients about expectations is essential. The most common issues experienced with any piercing are often as a result of a lack of aftercare. You have a responsibility to ensure that all clients understand the process and that they are given a copy of the after-piercing guidelines and a cleansing solution. It is common practice to build the after-piercing solution into the price of the piercing.

All certified training provided on authorised ear piercing systems will cover, in detail, the correct ear piercing procedure, from completing the consultation form, through to preparing the client, marking the ear, the correct piercing technique and detailed aftercare advice. The information covered will ensure the best and most hygienic codes of practice for ear piercing and compliance with local authorities. Ear Piercing Systems authorised for use in the UK, such as the Studex System 75 and Studex Plus, utilise fully disposable cartridges, ensuring hygiene and reducing any risk.

By including ear piercing on your treatment list you are continuing to build a relationship with your clients and then, in turn, possibly their children. A good ear piercing service will soon become popular – word of mouth is invaluable. Make sure that your clients are aware that you offer the service as it prevents them from having to look elsewhere for a service that you can provide quickly and profitably!"

Kathryn Reeve

Outcome 1: Maintain safe and effective methods of working when piercing ears

Ear-piercing is an **invasive treatment**, that is to say that the ear lobe is 'punctured' and the skin is broken, leaving a wound that is open to infection. Due to the potential for blood and serum loss there is a risk of cross-infection by the viruses AIDS and Hepatitis B. There are strict controls over the performance of this treatment. The practitioners, salon or premises must be registered with the local health authority. Only disposable types of equipment must be used and strict hygiene and waste disposal measures must be implemented. These controls apply to anyone performing this treatment, for example a mobile therapist or hairdresser.

Legislative requirements for ear-piercing

The **Local Government (Miscellaneous Provisions) Act 1982** controls the registration of the persons performing ear-piercing, electrolysis and tattooing at a premises within a local authority; this registration will also extend to other premises for those registered wishing to visit and perform the treatment elsewhere, a client's home for example. This act was amended by the **Local Government Act 2003** to allow a local authority to pass 'byelaws' or local laws that may be specific to that local authority, such as the specific hygiene requirements to do with the dealing of clinical or contaminated waste or the keeping of client records. The **London Local Authorities Act 1991** governs the performing of cosmetic piercing, electrolysis and tattooing in London boroughs, for example. More information on this and other relevant legislation can be found in Chapter 3 'Make sure your own actions reduce risks to health and safety'.

The consequence of not complying with legislation is an initial visit from an enforcement officer such as the Environmental Health Officer (EHO). They are responsible for maintaining standards of hygiene in public places and have the power to close the premises temporarily if hygiene is compromised or if they feel the public are at risk. They can visit without invitation and ask to see client records, inspect the premises and ask questions surrounding hygiene procedures. If the hygiene standards remain inadequate, the officer can remove the registration status. This would mean that ear-piercing could not be performed by the staff on or off the premises.

Key term

Invasive treatment – one which enters the skin through piercing or incision.

Hints and tips

When setting up your own business or changing jobs to a new area you should contact the local authority to ensure that your business and ear-piercing operatives are registered and comply with the local authority requirements.

Health and safety

Ear-piercing forms part of a service called '**cosmetic piercing**', which includes the piercing of areas of the body such as the tongue, nose, eyebrow and belly button. Piercing of these areas requires specialist skills, knowledge and training and therefore is not within your responsibility under the requirements of this unit.

Key term

Cosmetic piercing – the piercing of any part of the body for the purpose of ornamentation.

Test yourself

Test yourself on the Acts that apply to ear-piercing by answering the following questions. True or False? Decide for each of these statements:

1. The **Health and Safety (First Aid) Regulations 1981** states that every premises must have at least one fully qualified first aider.

2. The **Control of Substances Hazardous to Health Regulations 2002** includes the exposure to biological hazards such as bacteria, viruses and fungi.

3. The **Environmental Protection Act 1990** covers the disposal of clinical waste.

4. The **Local Government (Miscellaneous Provisions) Act 1982** requires only the salon to register if offering ear-piercing as a service.

5. The **Data Protection Act 1998** covers the security of both electronically kept and paper-based client records.

Setting up the work area

The treatment should be performed in an area with adequate ventilation and heating to ensure client comfort and yet minimise the risk of fainting. There should be plenty of light so you can see that you are performing the treatment safely and to the client's requirements. You may find a private area away from a busy reception more suitable if the client is particularly nervous.

When setting up the work area, consider the client's seated position. A chair that can be adjusted for height is important, as the client should be seated for treatment at a convenient height. They must be comfortable and able to sit upright with the head level and facing forwards to allow access to the ears on both sides. The correct positioning of the client will ensure accurate placement of the piercing and minimise injury to you through poor posture, for example backache from bending, or repetitive strain injury (RSI).

Industry hygiene and safety practices for ear-piercing

It is essential to maintain high standards of hygiene and professionalism, as with all beauty therapy treatments. This is important to prevent cross-infection, promote client confidence and salon reputation and ensure the client's return custom. As this is an invasive treatment, there is a risk of blood and serum contamination of materials and equipment.

The immediate work area should be prepared for treatment by wiping work surfaces with a disinfectant or sanitising solution, both before and after treatment. The trolley or work surface should be covered with disposable paper. A waste bin lined with a plastic liner for the disposing of clinical or contaminated waste should be available.

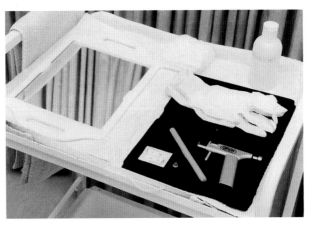

△ Ear-piercing equipment

Modern ear-piercing systems rely on being disposable to prevent cross-contamination of blood-borne viruses such as hepatitis. Either the ear-piercing gun itself is disposable, or the parts of the gun that could become infected are disposable. Where the system includes the type of gun with disposable parts, plastic mounting devices are used to protect the surfaces that would otherwise come into contact with the client. The parts are used once and then thrown away. Although this system prevents cross-contamination it is still important to wipe the ear-piercing gun with a disinfectant that contains either 'hypochlorite solution' (bleach) or surgical strength alcohol before and after use.

Stud earrings are commonly used to pierce the ears due to the reduced risk of infection compared with using the 'ring' or 'sleeper' type. The stud post appears larger in width than normal ear rings as this allows for slight shrinkage of the tissues during the healing process. They are sold in individually sealed pre-sterilised packs, which should only be opened just before use. The sealed packs often have an expiry date or coloured seal that indicates when the pack should no longer be considered sterile. If only one stud is used in the pack, the other should be disposed of in a waste bin.

The pack includes a disposable plastic 'cartridge' that allows the loading of the ear-piercing gun without touching the studs. A wide variety of studs is available – different shapes and those with small coloured stones in a range of colours, as well as the plain, round, gold type, in large or small sizes. For ear lobes that are more than 6 mm thick, long post studs are available for piercing. All studs should be made from a hypoallergenic material such as titanium, 14-carat gold or surgical stainless steel to avoid allergic reactions.

> ⭐ *Hints and tips*
> Nickel is a known allergen but can still be found in some jewellery. Always use only reputable suppliers that are aware of the use of hypoallergenic materials in ear-piercing studs.

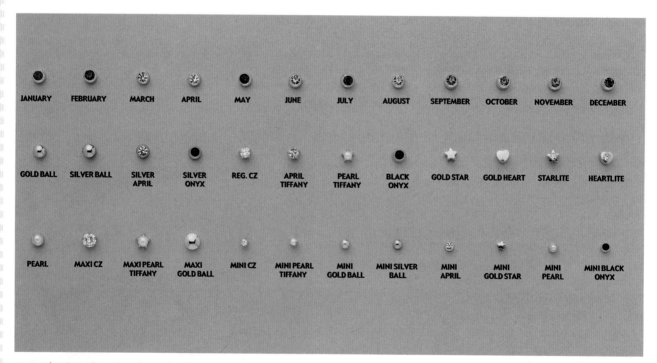

△ A selection of earrings for pierced ears

Before beginning treatment, hands should be washed thoroughly in hot soapy water or wiped with a suitable hand sanitizer containing surgical alcohol. Any open wounds, cuts and abrasions should be covered by a suitable waterproof dressing before applying a clean pair of powder-free nitrile or vinyl disposable gloves. Latex gloves should be avoided as they can produce allergic reactions in some clients. The use of personal protective equipment (PPE) prevents cross-contamination of infectious skin diseases and blood-borne viruses.

Outcome 2: Consult, plan and prepare for ear lobe piercing with clients

As with all treatments, it is important to perform a thorough consultation to ensure the client's suitability and safety for piercing and to determine their needs and expectations.

Consultation techniques

A good questioning technique is important to gain the information from the client that is necessary for safe and effective ear-piercing. It is important that you speak clearly. Questions should be worded to gain the relevant information while maintaining the client's privacy. To gain factual information, the questions can be closed ones, but where you need to gain more information, open questions are better. Listening is as important as speaking clearly if you are to write down the client's responses to your questions accurately on a record card and avoid any confusion later.

It is against the law to refuse treatment on grounds of age, gender, disability, culture or religious beliefs. There are some exceptions and your salon will advise you on this. Where reasonable adjustments can be made to the salon to provide access and to allow treatments, they should be made. Salons must meet the legal requirements outlined earlier in this chapter and the requirements of the industry standards.

The age of the client is important when treating 'minors' as you should gain a parent's or guardian's consent before piercing the ears of a child under the age of 16 years. Some establishments ask this of clients up to the age of 18, although there is no obligation to do so. Piercing the ears of a child of pre-school age is legal with parental or guardian consent, though some salons refuse to do this as part of their own salon policy. The parent or guardian should be present during the ear-piercing treatment when treating a minor. Treating minors without a parent's consent and/or without a parent being present may be construed as child abuse.

Only the soft tissue of the ear lobe is suitable for piercing. Piercing the cartilage leads to an overgrowth of cartilage and other tissue called **keloid scarring** and through inflammation of the cartilage tissue a condition called 'cauliflower ear'.

A visual and manual check of the area to be treated should also confirm its suitability for piercing. The ear should be checked for any signs of inflammation or infection. Wearing PPE, manually check the ear where it is to be pierced for keloid scarring from previous piercings or cysts.

 Hints and tips
More information on equal opportunity law is listed at the end of this chapter.

 Hints and tips
The age where one is considered a minor is variable in different parts of the UK. In England, Wales and Northern Ireland it is under the age of 18 years and in Scotland it is under the age of 17 years.

Key term

Keloid scarring – the excessive build up of scar tissue at the site of a wound.

 Health and safety

Special insurance and equipment is required to perform piercing of cartilage tissue such as that found in the nose and the ear and therefore are not in the scope of this unit.

 Activity

You are a salon owner and you are about to introduce ear-piercing into your salon. Prepare a suitable policy for your salon, including the procedures to decide suitability of clients for ear-piercing. Then design a poster that advertises the treatment and clearly reflects your salon policy.

Contraindications

It is important that you identify clients who can be treated safely and those for whom for ear-piercing is unsuitable. Contraindications are signs or indications why a treatment cannot continue (i.e they prevent a treatment) or that a modification to the treatment is required (i.e. they restrict the treatment).

▽ Contraindications that prevent treatment

Contra-indication	Why
Diabetes	Diabetics have poor healing ability so the risk of infection is high.
Epilepsy	The stress and shock of the treatment may induce a fit.
High or low blood pressure	The stress of treatment may cause light headedness or fainting.
Those clients prone to keloid scarring, e.g. black skins.	The formation of keloid scarring is likely with ear-piercing.
Allergies to metals	The allergic reaction may be severe and the risk of infection is high.
Inflammation of the ear or fever	This could indicate another illness.
Infections of the outer or inner ear	This could indicate another illness.
Local skin diseases and disorders	The risk of cross-contamination to you or another client is high.
Blood borne infections such as HIV/AIDS or Hepatitis	The risk of cross-contamination to you or another client is high.
Haemophilia	The blood does not clot and there would be persistent bleeding.
Those clients taking anti-coagulant drugs such as Warfarin	The blood does not clot and there would be persistent bleeding.

When a contraindication that prevents treatment is present you must use tact and diplomacy to inform the client that the service cannot be performed. The client should be advised to see a medical practitioner without naming the specific condition. You should be able to recognise a possible problem but must not diagnose it. Let the medical practitioner diagnose as they are qualified to do so. Clear and tactful communication is required to inform the client of the facts without causing them undue alarm or distress.

▽ Contraindications that restrict treatment

Contraindication	Modification
Swelling	If the swelling is of a known origin, the treatment should be delayed until it has gone.
Bruising	The treatment should be delayed and the client encouraged to return when the bruising has gone.
Cuts and abrasions	The treatment should be delayed and the client encouraged to return when healed.
Small ear lobe	Careful placement of the piercing would need to be discussed with the client.
Moles and warts	Careful placement of the piercing would need to be discussed with the client.
Previous piercing	Careful placement of the piercing would need to be discussed with the client. The distance between piercing should be approximately 1 cm.
Scar tissue	Careful placement of the piercing would need to be discussed with the client.

Client records

You should write clearly the details of the consultation onto the client's record card and ask the client (parent or guardian if the client is under 16) to read it for accuracy and sign to say they have understood and agree to the treatment being performed.

Information to be recorded on a client record card includes:

- personal details – name, address, telephone number, etc.
- date of treatment
- client, parent or guardian signature
- details of the treatment – number of previous piercings, position of piercing (indicated in a diagram), procedure and aftercare advice given.

Client records should be updated with accurate information on each visit so they can be referred to if necessary in the event of a contra-action occurring, or if legal action is taken against you. Even with the greatest of care and attention to procedure, an incident could occur and accurate records are invaluable to protect the business, the staff and the client. Failure to keep accurate and up-to-date client records can make your public liability insurance void.

Client records (whether kept by a salon electronically or in paper form) are protected by the **Data Protection Act 1998**. The records should be kept securely to prevent clients' personal information becoming available to those for whom it is unintended. If on computer, records must be 'password protected' or if paper-based, secured in a lockable cabinet.

Prepare the client for ear-piercing

Once you have performed the consultation you should have enough information to advise the client about the safe placement of the piercing and recommend the correct equipment, materials and products to achieve the required result. You should use your knowledge of the anatomy of the ear when discussing the placement of the ear-piercing.

The client should be allowed time to ask questions to clarify points. It is essential that the client is aware of the procedure, risks, cost, duration, healing time and aftercare before the treatment begins. This ensures the precise needs of the client are met and that the client fully understands the process. The commercially viable treatment time for an ear-piercing treatment is usually fifteen minutes. Treatment should be carried out within this time, as you should not keep your next client waiting.

Activity

Collect three price lists from local salons or other establishments that offer ear-piercing services and compare the prices and the times allocated for the treatment.

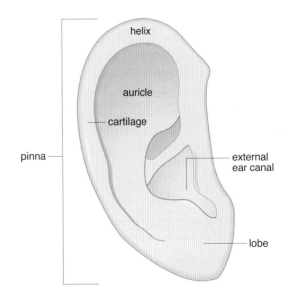

△ Structure of the ear

Equipment checklist

To perform an ear-piercing treatment you will need:

✔ ear-piercing gun that conforms to health and safety requirements
✔ sterile ear studs
✔ non-toxic marker pen
✔ medical wipes or swabs impregnated with surgical alcohol to cleanse the ears
✔ mirror
✔ clean cotton wool
✔ hand sanitizer
✔ waste bin lined with a yellow liner for contaminated waste
✔ sharps box for the disposal of unused studs
✔ head band or hair clips
✔ disposable powder-free nitrile or vinyl gloves
✔ aftercare lotion and instruction leaflet.

Back to basics

In order to promote professionalism, and to promote a healthy and safe working environment, the therapist must present the following. Use the boxes to check your personal appearance.

❑ A high standard of personal hygiene is presented.
❑ Fresh breath, free from cigarette or food odours.
❑ Clean, pressed work wear.
❑ Clean, low-heeled, enclosed shoes.
❑ Arms and hands free from jewellery (except wedding ring).
❑ Any earrings or necklaces are discreet.
❑ Make-up is discreet and expertly applied.
❑ Long hair is tied neatly away from the face and shoulders.
❑ Nails are short, smooth, clean and free of nail enamel.
❑ Tights, or socks with trousers, are worn.
❑ Cuts or open wounds are covered with a clean dressing.
❑ Hands are washed immediately before and after treatments.
❑ Calm and professional manner is maintained at all times.

The client may be nervous, so you must be reassuring and confident in your approach. The treatment should proceed as follows:

1. The client should be seated at a convenient height and position in good light.
2. Discuss the type and number of piercings required. No more than one pair of studs should be fitted at one time because the risk of infection and the discomfort is increased. If only one ear is to be pierced, the remaining stud from the sterile pack should be discarded.
3. Secure the hair away from the ear with clips or a headband as necessary.
4. With the aid of a mirror, discuss the exact position of the finished result, ensuring this is in the fleshy part of the ear. If other jewellery is worn it should be removed at this stage.
5. Put on a pair of powder-free nitrile or vinyl gloves as PPE.
6. Clean the ear back and front with a separate medical swab for each ear. Allow to dry.

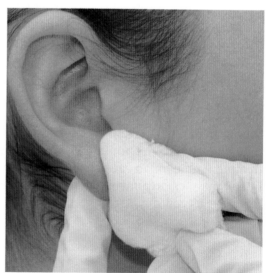

△ Clean the back and front of each ear with a separate medical swab

7. Place a small dot on each ear lobe using the non-toxic marker pen to indicate the position of the earrings. Remember the dot should be placed in the fleshy part of the ear and not too close to the edge as this may cause tearing if the earring is caught accidentally.

8. Check the intended position with the client using the mirror. If it is incorrect, remove the dot with a medical swab, then allow to dry before trying again. When both you and the client are happy, continue with the treatment.

Outcome 3: Pierce the ear lobes

1. Load the gun with the studs according to the manufacturer's instructions. Do not touch the studs and ensure that all disposable guards are in place.

2. Hold the ear to be pierced with your free hand and with the gun in a horizontal position place the stem of the stud over the mark made on the ear lobe. Squeeze the trigger gently so the stem is closer to the ear. If the position is not correct, reposition and repeat. Check the position over the mark and if correct squeeze firmly to release the gun and pierce the ear.

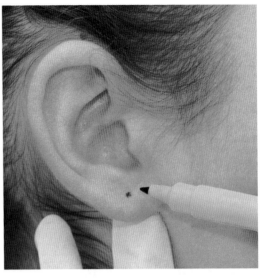
△ Mark the position with a non-toxic marker pen

 Remember...

Hold the piercing gun level parallel to the shoulder to ensure correct placement of the stud. Do not angle the gun up or down, inwards towards the head or outwards, as the stud will hang at that angle and not lie straight in the ear.

☆ *Hints and tips*
It is common for a person's ears not to be exactly the same shape and size. One may appear lower than the other or protrude more from the head. Any differences will be emphasised by the placement of an earring so take time to get the positioning correct and use the facial features as a guide if this helps.

3. Release the gun by gently pulling downwards, while still holding the ear with the other hand.

4. Repeat on the other ear if required.

5. If the gun malfunctions, the usual result is that the back of the stud is not secured to the stem. In this instance it is advisable to place the back into position by hand after wiping it with a clean medical swab. In the unlikely event that the ear is not pierced through, the stud should be removed, the area wiped with a medical swab, covered with a sterile dressing and the client asked to return when healed. This may take several weeks and they should be provided with aftercare lotion to bathe the area during the healing process. If any problems occur they should be advised to seek medical advice.

6. Show the finished result to the client in the mirror to gain her approval.

7. Instruct the client on accurate aftercare.

8. Remove the plastic cartridges and dispose of in the yellow waste bin.

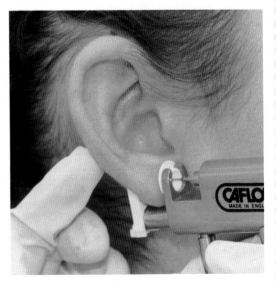
△ Piercing the ear with a piercing gun

9. Clean the gun with surgical spirit and store hygienically, for example in a UV cabinet, for the next use.

10. Dispose of any unused studs in a sharps box.

11. Remove all waste, including the gloves, from the area and place in a yellow bin liner in a covered bin.

12. Wash hands or use a hand sanitizer containing at least 70 per cent surgical grade alcohol.

The work area should be left clean and ready for use for the next client. This is part of working effectively as a team and ensures the smooth running of a beauty therapy business. The work area should be wiped with disinfectant or sanitising solution, furniture, equipment and materials replaced and waste disposed of appropriately.

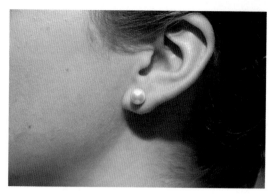

△ A just-pierced ear

Outcome 4: Provide aftercare advice

You are required to give advice and recommendations accurately following an ear-piercing treatment.

Contra-actions

Contra-actions are unwanted effects that occur after the treatment. Some are classed as normal for that treatment, others are not. Tingling and some redness and/or slight swelling in the area are normal effects after ear-piercing. Symptoms that are more unusual are:

 Dizziness/fainting or light-headedness – the shock of the treatment can cause these symptoms to some clients, particularly if they were nervous beforehand. They will accompany colour draining from the face and the client will appear pale. The client should be encouraged to remain seated and place their head between the knees, so that the head is lower than the heart, or if possible, ask the client to lie down on a couch and raise their feet with pillows so that the feet are higher than the heart. Encourage the client to relax by taking deep slow breaths and remain until the symptoms have passed.

 Infection – is often the result of not following the aftercare advice. The symptoms are inflammation, redness, swelling and the weeping of serum or pus. The client should contact the salon by telephone where relevant advice can be given and relevant notes made on the client's record card. If the problems continue you should instruct the client to see a medical practitioner.

 Allergic reaction – it is possible that although you have used hypo-allergenic studs an allergic reaction can occur; the symptoms of which will be swelling, irritation and redness. The client may be allergic to the aftercare lotion and should initially be instructed to stop using it and use a warm saline solution in its place. If this does not improve the symptoms it means the client is allergic to the studs and they should be removed and the wounds bathed with an appropriate antiseptic until healed. Clearly, ear-piercing is not suitable for this client.

✋ **Health and safety**

Remember that the waste from ear-piercing is classed as clinical or contaminated waste. This means that it should be placed in a yellow bin liner, which indicates that it needs special removal from the premises and taken for incineration. These special requirements should be requested through your local authority.

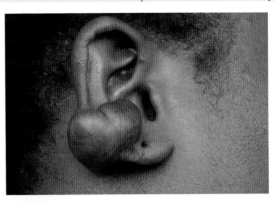

△ Keloid scarring

- **Keloid scarring** – is a condition where there is an overgrowth of the ear tissue resulting in a raised area of scar tissue. It is not painful or infected and if mild the studs can remain in place. In severe cases the studs would need to be removed and the client advised that ear-piercing is not a suitable treatment.

- **Extreme swelling** – in this case the ear lobe may swell to such an extent that the stud becomes 'embedded' in the tissue. You should put on PPE and adjust the back fastening so that it is more comfortable, wiping the area with aftercare lotion before and after touching the piercing. If the swelling is so severe the stud may need to be removed to allow the hole to heal and then re-pierced using a long post stud.

Aftercare advice

Advice on care of newly pierced ears is based on keeping the area meticulously clean. Advice should be given verbally and supported by a written aftercare leaflet. Aftercare lotions should be offered as a retail opportunity – they may be provided by your supplier as part of the ear-piercing system. They are a sanitising solution containing surgical grade alcohol or quaternary ammonium compounds. A fresh, warm saline solution can be used as an alternative or in the case of allergies.

The following points should be included in aftercare advice:

- Should any of the mentioned contra-actions occur, begin bathing with saline solution or aftercare solution.

- The studs should not be removed for six weeks to give the ears time to heal properly, preventing secondary infection. Premature removal will result in the hole closing up and/or infection.

- The ears should be bathed twice a day with the aftercare solution or warm saline solution. Undiluted antiseptic is not suitable for this as it is too strong and may cause irritation or chemical burns to the ear lobe.

- The hands should be washed before the ears are bathed.

- Touching the ears or studs between bathing should be avoided.

- After bathing, the studs should be turned to avoid the ear healing onto the stud. To do this, hold the back or 'butterfly' with one hand while turning the stud from the front with the other.

- Avoid spraying the ears with hairspray or perfume and ensure that shampoo and soap do not accumulate around the stud.

- After six weeks the studs can be changed with others of a good quality metal. Care should be taken with cheap fashion earrings as they are made of metals that cause irritation and should only be worn for short periods of time.

- The client should be advised that if no earrings are worn then the piercings are likely to heal over.

Hints and tips

It is advisable to note on the client's record card that you have provided an aftercare leaflet. This will prove useful if the salon needs to make an insurance claim.

Activity

Design an aftercare leaflet for use with clients who have had their ears pierced.

Cosmetic piercing

This is the term used to describe all body piercing, including ear-piercing. Body piercing is performed within a variety of civilisations and religions and for a variety of reasons, including spiritual and sexual, as well as a type of body adornment.

In the west, body piercing has become fashionable with often 'celebrity culture' leading the way. Tongue, eyebrow, nose and belly piercing are becoming commonplace and more clients are making enquiries about these types of service. More extreme body piercing (nipple and genitalia) are sometimes requested.

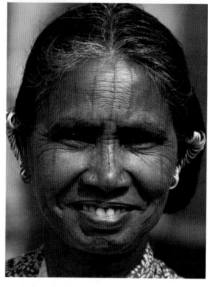
△ Cultural piercing

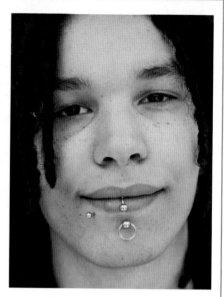
△ Facial piercing

Body piercing requires further training and knowledge and so is beyond the scope of this particular unit and your responsibility as a student of the qualification. However, there are private schools that offer training courses of between one and four days, depending on the types of piercing services you wish to learn.

Many body piercers do not like using a piercing gun but prefer instead the use of a needle with or without a hollow tube called a cannula. The needles come in a variety of sizes depending on the type of piercing and the result required. The needle pierces the skin after sterilising and anaesthetising and the cannula slides over the needle into the piercing. The jewellery is then inserted into the cannula before pulling it through the piercing where it is secured.

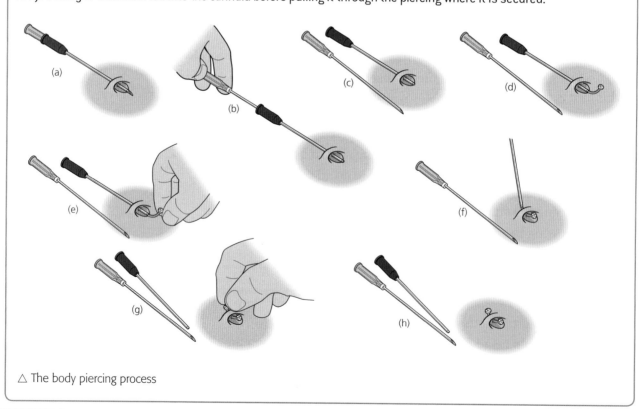

△ The body piercing process

Test yourself

Test yourself on ear-piercing by answering the following questions:

1. Which piece of legislation provides guidelines on hygiene practice for ear-piercing?

2. Why is only the soft tissue of the ear lobe suitable for piercing?

3. Why is it important to gain parental or guardian's consent when piercing the ears of a client under 16 years of age?

4. How often should the ears be cleaned and the stud rotated after piercing?

    a) once a day

    b) twice a day

    c) once a week

    d) twice a week.

5. How long should the studs be kept in the ears after piercing?

    a) two weeks

    b) four weeks

    c) six weeks

    d) eight weeks.

6. Which of these hygiene precautions must the therapist take when piercing ears?

    a) wash hands

    b) wear disposable gloves

    c) cover cuts and abrasions on the hands

    d) all of the above.

7. What information should be on a client's record card?

8. Why is it important that information on a record card is accurate and up to date?

9. Which part of the ear is recommended for piercing?

10. What action would you take if the ear-piercing gun malfunctions?

11. What action would you take if a client presented for ear-piercing treatment with a contra-indication that prevents treatment?

12. What action would you take if a client presented for ear-piercing treatment with a contra-action that restricts treatment?

13. Why is it important to allow time for the client to ask questions during the consultation?

14. Why is it important to wear disposable gloves when performing ear-piercing treatment?

15. How should you prepare the work area for ear-piercing treatment?

16. What should happen to an unused stud that is not required?

17. Why is only one pair of studs fitted at a time?

18. If the client experienced a contra-action to the treatment, what would be your advice?

19. What are the dangers with piercing the cartilage part of the ear?

20. Why is 'aftercare lotion' not suitable for use on everyone?

Are you ready for assessment?

 Remember...
Because ear piercing is an invasive procedure, hygiene procedures must be rigorously followed to prevent infection.

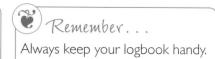 *Remember...*
Always keep your logbook handy.

The following checklist will help you to be fully prepared for your practical assessment.

The range of clients/treatments you must cover:

- Equipment used in ear piercing service.
- Various consultation techniques.
- Consider your actions if contraindications are present.
- Ear piercing techniques.
- Health and safety procedures.
- Give aftercare advice.

1. Practical observation

 Remember...
Your assessor will observe your performance on at least two occasions each involving a different client.

Your assessor will look at how you:

- prepare the treatment area ensuring that you carry out strict hygienic practice
- prepare the treatment area with suitable ear piercing equipment
- consult with the client and prepare a record card
- establish the needs of the client
- use products and equipment safely
- carry out the ear piercing in a commercially acceptable time
- check with the client that the result is to the client's satisfaction
- provide aftercare advice
- demonstrate professional practice throughout the service
- carry out all treatments with regard to health and safety.

2. Knowledge and understanding

What you must know:

- Organisational and legal requirements.
- How to work safely and effectively when providing ear piercing services.
- Consult, plan and prepare for treatment with clients.
- Contraindications and contra-actions.

- Anatomy and physiology.
- Ear piercing equipment, types of earrings and products used.
- Aftercare advice.

To ensure that you have the necessary knowledge and understanding of ear-piercing services your assessor will:

- ask you questions before, during and after carrying out the treatment
- ensure that you have completed project work and written exercises relating to the unit
- check that you have recorded in a log/diary treatments you have carried out with signed record cards showing that you have completed the required number of ear piercing services competently
- check that you have covered the range in your candidate logbook
- require you to take a test.

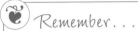
Remember...

Simulation is not a valid means of assessment for ear piercing service.

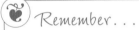
Remember...

Permission from a parent or guardian must be sought before piercing the ears of a child.

Sources of evidence

- Completed client record cards indicating the range of clients.
- Certificates of achievement from commercial courses.
- Photos/video.
- Aftercare leaflet you have produced.
- Client feedback.
- Project work on range of techniques used in piercing.

Chapter 16

Unit S1: Assist with spa operations

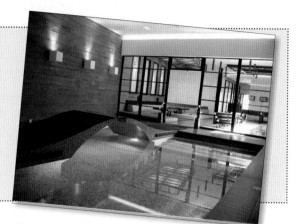

Learning objectives

This chapter covers Unit S1 Assist with spa operations, that is the maintenance of the quality and general condition and appearance of spa areas including the skills and knowledge needed.

> There are four outcomes for Unit S1 and they are:
>
> 1 Maintain safe and effective methods of working when assisting with spa operations.
> 2 Clean and set up spa work areas.
> 3 Check and maintain the spa work areas.
> 4 Shut down work areas.

You will need to be competent in all of these outcomes in assisting with spa operations to qualify for insurance and work within the spa environment.

Evidence requirements

Your assessor will need to observe you show competence for the above outcomes in the following work areas.

1 Work areas:
- wet areas
- treatment areas
- changing rooms
- relaxation areas
- service areas.

Introduction

Spa treatments have become increasingly popular with clients and are widely available. However, they are not a new phenomenon. The benefits of using heat and water for their therapeutic and relaxation effects were known in Roman and Egyptian times. The term 'spa' is believed to have originated from a Latin phrase *solus per aqua* which means 'health from water'.

Modern spa therapies include the traditional use of heat and water but with the addition of product application, wraps and flotation tanks for therapeutic effect.

Unit S1 is listed as an optional one, worth four credits. It appears in both the general and make-up routes of the NVQ qualification.

Meet the professional

"Working as a spa therapist on board a cruise liner was a real eye opener but I'm so glad I had the opportunity to do this. Long days at work and working six days a week on a commission and gratuity-based wage was really hard. The whole experience gave me a chance to meet other therapists from all over the world, to share different techniques and skills, and also to interact with a wide variety of clientele, and of course the chance to leave the ship and visit somewhere different every week!

Being a spa therapist provides fantastic rewards, perks and ongoing training, as well as sufficient product knowledge to perform treatments to the best of your ability. My passion for my job and standard of treatment combined with my enthusiasm in what I was doing meant my company saw my potential and I gained promotion – at first to Senior Therapist and then Treatment Supervisor. This was a great opportunity to gain more knowledge on how the department operates, understanding department targets, goals and financial figures. With the help and development from my manager I progressed to Assistant and then to Treatment Manager."

Kirsty Ellis

Spa treatments

Spa treatments include the following.

- **Steam** – a moist heat treatment applied in a specially designed room. Several people or individuals can be treated in a steam bath or cabinet.
- **Sauna** – a dry heat treatment applied using an insulated, log or pine-panelled cabin, for use by several people.
- **Hydrotherapy** – a general term used to describe the use of water to bring about therapeutic effects. Hot and cold water are used, often one after the other, or jets of water are used to massage while heating the body. Treatments for individuals or for several people, as in a **hydrotherapy pool**, are available.

 Hints and tips

Salt water is healing. The burns of fighter pilots whose aeroplanes were shot down over the sea during the Second World War healed more quickly due to the healing and sterilising properties of salt water.

- **Flotation** – the sensation of weightlessness created by this treatment induces a deep sense of relaxation and relieves aches and pains. **Wet flotation** involves being supported by water in either a small tank or a large pool containing high levels of mineral salts for therapeutic effect. **Flotation massage** is also available. **Dry flotation** involves the use of water but the client is separated from it by a vinyl waterproof sheet. No benefit is gained from contact with mineral salts but the treatment induces deep relaxation.

- **Body wrapping** – allows the skin to absorb products for different effects, which is then enhanced by wrapping the body in specially designed bandages or thermal reflective sheeting.

- **Relaxation rooms** – form an important part of the 'spa experience'. Large areas often with shaped, heated stone beds are provided for relaxation, where the temperature is similar to body temperature.

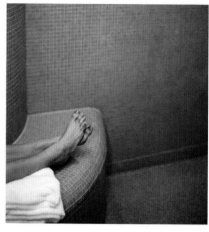
△ Steam room

Effects of spa treatments

The effects of individual spa treatments are specific and vary a great deal. However, they generally rely on the effects of changes in temperature, water, product application and relaxation on the well-being of the body and mind. The sections that follow give a summary of the general effects.

Effects brought about through temperature changes

Heat	Cold
Increases body temperature	Drop in body temperature
Induces perspiration	Perspiration is greatly reduced
Eliminates waste products	Waste removal slows
Increases blood circulation	Blood circulation slows
Produces an erythema	Skin pales as blood is diverted away from the surface
Lowers blood pressure	Lowers blood pressure
Raises pulse rate	Raises pulse rate
Increase in metabolic rate	Slows metabolic rate
Induces weight loss	Tightening and toning effect on the skin
Improves lymph flow	Reduces inflammation
Warms the tissues	Creates shortening of the muscle fibres and a temporary toning effect to the muscles
Relaxes muscles	Analgesic effect on nervous tissue reducing pain
Relieves minor pain and stiffness	Stimulating and invigorating
Gives a feeling of relaxation and well-being but also fatigue or exhaustion	Re-energising

Effects brought about through the application of water

Uses	Effects
To provide weightlessness and eliminate the effects of gravity	Reduces minor aches and pains
	Supports the body weight so complete body muscle relaxation
	Lowers pulse rate and blood pressure
	Reduces joint pain
	Alleviates back pain
	Aids injuries and conditions such as rheumatism and arthritis
	Reduces fatigue as it simulates sleep for conditions such as insomnia or jet lag
	Relieves stress and anxiety
	Aids respiratory conditions such as asthma
As resistance	Strengthens ligaments and tendons supporting joints
	Strengthens and tones muscles
	Improves fitness and body shape
As showers or jets	Has a massage effect on the tissues and its associated effects, i.e. increases blood circulation, etc.
	Deep relaxation of muscle tissue
	Increases the flexibility of the joints
	Improves lymphatic flow and drainage
	Reduces swelling
	Removes lactic acid accumulated after exercise
	Reduces stress
	Aids elimination so benefits cellulite and those on a detox programme

Effects brought about the application of products

As well as the creams, lotions and oils that can be applied as part of any treatment, spa treatments additionally rely on the special application methods to bring about beneficial effects.

During wet flotation the mineral salts in the water that help to support the body weight are also beneficial to the skin, improving its softness and helping skin conditions such as eczema and psoriasis.

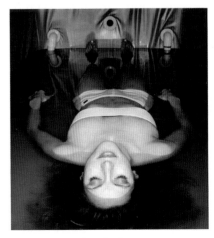

△ Flotation tank or bath

Mud used in body wrapping contain beneficial products such as seaweed extracts that are readily absorbed into the skin and can bring about a high degree of elimination of waste products, helping cellulite and **detoxification**.

Effects brought about through relaxation

Relaxation is the state of mind that may precede sleep. It is indicated by a change of frequency of waves in brain activity. Research has shown that this occurs during spa treatment. The psychological effects and benefits of spa treatments are:

- deep state of relaxation
- feeling of calm and well-being
- reduction in stress levels
- reduction in the symptoms of anxiety
- lowering of blood pressure (which over time reduces the likelihood of stroke or heart attack).

Rest is an integral part of the spa experience and special areas are set aside to facilitate relaxation.

> **Key term**
>
> **Detoxification** – the removal of excessive waste product accumulation, to return the body back to a state of homeostasis and therefore a more healthy condition.

Outcome 1: Maintain safe and effective methods of working when assisting with spa operations

The moisture and warmth of the spa environment enjoyed by the clients is an excellent breeding ground for micro-organisms. It is imperative that safe and effective working methods are employed during spa operations.

Safe and effective working methods when working in the spa industry

The spa industry expects a level of professionalism and effectiveness to ensure the safety of its clients.

Personal appearance and hygiene

As well as the normal high standards of appearance and personal hygiene stated previously in this book there are further considerations for working in the spa industry.

The hot and humid environment within a spa means that special attention must be given to personal hygiene, with the use of an effective antiperspirant. Professional work wear is best made of natural fibres such as cotton, rather than man-made fibres. If trousers are worn they should be cropped, as they are less likely to get wet.

Shoes should be flat, enclosed and have a non-slip sole to minimise the risk of slipping in the wet areas of the spa.

Jewellery should be kept to a minimum as the skin directly under jewellery may harbour micro-organisms and could lead to skin conditions such as dermatitis or fungal infection. Also, any metal will retain heat and could produce a mild burn.

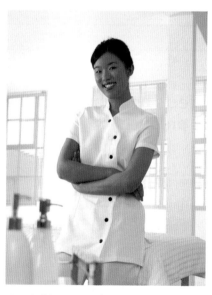

△ Suitable spa work wear

Make-up should be able to stand the extreme temperatures so waterproof products such as mascara are advisable.

Long hair needs to be secured firmly to sit off both the face and shoulder. Short hair should be styled in such a way that the use of hairspray is avoided. Hairspray can become soluble in water and is likely to enter the eyes if worn.

Personal protective equipment (PPE)

Appropriate clothing and equipment should be provided by the employer where there is a potentially hazardous task to be undertaken by an employee. In a spa this is largely applicable to the use, storage and disposal of cleaning solutions for use within the work areas of the spa. Depending on the size of the establishment it may be that this equipment is intended for the spa assistant rather than a cleaner.

The relevant PPE that should be provided by your employer includes powder-free nitrile or vinyl gloves, disposable apron and eye protection, and suitable footwear for use within the service areas of the spa. It is important that if PPE has been provided that you use it. The tasks you are undertaking warrant its use and you are legally obliged to follow organisational procedures and protect yourself while at work.

Legislative requirements for spa operations

General relevant legislation that states your health and safety responsibilities can be found in Chapter 3. As with all treatments, the local authority should be contacted to find out about any relevant local byelaws that apply.

There are important laws that set out the requirements concerning the provision of spa treatments.

The **Control of Substances Hazardous to Health Regulations 2002** are concerned with the use, storage and disposal of hazardous substances. In the case of spa treatments, this involves the assessment of the cleaning and sterilising agents such as chlorine that are used within spa operations. The employer should consider the **Manufacturer's Safety Data (MSD)** information provided for each substance and ascertain the necessary controls for safe use, storage and disposal. This will involve the provision of PPE, the writing of procedures and the dissemination of the information to employees. The MSD also provides the correct information for the disposal of such chemicals. It is not always possible to dispose of chemicals into a sink and the salon should find out about this, not only for the sake of the environment but to comply with legal requirements.

The **Managing Health and Safety in Swimming Pools (HSG179)** guidelines apply to the provision of spa treatments. The guidelines provide best practice procedures and standards for the operation of pools and spas, including identifying risks that may lead to drowning, chemical safety and general poolside safety.

 Health and safety

The **Personal Protective Equipment at Work Regulations 1992 (PPE)** state that the employer must assess the need for PPE within the workplace and provide the appropriate PPE for use by their employees.

 Health and safety

The **Health & Safety at Work Act 1974** states that an employee has a duty of care to act and behave responsibly whilst at work, comply with health and safety procedures as laid down by their employer and report any non-compliance or hazardous practices to the appropriate person.

 Health and safety

The **Environmental Protection Act 1990; Controlled Waste Regulations 1992** and **Special Waste Regulations 1996** can give further guidance as to your legal position.

Swimming Pool and Allied Trades Association (SPATA) is the trade association for the swimming pool and spa industry in the UK. Its members are pool builders, retailers, designers, service engineers and trade suppliers in the UK and overseas. It covers both domestic and commercial installations.

Test yourself

1. What piece of health and safety legislation is concerned with the assessment of work practices to identify risk and the associated hazards and set in place the controls to reduce the risk?

2. What piece of health and safety legislation is concerned with the displaying of health and safety policies and procedures?

Minimising risk of harm to self or others

Back problems, skin complaints such as contact dermatitis, and repetitive strain injuries are a risk for those working within the spa industry and care should be taken to prevent them. You have a legal obligation while at work to minimise any harmful situation, whether it be to yourself or to a colleague, client or visitor to the spa. This means that you must know how to identify potential risky situations and either control the risk if it is within the realms of your responsibility or report to someone who is responsible for that task.

Cross-infection

The risk of cross-infection or contamination in a spa organisation is high, due to the levels of moisture and heat present in the environment, which are ideal growing conditions for micro-organisms. You should employ the basic procedures for minimising cross-infection.

The best way to avoid cross-infection is to prevent anyone with an infectious condition from using the spa facilities. Strict application of contraindications by the therapist can greatly reduce the risk. Check the client for contraindications: anyone with ear, skin, respiratory, foot or other bodily infection should refrain from using the spa facilities. It may not be possible to identify infections as some conditions may yet to exhibit symptoms, so good hygiene practices are very important. The use of appropriate sterilising agents and the application of hygiene procedures at the correct time can minimise the risk of cross-infection even further. Where sterilisation is not practical, you should use disposable items such as couch roll, panties, spatulas, gloves, overshoes, aprons and oversleeves to place a barrier between the client and the surface or product, and between you and the client.

 Remember...

The terms **sterilisation** and **disinfection** are sometimes confused.

Key term

Sterilisation destroys all micro-organisms by the use of chemicals or high temperature.

Disinfection inhibits the growth of micro-organisms (except spores) that cause disease by the use chemical agents.

Antiseptic is a dilute disinfectant for use on the skin that slows the growth of bacteria.

 Health and safety

The **Working Time Regulations 1998** gives guidance as to the weekly hours worked and for the hours for those on night shifts. However, it does not specify how many breaks there should be, or how long. This is usually determined by the organisation for which you are working.

Dehydration and fatigue

The presence of heat in a spa, especially on a hot summer day, can increase the risk of dehydration and fatigue. It is important that plenty of fresh drinking water is available and that clients are encouraged to drink it frequently. You are responsible for yourself but also for clients so their fluid intake should be monitored. To combat fatigue, clients should be encouraged to rest in the relaxation areas away from the hotter areas of the spa. You must also ensure that you take regular breaks.

Posture

During the course of your working day it may be necessary to carry out tasks that could lead to poor posture or injury. You should be aware of your posture, particularly if lifting or performing a task for a period of time. Ensure that work surfaces are at the correct height for the task and ask for help to lift any objects that you consider to be too heavy. Working with inappropriate equipment at an inappropriate height or position can lead to postural problems, such as rounded shoulders, lower back pain and repetitive strain injury.

Refer to Chapter 3 on Health and Safety and Manual Handling Operations Regulations for correct lifting technique.

Contact dermatitis

With the prolonged exposure of the skin to moisture and chemicals, a condition known as **contact dermatitis** can occur. The moisture and chemicals breakdown the skin's natural resistance and it becomes sensitive to other products as well as those to which it was exposed. In severe cases this can lead to the end of a career in the spa and even the beauty industry, therefore it is important to use the PPE that is provided for you. It is also important to replace the natural skin barrier by the adequate use of suitable creams and lotions rubbed into the skin.

Reporting non-compliance

Your employer is responsible for the setting up of reporting procedures within your place of work. However, it is your responsibility to report incidents or accidents or cases of non-compliance of organisational procedures if you have come across them during your work. You should initially report to your line manager, who may be the senior therapist or the manager responsible for health and safety. Cases of injury or incident, however minor, need to be recorded in written form, either in an accident and incident book or on a report form designed for that purpose. These records should be kept for three years and can be used to review health and safety procedures.

> **Key term**
>
> **Contact dermatitis** – a skin condition caused by the exposure to an allergen or irritant. Skin appears red, dry and irritated and is accompanied by itching and, when severe, the skin will crack and bleed.

> **Health and safety**
>
> The **Manual Handling Operations Regulations 1992** requires your employer to identify hazards and to assess the risk involved with work activities and to put in place controls to reduce the risks. For example, the salon may provide lifting equipment and training in how to use it.

> **Health and safety**
>
> The **Reporting of Injuries, Diseases and Dangerous Occurrences Regulations 1995** (RIDDOR) gives guidelines for these reporting procedures including the information needed to be recorded and what to do in the case of a more serious accident or injury.

Outcome 2: Clean and set up spa work areas

Clients using a spa expect a high level of cleanliness and hygiene and do not expect to contract a disease or disorder. All staff are expected to contribute to the cleanliness of the spa but it is an important responsibility for the spa assistant.

Environmental conditions

The environment within the different areas of a spa vary depending on their function and use.

Wet areas

Wet areas include the sauna, spa pools, swimming pools, steam rooms, cold rooms, hydro baths, showers and wet flotation areas.

The lighting in the wet areas of a spa need to be bright in order to prevent accidents such as slipping. However, wet flotation areas have adjustable lighting that can be dimmed to provide relaxation once the client is in position – often lighting that represents stars in a night sky is used.

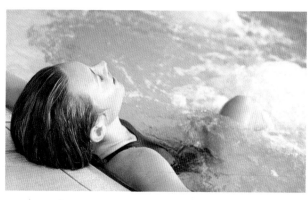
△ Spa pool

The temperature of a modern treatment sauna is between 60 and 90°C at the top of the sauna. Generally, women prefer a temperature between 60 and 70°C, and men prefer between 80 and 90°C.

Saunas are usually made of pine panels packed with insulating material, which retains the heat within the sauna. The heat is controlled by a thermostat, which should be placed outside the sauna to avoid clients attempting to adjust it.

Saunas produce a dry heat, which promotes a high degree of sweating and the elimination of waste products from the body. Very dry air can be uncomfortable to breathe so a water bucket and ladle are provided to pour onto the stones to produce steam.

Essential oils such as eucalyptus may be used in the water to create a pleasant smell and give therapeutic effects, but should only be added by someone qualified to do so. Pine wood is capable of absorbing the moisture from the air within the sauna and prevents the air becoming stale and smelling unpleasant. The air must be allowed to circulate around a sauna to permit an interchange of air within it.

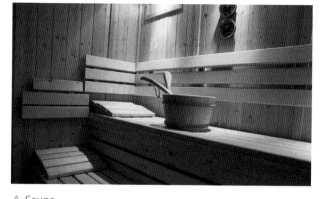
△ Sauna

A control panel away from the treatment area determines the temperature of a steam room at approximately 40°C. As several clients can use a steam room at once, the temperature cannot be adjusted to suit an individual. Instead, a thermometer is placed inside

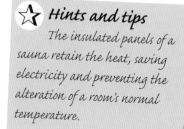
☆ *Hints and tips*
The insulated panels of a sauna retain the heat, saving electricity and preventing the alteration of a room's normal temperature.

or the temperature displayed to assist the client in judging their tolerance level. In general, men can tolerate a higher temperature than women. As the humidity is high (sometimes as much as 95 per cent) the temperature is usually lower than that of a sauna.

The temperature and timing controls for a steam bath are usually found on the outside of the equipment. These can be adjusted to suit an individual's tolerance level and are used to achieve a working temperature of between 50 and 55°C. The humidity within a steam bath is also high, as much as 95 per cent.

Spa pool water temperature should not exceed 40°C as the water's turbulence will raise the body temperature. At this temperature, exposure should be limited to 15 minutes before cooling down. After cooling down, further exposure can occur but for a shorter period. If prolonged exposure is desired, the water temperature should be reduced to normal body temperature (37°C).

Wet flotation tanks should also contain warm water so as to be pleasant and aid relaxation, whereas in dry tanks the client lies on a waterbed or airbed wrapped in thermal blankets and so a more comfortable room temperature is needed for comfort. The temperature of the water should be similar to that of body temperature – between 34 and 36°C.

Spa treatments naturally produce a high level of humidity, meaning that the air has up to 95 per cent saturation level of water vapour. Removing the warm, humid air and replacing it with fresh air greatly reduces the risk of cross-infection and reduces condensation. This is called air exchange.

This high level of humidity requires approximately 17–20 cubic metres of fresh air exchange per hour for each person using the room. The frequency at which the air should be exchanged is calculated by cubic metres of air, multiplied by the number of people using the facility, divided by the volume of the room.

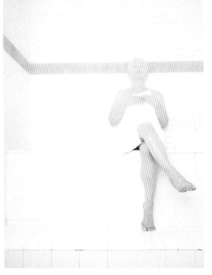
△ Steam room

Example

In a steam room that measures 3 m high × 4 m wide × 10 m long there is the facility for 14 people.

The calculations are:
Cubic metres of air: 17
Maximum number of people: 14
17 × 14 = 238
Volume of the room: 3 m × 4 m × 10 m = 120
Cubic metres of air x the number of people ÷ the volume of the room
238 ÷ 120 = approx. 2
The number of air changes needed per hour is 2.

The best method of ventilation is the use of air exchange units or air conditioning. Modern units filter dust and other airborne particles, including micro-organisms. They also warm or cool air as desired and can moisten or dry air by the use of a control panel.

Treatment areas

The treatment rooms are used to perform specific spa treatments and more traditional beauty therapy treatments such as facials and manicures. They have adjustable lighting that can be dimmed to promote relaxation, yet provide sufficient lighting at times when needed to allow the therapist to perform the treatment safely and effectively. The temperature should be comfortable for the client but not too hot as to cause fatigue and dehydration in the therapist. The client can be wrapped using sheets, blankets or quilts as appropriate to keep them warm. Higher room temperatures are needed during 'wet treatments' such as power showers so that the client does not feel cold. Humidity levels within the treatment rooms should be lower than in the wet areas (about 50–70 per cent) as high levels can increase fatigue and leave therapists prone to air- and water-borne infections. Ventilation is important to allow sufficient air exchange but without being draughty for the client.

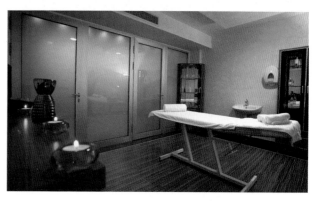
△ Spa treatment room

Health and safety

The Workplace (Health, Safety and Welfare) Regulations 1992 states the requirements for adequate working conditions such as ventilation, lighting and temperature, etc., for employees within the workplace.

Changing rooms

Changing rooms are usually bright areas with lockers to secure personal belongings and facilities such as mirrors and hairdryers. Changing rooms should be pleasantly warm as the client may be wet and will feel chilly if the temperature is too low. Ventilation should be sufficient to maintain the hygiene, safety and comfort of the client. There is seating for those who may need it and products such as cleansers, shampoo, body lotions and other consumables such as cotton wool and tissues, as well as hair-drying facilities.

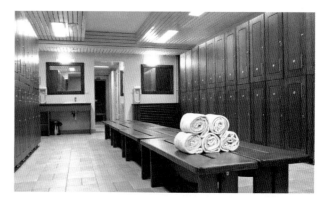
△ Typical changing area

Relaxation areas

The lighting in relaxation areas is often soft. There may be relaxation music playing.

The temperature is warm, close to body temperature to allow the body to recover from the treatment. During recovery, the blood pressure, pulse rate and body temperature can return to normal levels. Rest combats fatigue and allows time for the body to gain the benefit from the effects of the spa

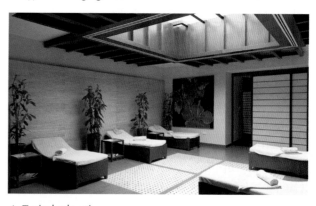
△ Typical relaxation area

treatment. Magazines and refreshments such as water and fruit juice are available for consumption. Clients should use these areas both during and near the end of their session to complete their spa experience.

Service areas

The lighting for these areas is bright and controlled within each room so that the facility can be used safely and effectively but switched off when not in use. **Service areas** are not normally heated and simple ventilation such as opening a window is adequate as use of the room is not prolonged.

Cleaning of spa work areas

General sterilisation methods use very high temperatures or strong chemicals, so are not suitable for use on many materials. Sterilisation methods are covered in Chapter 1.

The main risk of cross-infection within the spa are: **air-borne micro-organisms** such as viral infections responsible for colds and flu, which are spread in minute droplets of water expelled into the air where they can be breathed in by another person; **water-borne infections** that can be spread by direct or indirect contact with infected surfaces or by being immersed in contaminated water. This is more likely where water is allowed to stagnate.

There is a risk that air- and water-borne infections can also be spread through the consumption of food and drink.

Bacterial, viral and fungal skin infections such as impetigo, verrucae and athlete's foot can also be spread through direct or indirect contact with surfaces and equipment.

Other more serious air-borne or water-borne infections include:

- **Legionnaire's disease** – a bacterial infection, the symptoms of which are similar to flu, but in fact is a form of pneumonia. It is transmitted through water droplets in the air in which the bacteria are suspended. The bacteria need warmth and a food source such as sludge, scale, rust or algae so stagnant water is a high risk factor. Regular cleaning and maintenance of the spa wet areas and circulation of water in the spa pool greatly reduces the risk of contracting the disease.

- **Escherichia coli** (E. coli) – a bacterial infection, the symptoms of which are severe stomach cramps and diarrhoea. It is spread through drinking contaminated water as well as eating contaminated food. Fresh drinking water provided in a spa should be stored in a closed receptacle and food should be prepared only in designated areas of the spa to reduce the risk of transmission.

By following a few basic procedures and controls, the risk of contracting such diseases are minimised.

- Clients should be asked about any infectious conditions they may have and politely asked to shower before they use the spa facilities. They should wear clean swimwear or disposable

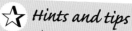

Hints and tips

The music or sounds played in relaxation areas have a low number of beats per minute to slow the heart rate.

Key term

Service area is a term used to describe different areas of a spa that 'service' the main areas of the spa. This includes the 'plant' rooms from where the controls for the equipment and facilities are operated, stock rooms, laundry facilities and waste storage areas.

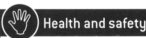

Health and safety

Usual methods of sterilisation are much too harsh to use on the skin. However, an antiseptic designed for skin use is safe and will inhibit the growth of micro-organisms.

underwear as appropriate and cover any cuts and/or abrasions with a waterproof dressing.

- Clean, fresh laundry should be provided for each client, including a gown for personal use while visiting the spa. Laundry should be washed at the highest temperature possible with a suitable detergent.

- When sterilising procedures cannot be followed disposable products should be used, such as absorbent paper on seats as well as towels and disposable foot wear. These act as a barrier between the client and a surface, which is especially useful when cleaning the surface after each contact is impossible.

- The possibility of external pollutants entering the spa on shoes and clothing can be avoided by providing changing facilities for both clients and staff. Therapists should not wear their work wear or shoes outside of the spa. If during the course of the day it is necessary to venture outside, special disposable shoe covers should be worn. Any visitors to the spa should also cover their shoes.

- No food or drink should be consumed within the spa, only in specially designated areas, such as the relaxation room. Water and fruit juice can be offered but should be provided by and be kept under the control of the organisation. Such drinks should be kept in a refrigerator or sealed drinks dispenser and not left out in the spa areas. Any unused beverages should be disposed of at the end of the day.

- Stagnant water is an ideal breeding ground for micro-organisms. Pools of water from condensation or spillage must not be allowed to remain but should be mopped up immediately.

- Washing hands in hot soapy water before and after each client and after visiting the toilet is a simple yet effective way of reducing cross-infection. Wash hands after handling chemicals, even if gloves have been worn, and before handling beverages.

- The surfaces, floors and walls of the **work areas** of a spa should be designed to be easily cleaned with an appropriate disinfectant. Materials such as ceramic tiles, glass or marble are easy to clean with the appropriate disinfectant or other suitable chemical agent. All surfaces (floors, walls, benches, showers, etc.) should be washed down daily, or more frequently if in constant use, with an appropriate disinfectant that leaves no residue or smell. Follow the manufacturer's instructions and wear personal protective equipment such as gloves, apron, mask and goggles as appropriate.

The cleaning of equipment within **wet areas** is more specific, as follows:

1. The sauna should be scrub-washed regularly, preferably with plain water or suitable cleansing agent to avoid noxious fumes when the sauna is reheated.

2. The water in the sauna bucket should be changed to avoid stagnation.

3. Towels should be provided to place on seating within the sauna, steam room or bath.

4. The steam bath or cabinet should be wiped with a disinfectant solution after each client.

5. Hydrotherapy pool equipment requires regular circulation of the water to ensure the correct use of commercially installed filtration plants. The number of circulations before a hygienic level is achieved depends on the size of the spa pool. Be guided by the manufacturer's instructions.

6. Chemical treatment of water in swimming and hydrotherapy pools with chlorine or bromine is essential. The latest commercial installations incorporate automatic chemical treatment machinery, which can test regularity at short intervals. However, this should not replace manual testing and the appropriate records being kept.

7. The spa pool should be drained occasionally and the acrylic surface wiped with a cleaning agent recommended by the manufacturer to avoid destroying the surface.

8. Spa baths are drained and cleaned for each individual user and therefore in general, the water does not need to be treated. Most spa baths and flotation tanks are made of an acrylic material so the surface must be wiped after each use with a cleaner recommended by the manufacturer to avoid contamination of the circulating water machinery.

Setting up the spa work areas

Preparing the different spa work areas involves the use of general procedures and those specific for each type of equipment. **General procedures** include ensuring an adequate supply of towels and gowns, consumables such as tissue, cotton wool, cleansers, shampoo in changing areas and showers, products such as cleansers, mineral mud, body lotions in the treatment rooms and magazines and fresh water or fruit juices in the relaxation areas.

Each spa organisation will have its own routine to follow but the procedures must comply with legal requirements to ensure hygiene, health and safety levels. Regular stock controls should be in place to ensure availability and adequate consumables and laundry supply and should be gauged by the number of clients booked for that day, with extra in case of emergency and late bookings.

Specific procedures for the individual facilities involve the protection of surfaces with towels and paper in accordance with organisational guidelines and heating up equipment to efficient operational temperature.

Spa pools do not require preheating – this would be very expensive. Instead, a thermostat similar to that of an immersion heater in a domestic house maintains the pool's temperature.

However, the water is not circulated overnight and so must be started at the beginning of each working day. The water should be allowed to circulate the correct number of times, depending on the size of the pool, to allow sufficient filtration to have occurred before the first client can enter it. It is important to be guided by the manufacturer's instructions for use.

Hints and tips

The aim of the chlorine or bromine chemicals is to produce a stable chemical condition that acts as a disinfectant.

Health and safety

Using too much chemical in pools and treatment facilities can cause eye problems such as stinging and irritation, dry skin and stomach upsets if consumed, as well as leaving an unpleasant smell on the skin surface.

Hints and tips

It is common practice for gowns and towels to be placed within each locker ready for use by the clients at the start of their spa experience.

Below is an indication of the possible start-up times for some equipment. The exact times will vary according to the size of the piece of equipment.

Equipment	Warm-up period
Steam room	20–30 minutes
Steam bath/cabinet	10–15 minutes
Sauna	20–30 minutes

Body wrapping preparation involves preparing the couch with towels and thermal sheeting, placing bandages into special heaters or warming products in a water bath.

Use and storage of cleaning materials

Many of the chemicals used to perform cleaning and sterilising procedures are hazardous and are controlled by the **Control of Substances Hazard to Health Regulations 2002**. General safety procedures to follow when using and storing chemicals are as follows:

1. Read the manufacturer's guidelines for use and dilution.
2. Follow the controls described on the manufacturer's safety data (MSD) sheet.
3. Wear recommended PPE such as gloves and goggles.
4. Store chemicals as recommended on the MSD. Keep separate any chemicals that might react together and place flammable materials in a fire-proof cabinet.
5. Chemicals should be stored with clear signage to avoid confusion and misuse.

Cleaning records

Strict records of cleaning regimes should be kept in order to maintain hygiene levels and satisfy environmental health officers. A simple method for a small spa is to have a chart on the wall of each facility so that the person responsible signs in the appropriate space when the cleaning regime has been carried out. In larger organisations a book containing all the daily records associated with cleaning, maintenance and usage may be kept together. Most local authorities require strict procedures to be followed in public spas and swimming pools and you should follow local authority guidelines and the instructions given by your line manager and those in authority.

Signage

Where applicable, health and safety warning signs should be posted in the relevant position to be clearly seen and noted by those for whom they are intended; this means clients as well as staff. As an employee you have a responsibility to not tamper with the signs, act upon them as instructed and report if the signs cannot be seen or have been defaced. You should also encourage clients and colleagues to act upon the sign's instruction and/or point out the sign or hazard as applicable.

Health and safety

Control of Substances Hazard to Health Regulations 2002 (SR24) available on the Health and Safety Executive website (www.hse.gov.uk) gives specific advice for the storage of chemicals, which should be followed.

For more information on health and safety signs, see Chapter 3.

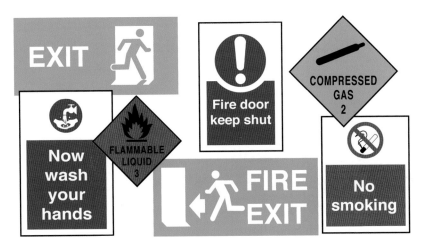

△ Health and safety signs

> **Health and safety**
>
> **The Health and Safety (Safety Signs and Signals) Regulations 1996** standardises health and safety signs so that they are uniform throughout the European Union. The regulations state that a relevant health and safety sign should be displayed where a hazard has been identified and the risk cannot be controlled by any other means.

Outcome 3: Check and maintain work areas

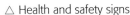

To maintain hygiene and safety standards to legal and organisational standards throughout the day, routine checks should be employed.

Client checks

Contraindications

The client should be checked for contraindications before using the spa facilities. This normally involves completing a questionnaire at the spa's reception. The contraindications for the use of the spa are divided into those requiring medical referral and those that may restrict the use of the facilities.

> **Activity**
>
> With a partner decide who is to be the client and perform a consultation for a spa visit. You can decide which facilities and treatments you would like to have.

Those requiring medical referral	Those restricting use
Cardiovascular conditions, e.g. angina, heart attack	Pregnancy
High or low blood pressure	Headache or migraine sufferers
Blood vessel conditions such as varicose veins, thrombosis, phlebitis	Within 2–3 hours of a heavy meal or if no food has been eaten for several hours
Swelling of a systemic origin	Persons under the influence of drugs or alcohol
Respiratory disorders – colds, flu, bronchitis, asthma	Recent scar tissue
Skin diseases such as athlete's foot and verrucae	During the first two days of menstruation
Fever or high temperature	Severe exhaustion
Diabetes	Severe bruising
Epilepsy	Cuts and abrasions
Loss of skin sensation	Sunburn

BEAUTY THERAPY **Level 2** NVQ/SVQ Diploma

Test yourself

What is the correct action to take if a client has booked in to use the spa but during the consultation she reveals that he/she

    a) has a cut on their leg

    b) has high blood pressure

    c) has verrucae on the ball of one foot

    d) is 15 years of age.

To maintain a professional and safe spa environment it is important to update client records with accurate information after every visit. Accurate records ensure the safety of the individual without repeating information. This is particularly important if a different therapist is responsible for the client on another visit. A high level of service is therefore assured.

These records must be confidential. If logged in a paper-based system they must be stored under lock and key and if on a computer, they are subject to the **Data Protection Act 1998**.

For much of their visit to a spa the client will not be with a therapist and therefore the comfort and well-being of the client should be checked frequently to ensure that they are at ease, feel relaxed and comfortable. Regular checks on consumable and towel use will ensure a regular supply.

Checks should be made as to the client's use of the spa facilities and they should be encouraged to rest and drink water or fruit juice to rehydrate, especially after prolonged use of the wet areas. Care should be taken with all clients, but especially those who presented with a contraindication who have gained medical permission to use the spa. Below is a summary of the service times to use as a guide.

Spa facility	Recommended time for use (maximum)
Steam room	15–20 minutes
Steam cabinet or bath	25 minutes
Sauna	30 minutes
Hydrotherapy pools and baths	10–15 minutes
Wet flotation	30–45 minutes
Dry flotation	20–30 minutes

 Health and safety

Overuse of the wet area of the spa can result in contra-actions such as fatigue, dehydration and headaches.

Contra-actions to spa services

Contra-action	Cause	Action
Exhaustion or fatigue	Prolonged heat exposure	Rest
Dehydration	Prolonged sweating	Rehydrate with water or fruit juice
Nausea	Lowering of the body salts through sweating	Replace body salts and fluid with a 'sports drink'
Fainting/light headedness	Heat raises the blood pressure	The head should be lower than the heart so lie the client down and raise the feet until the feeling passes
Cramp	Lowering of the body salts through sweating	Stretch the affected muscle and replace body salts and fluid with a 'sports drink'
Burns or scalds	Touching of heating elements or steam source	Flush area with cold water for at least 10 minutes and if severe seek medical assistance
Nose bleed	Dry heat in the sauna breaks the capillaries in the lining of the nose	With the head forward, pinch the bridge of the nose until bleeding stops. If it continues seek medical assistance
Allergic reaction	Exposure to allergens in products or cleaning materials used	Remove allergen and flush areas with cool water
Respiratory problems	High humidity can bring on asthma	Remove client from high humidity areas and allow them to administer their medication

Work area checks

The condition of the spa work areas should be checked throughout the day depending on usage. This could mean hourly if there are a large number of clients. Replenish laundry, products and drinking fluids as required.

Checks for hazards such as water spillage or condensation and the incorrect use of spa facilities by the clients should be ongoing. Hazards should be dealt with immediately by the appropriate course of action laid down in your organisational policies and procedures.

Areas should be checked for cleanliness and the appropriate action taken and records updated as necessary.

Written instructions intended for the client should be clearly displayed, legible and posted in the relevant position.

Equipment checks

To maintain spa equipment the following checks are necessary.

Operational maintenance

Efficient operational maintenance procedures ensure the smooth, safe and hygienic running of a spa and involve electrical and cleaning checks and maintenance of stock and water levels.

Electrical checks should be made by a qualified electrician as laid down in the **Electricity at Work Regulations 1992**, with frequent checks by the therapist for exposed wires and broken plugs. If faulty, the equipment should not be used. All electrical appliances should be switched off and disconnected from the mains when not in use. Due to the humid environment presented, a qualified person should install and maintain the electrical equipment in a spa.

At the beginning of the day the correct function and the temperature of the equipment should be checked. The temperature should be checked at regular intervals during the day with a thermometer being placed in situation. Any faults should be reported and the equipment labelled 'faulty' and use discontinued.

Water levels are checked visually and these checks apply to steam and hydrotherapy equipment. A spa pool's water should be clear so that the bottom of the pool can be seen before the jets are running. Water must be maintained at the correct level so adequate filtration can take place. The water in pools should be drained and replaced according to the schedule laid down by the manufacturer. Filter systems should be checked for operation but a professional fitter must perform maintenance.

> **Remember...**
>
> Check for cleanliness, health and safety and hygiene so levels are maintained throughout the day. Consider the frequency of use, levels of condensation and ventilation and ensure adequate supply of fresh towels, consumables and products.

Chemical testing

Modern professional hydrotherapy equipment that seats more than one person has suitable chemical testing equipment already fitted. However, this does not replace the twice-daily manual checks using a testing kit recommended by the manufacturer. This is important in the case of testing equipment failure.

These take the form of simple pH and chlorine level tests. It is important to maintain the correct level of pH to provide adequate protection from cross-infection and hygiene effectiveness with no detrimental effects. A pH 6 gives maximum disinfectant power but is unpleasant to bathe in. A pH 9 means that only a small percentage of chlorine or bromine is free to act as a disinfectant. An acceptable level is approximately pH 7.4–7.6.

Test the water in the spa or swimming pool with a reliable test kit and add the necessary chemicals according to the test results and the manufacturer's instructions. In the hot water environment of spas and hot tubs, disinfectants may rapidly break up and spread out, requiring more frequent water testing. Follow the manufacturer's instructions in this regard. The more people who use the facility, the more frequently the water should be tested.

Health and safety

When handling chemicals:

- Always read and follow the manufacturer's instructions carefully.
- Never mix two chemicals together.
- Use a clean scoop for each chemical.
- Avoid combining material from 'old' and 'new' containers.
- Always add the chemicals directly to the spa or hot tub water, either in a suitable feeder, distributed across the surface of the water, or diluted and poured into the water.
- When preparing water solutions for feeder application, pour the chemical slowly into the appropriate amount of water, stirring constantly to provide mixing and dilution.
- Always add chemicals to water. Never add water to chemicals.
- Never add chemicals to the water while people are using the facility.
- Carefully clean up any spilled chemicals with large amounts of water, to dilute and wash away.
- Disinfectant and pH adjustment chemicals can usually be disposed of in drains with large quantities of water but if in doubt follow the manufacturer's instructions.
- Wash out empty disinfectant containers before disposal to eliminate danger of fire, explosion or poisoning.
- Do not inhale dust or fumes from any chemicals. If necessary, use proper protective devices for breathing, handling and eye protection.
- Promptly wash off the skin any accidental splashes.
- Never reuse old chemical containers.
- If you have any questions regarding safe handling, storage or use of spa or hot tub chemicals, consult the MSD sheet or contact the manufacturer.

Spa operational records

You have a legal obligation to keep up-to-date, legible and accurate records for the opening, maintenance and closing of the spa. This includes water and chemical levels, frequency of testing and general maintenance and cleaning regimes. The local authority environmental health officer will inspect these records, which should be kept for a minimum of three years. They should be easily accessible and written clearly so they cannot be misinterpreted.

Opening, maintenance and closing records are performed daily and vary with each organisation but these records usually consider health and safety, cleanliness and stock levels. They often take the form of a chart and should list the key checks with space for date, time and initials of the person performing the checks. These records can feed into other records relating to stock controls and ordering, health and safety records and maintenance/repair records. Cleanliness check records are often displayed for the public to see and include a contact number or person to report unclean facilities to. Other records are for the use of staff so that important checks are not missed and anomalies are rectified by the appropriate person.

Activity

Design your own spa operational record for use within the wet area of the spa.

Reporting

Following the discovery of a piece of faulty equipment, a clear label advising discontinued use should be attached and the fault reported to a senior member of staff. This should be entered into the equipment log and a professional contacted to undertake a repair if possible. The reporting of faulty equipment is a legal requirement and such reports should be made available for inspection if desired.

Chemical concentration problems or temperature fluctuations should be reported to your line manager or other person responsible so that they can be rectified.

The unavailability of laundry, products and consumables should also be reported to your line manager or other relevant senior member of staff so provision can be made for their replacement. This can involve altering stock levels and reviewing laundry procedures.

Outcome 4: Shut down work areas

The shutting down of the spa work areas involves cleaning, the removal of waste products and dirty laundry, the restocking of products and consumables and reporting of any required maintenance procedures – basically, preparing the work areas in readiness for the next use. These procedures should fulfil the legal requirements described earlier and those of the organisation.

Hygiene procedures

At the end of each day it is important that all equipment is cleaned according to the manufacturer's instructions using the appropriate disinfectant. Water and chemical levels should be checked, as well as cleaning of general surfaces such as walls and floors.

Removal of condensation/water

If left to stagnate, water is a breeding ground for micro-organisms and can lead to the growth of unsightly mould, so it should be mopped up from floors, walls and equipment at the end of every day.

Circulation of air

Fresh air should be allowed to circulate to provide good ventilation after the spa area has ceased trading for the day. Steam rooms and baths should have doors left ajar to allow the air to enter and prevent musty smells and the spread of airborne diseases.

Disposal of waste

Correct disposal of waste is a legal obligation of the therapist and includes making special provision for the disposal of contaminated waste in a yellow bin liner for incineration. Non-contaminated waste should be placed into black bin liners and placed in an agreed place for collection, away from the spa treatment area.

Liaison with colleagues

All of these procedures should be performed together as a team and require liaison with the other members of staff to avoid duplication and to ensure that all the necessary tasks are carried out.

When the tasks are completed, a relevant person such as the manager should be notified. They will then confirm the procedure has met legal, organisational and manufacturers' requirements.

Want to know more?

There is a wide and varied range of spa treatments available at spa venues in the UK and abroad. Many were inspired by the holistic and natural nature of products as an alternative to more invasive treatments such as Botox injections and cosmetic peels.

More information about the treatments and about education, training and employment can be found on the following websites:

☞ British International Spa Association http://www.spaassociation.org.uk/
☞ European Spas Association http://www.espa-ehv.com/
☞ International Spa Association http://www.experienceispa.com/

Test yourself

1. Modern saunas are made of:
   a) logs
   b) pine
   c) fibreglass
   d) plastic.

2. Steam baths are usually made of:
   a) wood
   b) enamel
   c) fibreglass
   d) plastic.

3. What are commonly found near steam rooms to cool clients down?
   a) swimming pools
   b) plunge pools
   c) spa pools
   d) cold towels.

4. The humidity level in a steam bath is:
   a) higher than a sauna
   b) lower than a sauna
   c) the same as a sauna
   d) the same as a spa pool.

5. The jets within a spa have a similar effect on the body tissues as:
   a) massage
   b) sauna
   c) a steam room
   d) a flotation pool.

6. The area around a spa should be:
   a) wet
   b) open and airy
   c) non-slip
   d) dry.

7. Before a client uses spa treatment equipment they should:
   a) shower and remove jewellery
   b) have a pedicure
   c) have a leg wax
   d) sit and rest.

8. Spa treatments can affect the muscles by:
   a) relaxing muscles
   b) building muscle tone
   c) strengthening muscle fibres
   d) building muscle bulk.

9. The chemical added to a communal spa is:
   a) surgical spirit
   b) chlorine
   c) cidex
   d) alcohol.

10. Aftercare advice for spa treatments should recommend:
    a) exercise and more heat treatments
    b) always follow with a cup of tea
    c) rest and drink plenty of water
    d) exercise.

Are you ready for assessment?

 Remember . . .
It is important to ensure that the client's modesty and privacy are respected at all times.

 Remember . . .
Always keep your logbook handy.

The following checklist will help you to be fully prepared for your assessment.

The range of clients/treatments you must cover:

- Equipment used in spa service
- Work areas: wet areas, service areas, changing rooms, relaxation areas
- Range of spa services: sauna, relaxation room, steam service, hydrotherapy, flotation, body wrap
- Oversee clients during treatment
- Consider your actions if the client has any contra actions during treatment
- Effects of spa therapy services
- Health and safety procedures
- Spa services preparation, cleaning and closing down

1. Practical observation

 Remember . . .
Your assessor will observe you on at least four separate occasions which must include wet areas and changing rooms.

Your assessor will look at how you:

- prepare the spa area and ensure that you carry out strict hygienic practice
- maintain safe and effective working practices
- prepare and clean work areas using appropriate cleaning materials
- assist with treatments as required by a senior therapist
- ensure clients' modesty and privacy is maintained throughout the spa service
- check with the client that they are comfortable and no contra-actions to the treatment occur
- clean and maintain areas after spa services and shutting down work areas
- demonstrate a professional approach throughout the service.

2. **Knowledge and understanding**

What you must know:

- Organisational and legal requirements.
- How to work safely and effectively when providing spa services.
- How to prepare for spa treatment with clients.
- Contraindications and contra-actions.
- Anatomy and physiology.
- Spa services equipment, range of treatments and products used.
- Aftercare advice.

To ensure that you have the necessary knowledge and understanding of spa services your assessor will:

- ask you questions before, during and after assisting with the spa treatment
- ensure that you have completed project work and written exercises relating to the unit
- check that you have recorded in a log/diary treatments you have assisted with
- signed record cards showing that you have completed the required number of services competently
- check that you have covered the range in your candidate logbook
- require you to take a test.

Sources of evidence

- Completed client record cards endorsed by a senior therapist
- Certificates of achievement from commercial courses
- Photos/video
- Reports when assisting senior staff
- Client feedback
- Project work on spa treatments

 Remember . . .

An assisting role requires you to follow instructions from senior staff and carry out cleaning, checking equipment and overseeing client's well being during spa services to the required standard.

Chapter 17
Unit G18: Promote additional products and services to clients

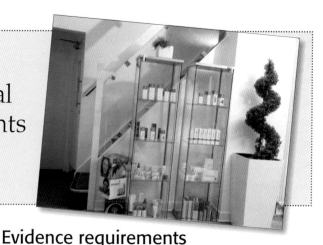

Learning objectives

This chapter covers Unit G18 'Promote additional products and services to clients'. It is about identifying additional products and services, and providing information to clients about them.

There are three learning outcomes for Unit G18 and they are:

1 Identify additional services or products that are available.

2 Inform clients about additional services or products.

3 Gain client commitment to using additional services or products.

You will need to be competent in all of these outcomes to identify and inform clients about products and services.

Evidence requirements

You will need to show that you can:

- follow salon procedures for offering additional services or products to clients
- create opportunities for encouraging clients to use additional services or products
- identify your client's needs by seeking information directly
- identify your client's needs from spontaneous client comments.

Unit G18 'Promote additional products and services is a mandatory unit for Level 2 Beauty Therapy: both General and Make-up routes and Level 2 Nail Services. It is worth six credits.

Meet the professional

"If you know your treatments and products, promoting them should be second nature. Posters are a great way to promote new ones. Product manufacturers have some eye-catching marketing and publicity material. If you have window space, use it! Change your posters regularly to maintain the interest of existing clients and to attract new ones. Build an electronic client database – if you have a client's permission to contact them, you can offer them special introductory offers and other promotions.

If possible, take 'before' and 'after' photographs of treatments and place them in reception for clients to see. And try out the products yourself. I recently applied 'foils' to all my beauty therapists' toes. This was a great advertisement and amazingly effective, increasing bookings for foiling threefold!"

Jacqui Bostock

Introduction

In order for any salon business to survive and make a profit, customers must be encouraged to return. The responsibility for making this happen falls on everyone within the business. Effective marketing and promotion by management will attract new clients into the salon, but all staff are responsible for providing the right circumstances to ensure return custom. This involves professionalism, good communication, a comfortable environment, client care, good quality treatments and a friendly atmosphere.

Once a client has become loyal to the salon, their interest in new or different treatments should be encouraged. Promotion of the salon's product range should complement the treatment without the client feeling pressurised into buying.

Outcome 1: Identify additional services or products that are available

Updating and developing professional skills

Everyone in the organisation has a responsibility to promote additional products and services but the therapist is in a prime position to do so. You should ensure that your knowledge is up to date. One of the ways to do this is to undertake continuous professional development (CPD), which will ensure that you have the skills and knowledge to carry out your job safely, efficiently and competently.

To promote products and services well, you need to:

- **Know what is available** – this will mean attending seminars and training days and reading
trade magazines and promotional material from manufacturers.

- **Understand effects, benefits and features** – you need to be able to describe how the service or product will aid the client in fulfilling the requirement or correcting the problem they have discussed with you. You must ensure that the information given is correct. Inaccurate advice results in a dissatisfied client and may result in prosecution.

- **Work as a team** – a well-run salon depends on staff supporting each other. Sharing good practice is one way that the team can promote services to clients. When a member of staff attends a course on a new product or treatment, they can share their new knowledge in a training session held for all the staff.

- **Know your limitations** – referral procedures are firmly established within an organisation regarding contraindications, but there are times when a client's wishes are beyond the responsibility of the therapist. For example, a client with severe acne may need referral to a doctor. You must also be aware of the limitations of products and treatments and avoid making claims that solutions are likely when they are not possible.

- **Show commitment and enthusiasm in your industry** – the beauty industry thrives on change. Each season brings a new look or a different trend in hair and make-up design. The therapist should keep up to date with these trends through trade magazines and trade shows.

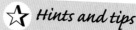

> ⭐ *Hints and tips*
>
> *It is not enough just to go through the process of treating the client. You should offer a personal service with professional advice. Clients should feel able to discuss and make informed decisions about treatments and products.*

Promoting additional products and services

The need for promotion has two aspects. The salon's need as a business is first to survive and then to make a profit.

The therapist's time is an expensive commodity. They need to be paid even when not performing treatments, so ensuring that therapists are kept busy makes economic sense. Therapists are often paid commission on products and services sold to clients. Many salons aim for approximately one-third of profits to come from product sales.

Establishing the client's needs and expectations

Of course, the priority must always be the needs of the client. Whether they are a new client or an existing one, they should be considered in the same way.

The additional product or service may be:

- **New to the client** – during conversation the client may express an interest in a new or different product or service they have seen advertised. The therapist may suggest a new product or service when a problem or requirement presents itself. For example, if the client announces that her daughter is getting married, it is an ideal time to promote the wedding service offered by the salon.

- **Replacing an existing one** – the process of regular analysis of the client's condition allows the therapist to highlight another product or service.

- **More of the same** – a repeat analysis and discussion may determine that the treatment and products recommended are still suitable. Do not change a product or service that a client is happy with and that is fulfilling their need.

Sometimes, a client may require a referral. The service or product may not be available from the salon or their usual therapist may be unavailable. Referral to another professional person to fulfil the client's needs may be necessary. This should be done without bias and professionalism must be maintained. For example, you may refer a client to a chiropodist after a pedicure, or to a registered practitioner for Botox or fillers.

> Remember...
> Communication is the key to establishing the client's needs and expectations.

Discussion should be based around the client's perception of their requirement. You should be prepared to advise and recommend products and services where the client has unrealistic expectations. This is important if you are to fulfil the client's needs accurately. If you send them away happy it is much more likely that they will return and tell their friends about the salon. Recommending the wrong service or product could mean that the client does not return and they may share their disappointment with their friends.

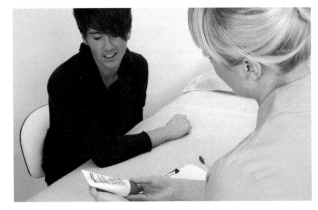

△ The consultation is the right time to discuss the client's needs and expectations

The timing and location of the discussion are important too. The client may have walked into the salon without an appointment to make an enquiry. It is important to provide privacy for the discussion as the enquiry may involve a treatment of a private nature and the client may not wish to discuss this in a busy reception area.

Choosing the right opportunity

There are several points during contact with a client when therapists can inform them of the services and products available to them. You need to choose the most appropriate.

When clients arrive in reception

Carefully select magazines for clients to read in the reception area. Many magazines now carry regular beauty features extolling the virtues of the latest new treatments. Ensure that you are able to tell clients when new treatments will be available. Keep a record of clients' interests in new treatments. This will act as a prompt for the salon to contact them when the new treatment becomes available. The reception area should have:

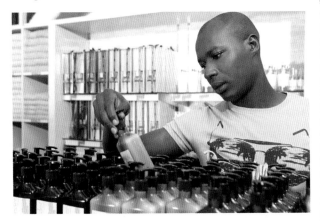

- well organised and attractive product displays
- product leaflets available
- promotional leaflets available
- promotion posters carefully placed around the salon and on the window
- an attractive and up-to-date window display.

(You will find more about reception in Chapter 2.)

△ Keep your displays up to date and change regularly to reflect different seasons and trends.

During the consultation

For clients who have booked appointments, the consultation is the correct time to discuss their needs and expectations. When contraindications have been considered and it has been established that the treatment can safely go ahead, the emphasis should turn to providing the most suitable treatment for the client.

Even with regular clients, you should always carry out a consultation. It is a mistake to assume that a regular client is still in need of the treatment or product prescribed on a previous visit.

During the treatment

This is the point at which the therapist makes choices based on the consultation and is the ideal time to recommend further treatments or products. Adding variety to a client's treatment regime will prevent the client becoming bored, increase their interest in their treatments and help to ensure that the therapist stays alert to their client's needs.

When evaluating the results of the treatment

Regular review of progress in the treatment area and asking questions that follow up on the aftercare advice and/or treatment provides the therapist with the relevant information to judge whether or not any change is necessary.

When offering home care advice

Giving advice to the client on the use of products and treatments is an ideal time to reinforce what has already been discussed during the treatment. Try not to repeat advice but emphasise the main points, focussing the client on the main features and benefits of two or three products.

Always complete a treatment with the question 'would you like to make another appointment?'

Outcome 2: Inform clients about additional services or products

Marketing and promotion

The reasons for a promotion may be to:

- announce a new product or service
- attract new clients
- announce a change to the business
- make a special offer
- invite enquiries
- announce the location of stockists
- educate new and existing clientele
- maintain sales
- challenge competition
- remind existing clientele about a product or service.

Linking treatments

Linking treatments provides the opportunity to offer additional services or products.

> **Key term**
>
> **Marketing** – creating a demand for what the salon has to sell.
>
> **Promotion** – making known what the salon sells and what each client may want to buy.

Treatment	Link to other treatments
Facial	Lash and brow tint
	Brow shaping
	Make-up lesson or make-up for a special occasion
	Specialist face mask or referral to senior therapist for specialist facial treatment such as Botox
	Homecare products
Manicure	Nail extensions
	Nail art
	Special hand treatments, such as paraffin wax
	Retail nail products and nail polish
	Pedicure
Pedicure	Waxing
	Specialist treatments
	Retail nail products and nail polish
Waxing	Other areas for waxing
	Pedicure

There are four steps to effective marketing and promotion for a salon. These are:

- advertising
- selling
- publicity
- sales promotion.

Advertising

Advertising can be described as non-personal communication in a mass medium (such as newspapers, magazines, radio, television, billboards and the internet) that has a cost attached. Radio and television adverts may certainly feel out of the reach of a local salon, but local radio stations may be able to promote a special event more widely than an advert in the local paper and so should not be dismissed on cost alone.

Placing an advert in a newspaper or trade magazine is expensive, so careful choice of media is essential. For example, the readership of a trade journal may not be your intended audience, as it is clients you are seeking to attract. Leaflets or a mailshot can be a cheaper option but you should still consider your target group carefully. A window display to promote a new service or product range can

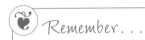
Remember...

Seasonal treatments can be linked, for example waxing and pedicures for summer.

work if the salon's position encourages 'walk-in' trade. Organising a demonstration to local groups is an effective way of letting people know what you have to offer.

Selling

This usually involves the therapist in face-to-face communication with the client. Excellent communication skills are therefore essential for effective selling techniques. A therapist may feel uncomfortable selling in this way but they are in a perfect position to do so. Questioning techniques using open-ended questions to obtain accurate information from the client is only one part of effective communication. Listening to the information and watching for non-verbal communication signs ensures that accurate and appropriate advice is given to match the client's needs and expectations to the appropriate product and service. Gain commitment from the client to the discussion by asking a closed question, for example, 'Would you like to try the moisturiser I have used today?'

You can find out more about effective communication techniques in Chapter 1.

Publicity

Publicity can be described as non-personal communication in a mass medium (such as a newspaper) that is not paid for. It can be in the form of a favourable editorial comment or news story. However, word of mouth is possibly the best form of publicity. If a client has received a good service in all aspects of their visits to the salon, they are likely to inform friends and relatives. This can generate significant extra trade.

Activity

Think about what attracts you in publicity and marketing material. What catches your attention and why?

Sales promotion

These are persuasive activities that may involve displays, demonstrations, exhibitions, competitions, vouchers, gift tokens, free gifts and sampling.

Sales promotion should give products and services a short period of added value and can be used to improve sales. Techniques used are:

- **Introductory trial** – a special reduced cost to encourage clients to try a new product or service. This is frequently used when a salon is introducing a new service. After the trial period the price of the service returns to normal.

- **Building customer loyalty** – a reduced rate on treatments for a number of sessions or block bookings rather than payment for single sessions.

- **Combined services** – a reduced rate is offered on an additional service when booked with another. For example: book a facial and get a manicure for half the usual price.

- **Sampling** – samples of products are given to encourage clients to try new product ranges or a new one within an existing range. This is a useful promotion when linked with the products used within the treatment or as aftercare.

- **Vouchers** – this technique can include gift vouchers to be redeemed at a later date or money-off vouchers redeemable against services or products.
- **Free gifts** – to be used with caution but can encourage additional purchases. For example: 'If you buy a cleanser and toner you will receive a free trial-size moisturiser.'
- **Competitions** – when a salon or supplier donates a prize such as a product or treatment, either within the salon or at a related event, for example a health page in the local newspaper. This promotes additional interest in the salon or service.
- **Trade incentives** – often, suppliers will offer special discounts and incentives in order to encourage salons to 'stock up'. Although these can result in an excellent return for the money spent by the salon, care should be taken in these situations. If the reduction by the supplier is given in order to sell stock in old packaging, for example, the salon may have difficulty selling the products to clients without reducing the price, cancelling any benefits that may have been gained.
- **Talks and demonstrations** – given in offices, at women's clubs, on local radio or to newspapers, these are an effective way of promoting services and are often given in return for prizes of free treatments.
- **Editorials** – these take the form of unbiased reports on treatments or products. They are very effective as a means of publicity.

Ethical selling

Ethical selling relies on the professionalism of the therapist to only promote products and services that are going to benefit the client. This should concentrate on providing solutions to the client's problems and requirements and must not be based on the latest trends, the services the therapist prefers to perform or the amount of stock in the stockroom! The therapist is in an ideal position to advise a client on the best suitable product or service.

Selling procedures

There are many ways that therapists can encourage sales.

- **Create the desire** – in the form of promotions, displays, posters, demonstrations, talks, etc. All this should create an exciting visual image in the salon, aimed at persuading current clients to try new or different products and services, and to entice new clients.
- **Establish the need** – with good consultation, analysis and communication skills, the therapist can determine the most suitable product and/or service.
- **Prescribe and educate** – the therapist should use their knowledge of the services and products on offer to fulfil the need established at the consultation. This is a time when the client can be educated to guide them away from misconceptions or unrealistic expectations.

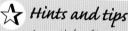 **Hints and tips**

An article of just one page can result in much more business than several pages of advertising. Work on building a good relationship with the local press.

Key term

Ethical selling – promotion of products and services that will be of benefit the client.

 Remember...

Ensure you have sufficient stock available to support the promotional event to avoid client disappointment.

🌸 **Closing the sale** – to close the sale effectively the therapist must remember that they are the professionals and should have faith in their recommendations. Repeat the benefits the client will gain by taking up your recommendation. Offer a choice to overcome problems presented by the client and give them the chance to try the products or service by suggesting they try introductory offers, samples or trial sizes. Place the client in the position of ownership with phrases such as, 'When you have the treatment your nail condition will improve'. Finally, ask, 'Would you like to book for that treatment?' or 'Would you like to try that product?'

Remember...

Home care products are an important aspect of selling, ensuring that the client maintains the beneficial effects of salon treatments.

Legislation

Any person who buys goods or services is protected by the law to ensure that:

🌸 goods are not faulty

🌸 goods are of good quality

🌸 there is an accurate description of the goods or service

🌸 the client is treated fairly and respectfully.

The following legislation relates to sales and promotion of products and services.

Key term

Equal opportunities – the rights of all individuals to respect, without discrimination on any grounds: race, language, colour, disability, sex or religion.

1. **The Sale of Goods Act 1979**

   This was the first of the laws that required goods to be accurately described without misleading the customer. The law takes into account the:

   🌸 suitability of the goods for a particular purpose

   🌸 quality

   🌸 description.

2. **The Supply of Goods and Services Act 1982**

   This went further than the 1979 Act to include standards of service, which should be:

   🌸 of reasonable quality

   🌸 described accurately

   🌸 fit for the intended purpose.

   The Act also required that the service provided to a customer should be:

   🌸 carried out with reasonable skill and care

   🌸 within a reasonable time

   🌸 for a reasonable cost.

3. **The Sale and Supply of Goods Act 1994**

   This amends the previous Acts by introducing guidelines on defining the quality of goods.

4. **The Consumer Protection Act 1987**

   The European Community legislation provides consumers with protection when buying goods or services to ensure that products used on the client during treatment or retail products sold to the client are safe.

5. **The Cosmetics Products (Safety) Regulations 2004**

   These regulations are part of the Consumer Protection legislation. The regulations expect that the formulations of toiletries and cosmetics are safe and used for their intended purpose as a cosmetic, labelling is accurate, and complies with European Union directives.

6. **Consumer Protection from Unfair Trading Regulations 2008 and Business Protection Misleading Regulations 2008**

   These regulations replace most of the former Trades Description Acts of 1968 and 1972. The regulations state that traders in all sectors are not allowed to operate unfair commercial practices against consumers, such as marketing and selling that is misleading.

   The regulations protect the client from misleading descriptions or claims relating to treatments and retail products. For example, to claim that a treatment is a miracle cure that will prevent skin from ageing will be regarded as misleading.

7. **The Data Protection Act 1984**

   The increase in the use of computers by businesses to store information about their clients has brought about a need for legislation to protect clients' personal information.

   The Data Protection Act requires the business to be registered and to comply with rules on storage and security of data. Salons should:

   - only hold information that is relevant

   - allow individuals access to information held on them

   - prevent unauthorised access to information.

8. **Equal opportunities**

   Equal opportunities legislation relates to the rights of all individuals to respect, without discrimination on any grounds, whether race, language, colour, disability, sex or religion. When working with the general public, the therapist has a duty to treat all clients respectfully and equally.

   The Equality Act became law in October 2010. The new Act replaces previous legislation (such as the Race Relations Act 1976 and the Disability Discrimination Act 1995). The legislation ensures consistency in what you need to do to operate a fair environment and to comply with the law.

   It also relates to promoting good race relations between people in their communities and respecting each other's differences. The UK has a very diverse population. The salon employer has a duty to treat all employees equally and to promote good race relations through the services offered to clients in meeting the needs of the ethnic mix of the community the salon serves. This includes:

   - a range of treatments

   - retail products – make-up and skin care range for all skin colours and types

   - promotional materials to include images that are relevant to the local community.

Treating a person differently because they have a disability is unlawful. The employer and the therapists should make every effort to meet the needs of all clients who come to the salon for treatment, regardless of their disability. However, a small business may not have the resources to accommodate a client with physical disabilities. (For example, if your business is on an upper floor then some clients with disabilities may not be able to access your services in the salon.)

Beauty therapy has traditionally been a female profession with few male therapists or clients. However, the trend for men to be more aware of skin care has resulted in an increase in the number of male clients in the salon, and the increase in male make-up and skin care consultants has brought male students into training. The legislation ensures that both sexes are treated equally, for example equality in employment prospects and pay for both males and females.

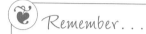

Remember . . .

Remember your target markets when preparing publicity and marketing materials.

The therapist and the law

The implications of the legislation for the therapist are clear. The customer or client has a right under the law to expect quality in respect of:

- the service they receive
- the products used during treatment
- the cosmetics or products that they purchase.

The therapist should be aware that not giving accurate information to the client, or claiming that a product or treatment can do something that it clearly does not, is misleading and the client can demand their money back. If incorrect information is given, a product could be regarded as unfit for the purpose intended or not accurately described. The client must be reassured that information given during the consultation process is confidential and secure.

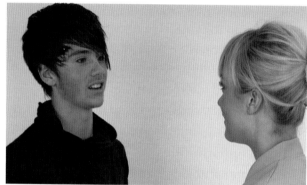

△ The trend for men to be more aware of skin care has resulted in an increase in the number of male clients

Outcome 3: Gain client commitment to using additional services or products

Meeting clients' needs and expectations

Clients often have unrealistic expectations. It may be that they expect a result based on what they have seen in a magazine, or they may feel that only one treatment will be enough to put right a problem (such as damaged nails and cuticles).

Gaining feedback

The salon manager needs to ensure that clients are satisfied with the services being offered. It is good practice to carry out surveys from time to time, using questionnaires or comments cards. The salon may decide to glean information from new and existing clientele by means of a market research questionnaire. This can be placed on the reception desk, where clients are invited to complete it. New ideas and promotions can be based on the information gained. Anonymous feedback may give a more accurate response, as some people are reluctant to make negative comments face to face.

Clients' comments can be collected in the following ways:

- A suggestions box will encourage people to make comments.
- Comments cards can be left in the waiting area of reception. These cards could be like the ones you find at your table in some fast-food restaurants – simple and easy to complete.
- The therapist should make a point of asking the client at the end of the appointment whether they enjoyed the treatment and were satisfied with the result.
- The manager should use observation on a daily basis to gain information by checking the efficiency of appointment schedules, health and safety practice, client care or client satisfaction.
- Staff can contribute by listening to their clients and informing senior staff or the manager of any dissatisfaction or by making suggestions for improvement.
- Surveys or questionnaires can help to maintain and improve salon services as well as provide staff with valuable feedback on how they are doing within the team.

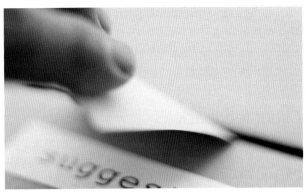

△ A suggestions box will encourage people to give feedback.

The manager will want to know that clients are being dealt with efficiently and that staff are meeting the targets of the business. Some clients may use the opportunity to complain and criticise rather than make helpful suggestions. However, if there is a common thread running through the comments, it may indicate a need for action.

The salon manager may also wish to gain client feedback before a staff appraisal.

Checking client understanding of the treatments or products

All clients should be given the opportunity to discuss the subsequent treatments that are required. Any follow-up to the treatment should be explained in terms of the benefits and the time and cost involved.

Any discussion should be based on the client's interest, not on the need to sell products or services. If the client feels under pressure to buy, it can cause her not to return to the salon.

The client may enquire about how products they may wish to purchase are applied. A full explanation should be given. Allow the client to hold the product or use a tester. Provide a leaflet for the client to take away, explaining how the products are used and their ingredients and benefits. Always provide the client with a list of the products and treatments available at the salon.

Knowing when to close the discussion is very important and is based on the client having understood the discussion. Simply asking

 Remember . . .

Remember to have the salon name and telephone number/ email address on all promotional materials that are offered to the client.

the client a few questions, such as 'How will you apply the cream?' and explaining the treatment plan and recommendations for future visits will help bring the salon visit to a close. An enthusiastic and interested therapist will have the confidence to recommend products and services.

Client feedback

Client satisfaction is paramount for returning business. The therapist will ask their client about the enjoyment and results of services at the end of the treatment but it may be other aspects of salon services that are not up to scratch.

For example, when selling products it is essential that stock levels are adequate to meet the needs of the client. This is a difficult task, as carrying too much stock is not cost effective. Careful monitoring of what products sell and ensuring prompt delivery from suppliers is essential.

It is always necessary to balance the needs of the client with what is viable for the business. To achieve this balance, feedback from both clients and staff is essential. However, it is no good requesting suggestions and comments unless the information gained is acted upon.

Urgent action will be required where matters of health and safety, security or client distress are encountered. Non-urgent matters may be used to develop an improvement plan.

Comments from clients that will require urgent attention may include:

- 'The carpet is worn on the steps and I nearly tripped.'
- 'The temperature control on the shower is broken, causing very hot water to come through.'
- 'The towels used for my treatment did not smell fresh.'
- 'The therapist was rude and abrupt when I phoned.'
- 'I was given the wrong change again today.'
- 'There is still no cleanser available for my skin type.'

Feedback of this nature must be dealt with immediately.

Clients may also make comments on aspects of the service that are desirable but not matters of urgency:

- 'I have read about a new face cream – are you going to stock it?'
- 'I wish you stayed open until 8.00 p.m. on Friday instead of Thursday.'
- 'I would rather have fresh coffee than instant.'

It is not always possible to act on every piece of client feedback. The salon manager will have to consider whether suggestions for improvement are sensible and whether the business can afford to implement them. There may be implications for:

- financial investment in the salon for new equipment, products or staff
- staff training
- refurbishment.

Activity

Design a short questionnaire that could be given to clients to gain information on how satisfied they are with their salon visits.

Use the following headings to help you:

- First impressions of the salon and staff
- Salon appearance/decor
- Hospitality and comfort
- Enjoyment of treatment(s)
- Value for money.

If possible, use your questionnaire to collect some views. You will need to design it so that it looks professional and plan how it is to be issued to the clients. You will need to collect in the completed questionnaires and analyse the results. You may be able to make recommendations for improvement to the services your salon offers.

As many clients as possible should complete the questionnaire to ensure that sufficient information is collected and the findings are of value.

Remember...

During training, it is important for you to gain feedback from clients on your own performance. You may be asked by your assessor to keep a diary or log to record the treatments you do and the views of your clients.

Test yourself

Test yourself on promoting additional products and services by answering the following questions:

1. Think of five reasons for a promotional campaign.
2. What are the therapist's responsibilities to the client?
3. List the ways in which clients' comments can be collected.
4. What is the name of the Act that came into force in October 2010?
5. What is the purpose of the Cosmetics Products (Safety) Regulations 2004?

Are you ready for assessment?

 Remember . . .
Always keep your logbook handy. Your logbook contains details of the evidence requirements for each unit and is an important record of your achievements.

 Remember . . .
The profitability of the salon depends on you promoting services and products which will encourage the client to return to the salon for further treatment.

The following checklist will help you to be fully prepared for your practical assessment

1. **Practical observation**

   Your assessor will observe you as you:
   - identify additional services or products that are available
   - inform clients about additional services or products
   - gain client commitment to using additional services or products.

2. **Knowledge and understanding**

   What you must know:

   Salon requirements
   - How your salon encourages the use of additional services or products.

   Service and product promotion
   - How the use of additional services or products will benefit the business.
   - The main factors that influence clients to use your services or products.
   - How to introduce additional services or products to clients.
   - How to give information to clients about services or products.

   To ensure that you have the necessary knowledge and understanding of promoting services or products your assessor will:
   - ask you questions before, during and after carrying out the procedure

 Remember . . .
Your assessor will observe your performance on at least three occasions.

- ensure that you have completed project work and written exercises relating to the unit
- ensure you have completed a test
- check that you have recorded in a log/diary or the client record card sales you have made
- look at evidence of sales and promotion in your portfolio.

3. **Sources of evidence**

- Observation by your assessor of a client consultation where you recommend products which supplement the treatment or types of complementary specialist treatments, for example offering a paraffin wax treatment to your manicure client.
- Observation by your assessor of discussion with your client following treatment to evaluate the service and recommend home care products and future salon treatments.
- Clients' record cards, where you can record recommendations for future treatments and what products you have sold.
- Design a leaflet or poster for the salon promoting a new product or treatment.

Remember...

All promotional posters and leaflets must be well designed and produced to project the right image.

- Design an aftercare leaflet for the client to take away with them, suggesting further treatments and products and tools they can use at home to continue the benefits of salon treatment, for example night cream.
- Certificate from commercial training seminars on promotion and selling.
- Design a client questionnaire to establish their understanding of what products and treatments are available in the salon.

Part 3: In the team

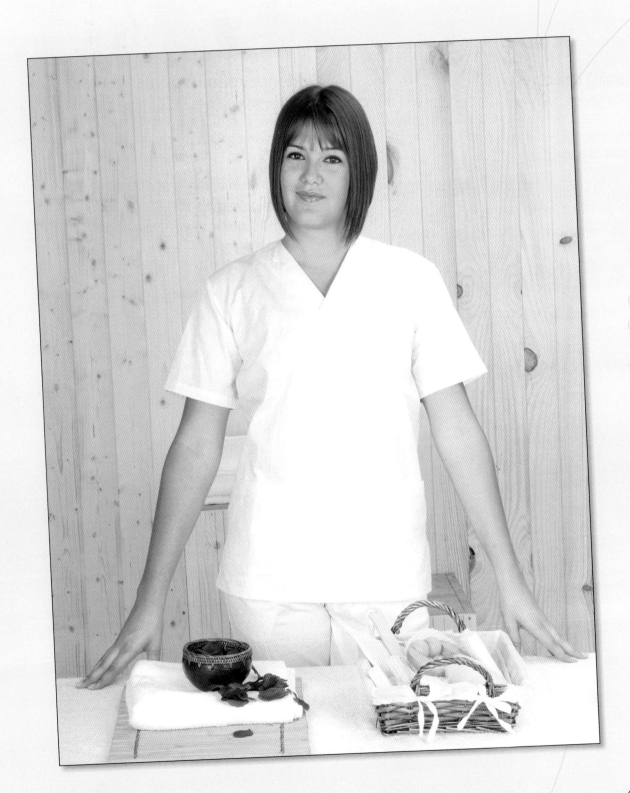

Chapter 18

Unit G8: Develop and maintain your effectiveness at work

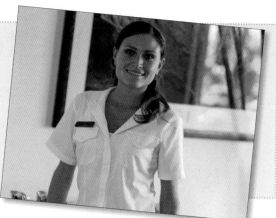

Learning objectives

This chapter covers Unit G8 'Develop and maintain your effectiveness at work'. It is about improving your personal performance and working effectively as part of a team.

There are two learning outcomes for Unit G8 and they are:

1 Improve your personal performance at work.
2 Work effectively as part of a team.

You will need to be competent in both of these outcomes.

Evidence requirements

Your assessor will need to observe you being effective as part of a team on at least one occasion. You must also gather documentation to support this observation. From the range, you must:

1 Participate in the following opportunities to learn:
   - from colleagues and other relevant people
   - active participation in training and development activities
   - active participation in salon activities.

2 Agree and review your progress towards these targets:
   - for productivity
   - for personal development.

3 Offer assistance:
   - on a one-to-one basis
   - in a group.

Introduction

The success of any business depends on the way in which the staff work together to meet the aims of the business. Working as part of a team helps to spread the workload, promote good relationships with colleagues and ensure that the business runs smoothly.

Everyone needs to know their roles and responsibilities within the salon to ensure that tasks are satisfactorily completed. Having your roles and responsibilities set out means that you can review how effective you are and plan for your future development.

Unit G8 'Develop and maintain your effectiveness at work' is a core mandatory unit within Level 2 NVQ Beauty Therapy on both General and Make-up routes and a mandatory unit in the Level 2 NVQ Nail Services qualifications.

Meet the professional

"To stay on top you need to keep up to date. This can be quite difficult to achieve: it is time consuming, can be expensive and takes dedication.

You have to be passionate about providing the perfect service every time. You will need to visit shows and exhibitions, go on courses and above all else go for treatments yourself! You will definitely learn a lot by having the treatment and experiencing it from a client's perspective!

If your boss is not very forthcoming with organising events and courses then ask them."

Remember...

Enthusiasm shows that you are interested in your career.

Outcome 1: Improve your own personal performance at work

As an employee you should have a job description that outlines your work role and how your work contributes to the overall work of the team. This needs to be reviewed as you gain experience.

Your job description states your job title and describes your role and responsibilities. It is necessary to ensure that you are aware of the areas that are your responsibility. It is equally important to know where your responsibility ends (i.e. what you are not expected to do). Further details of your job, such as hours of work, pay and holidays, form part of your contract of employment.

Your job title will give you an indication of the level of your job (for example, assistant, senior therapist). Your job role consists of the duties and responsibilities defined in the **job description**.

Below is a list of typical job roles and responsibilities for various positions within a beauty salon.

Salon Owner:

- Part-time therapist with regular clients.
- Works in the salon on Thursdays and Fridays.
- Only member of staff trained in advanced epilation, so has clients from the hospital.
- *Responsible for*: running the business, checking takings/till, banking, paying the wages, ordering stock, health and safety, staff appraisals, staff training

Manager/Senior Therapist:

- Full-time, six years' experience, works every day except Thursdays (unless the boss is away).
- Does all treatments and has regular clients.
- *Responsible for*: the day-to-day running of the salon and supervising the staff, client records, appointment book, allocating salon duties, stock checks, health and safety checks, staff rotas and holidays, daily cashing up.
- *Responsible to*: Salon Owner.

Beauty Therapist:

- Full-time, two years' experience.
- Building up her clientele, when not busy assists the Senior Therapist.
- *Responsible for*: daily hygiene practices and salon appearance, retail display, retail sales figures.
- *Responsible to*: Senior Therapist and Salon Owner.

Assistant Beauty Therapist:

- Part-time, recently qualified to NVQ Level 2, taking NVQ Level 3 course part-time at college.
- Manicurist and nail technician, waxing and make-up.
- Assists all the therapists by preparing treatment rooms, equipment and products.
- *Responsible for*: general cleaning duties including laundry, reception duties.
- *Responsible to*: Senior Therapist.

Key term

Job description: an outline of your work role and how you will contribute to the overall work of the team.

Activity

List what you consider to be your roles and responsibility in the salon.

Activity

If you have already been in employment, you will have had a job description and a contract of employment. Share your experience with someone in the group who may not have been in employment by discussing:

- ❖ your job title
- ❖ the job description
- ❖ the tasks you were expected to carry out
- ❖ who you were responsible to.

Activity

In your group, use the proforma on p. 428 to design a job description for a member of staff in a beauty therapy salon. To enable you to do this you will need to look at the staff in your salon or your work placement and list their main responsibilities. Use the lists shown earlier to help you.

Name: _____

Job title: _____

Place of work: _____

General description of the job:

_____

_____

_____

_____

Responsible to:

-

Responsible for:

-
-
-
-

Main beauty therapy tasks (treatments):

-
-
-
-
-

Other tasks (general salon duties):

-
-
-
-
-
-

△ An example of a job description proforma

Trainee beauty therapist:

- Full-time, attends college one day per week for NVQ Level 1 and 2.
- Assists all staff in the salon, observes treatments as appropriate.
- *Responsible for*: greeting clients, providing coffee, general cleaning duties.
- *Reports to*: all therapists, with training from the Senior Therapist.

Appraisal and personal development

Throughout your time at school, college or work you will have been involved in reviewing and checking your performance and achievements. At school or college you will have discussed your progress with your tutor and set targets for future learning that were then set out in an action plan. At work, we check our performance through staff reviews or 'appraisals'.

Remember . . .

An appraisal is designed to improve your performance and to praise what has been achieved.

Before an appraisal, it is important to prepare by asking yourself some questions. Asking 'Where do I want to be?' will help you identify your future aims. Setting out your aims in relation to your career and future training needs is important.

Asking 'How am I going to get there?' will help you identify how you are going to achieve your goals and who can help you achieve them.

During a staff appraisal, the salon manager will discuss with you your strengths and weaknesses in relation to your performance in the salon. You must be prepared to discuss how to improve your weaker areas.

The manager may have ideas for your future that are different from yours. It is important that an appraisal is a joint discussion that results in agreement on the goals and targets to be achieved.

Targets arising from your appraisal should be SMART:

- **S**pecific – clear
- **M**easurable – determines progress towards targets and when achieved
- **A**greed – clearly understood by both the therapist and the employer
- **R**ealistic – achievable
- **T**imely – within an agreed timeframe.

It is essential to put your goals and targets in writing so that you can check them to monitor your progress. Once you have identified your goals then you need to think about what you need to do to achieve them.

Appraisal is sometimes referred to as a 'review cycle' because each time the targets are reviewed and are achieved, the process starts again with new or modified goals and targets.

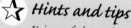
⭐ *Hints and tips*
It is useful to ask yourself the following questions:
☆ Where am I now?
☆ Where do I want to be?
☆ How am I going to get there?

During an appraisal interview you will be encouraged to plan your training and development needs. An action plan is agreed, setting out your targets and the support you will need to achieve them. An action plan should include short-term targets (for example, to practise using the nail foiling system so you are able to work on clients by next month) and long-term targets (for example to achieve the Beauty Therapy NVQ Level 2 by July).

The date to review your targets will be agreed on the action plan and a copy retained by your appraiser. You will need to refer to the action plan to ensure that you stay on course to achieve your targets. Setting targets will give you the encouragement and motivation to work hard to achieve your goals.

Managers in business use staff reviews or appraisals to evaluate the effectiveness of the whole team. During an appraisal, you and your manager (in an interview situation) review your progress and contribution to the performance of the salon against the targets of the business and your personal goals. As well as thinking about your past performance, you will also look to the future. This will involve setting targets for your personal development, including training.

Appraisal is not just about identifying problems and planning how to solve them. It needs to be a positive process, providing you and the manager with the opportunity to discuss all aspects of your job role.

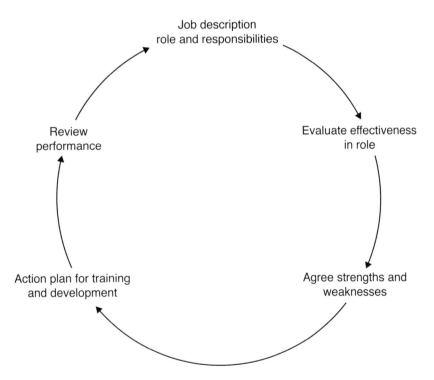

Purpose of appraisal: – review role and responsibilities
– identify areas for improvement
– identify training needs
– review progress

△ An appraisal review cycle

Doing a SWOT analysis

To help you answer the question, 'Where am I now?' you will need to spend some time looking at your strengths and weaknesses. This is not always an easy thing to do as we are often more comfortable talking about our weaknesses rather than stressing our strengths. A useful exercise is to carry out a SWOT analysis. SWOT stands for **S**trengths, **W**eaknesses, **O**pportunities and **T**hreats.

1. Begin by making a list of the broad areas of your job, such as assisting therapists with treatments and reception duties.

2. Then ask yourself, 'What do I do well and with confidence?' This will usually indicate your **strengths**.

3. Then ask yourself, 'What do I find difficult?' This will be tasks that you are more wary off – things that make you feel anxious. This will give you an indication of your **weaknesses**.

4. **Opportunities** will need to be considered through discussion with your manager during your appraisal. This refers to things to consider when setting targets. So, if you identify a weakness such as using nail foils, this will require training. Training is an opportunity, and will depend on the manager making the time available for you to go on a course or for someone to spend time with you in the salon for training.

5. The **threats** refer to any restrictions on realising the opportunities discussed above. For example, the cost of training staff to use a new range of products and whether it would be cost-effective to take time for this particular training need when there may be other priorities, would be a threat.

The SWOT analysis or any method of assessing your strengths and weaknesses will help you to monitor your progress and set your personal goals for the future.

strengths	**weaknesses**
– smart appearance	– not confident using electrical treatments
– good communication skills	– need to be quicker with treatments
– enjoy working with people	– find it difficult to choose products from the range available for individual clients
opportunities	**threats**
– attending course at college for NVQ Level 3 in September	– employed part-time with little job security
– go to the trade shows in London to gain information about new products, new treatments and equipment	– work in a small salon with only two other therapists who are also part-time so do not get much time together

△ An example of a SWOT analysis

Training and development

Beauty therapy is a fast-growing industry that requires the beauty therapist to be skilled in a wide range of treatments. The beauty therapist needs to keep up to date with new techniques, treatments and products, health and safety legislation and emerging technology.

Training needs of the staff will vary depending on their position, role and responsibilities within the salon. Training can include:

- nationally recognised qualifications such as NVQs or equivalent vocational qualifications (National Diploma)
- manufacturers' courses and information
- keeping informed of the latest technology and trends through trade journals and professional bodies
- in-house training to meet the needs of the salon (for example using a new product range)
- job shadowing – allowing less experienced staff, possibly trainees, to observe treatments being carried out by senior therapists
- management training for senior staff.

Trade magazines and newsletters from professional bodies should be available in your salon as they are particularly useful for learning about the latest research and development in skin care, cosmetics and treatments. Trade fairs offer the very latest in products and equipment with demonstrations, leaflets and free samples available. The internet can also provide valuable information.

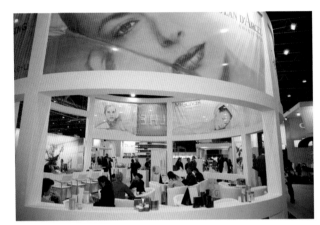

△ Visiting trade fairs allows the therapist to keep up to date with the latest products and equipment available in the beauty industry

 Remember . . .

You may not be able to offer some treatments (such as Botox® or fillers) but you should still be aware of them as it will affect the way you handle the skin and adapt the treatment plan. Always ask when carrying out consultation treatment. Do not rely on the client to tell you.

Treatment times

It is very important that you are aware of the expected treatment times when making client bookings.

The minimum service times for treatments are:

Facial	60 minutes
Eyebrow shape	15 minutes
Eyebrow tint	10 minutes
Eyelash tint	20 minutes
Artificial lashes	20 minutes
Partial set of lashes	10 minutes
Eyebrow wax	15 minutes

Underarm wax*	15 minutes
Half leg wax*	30 minutes
Bikini wax*	15 minutes
Full leg wax*	45 minutes
Upper lip wax *	10 minutes
Chin wax*	10 minutes
Manicure*	45 minutes
Pedicure*	50 minutes
Make-up (day)	30 minutes
Make-up (evening/bridal)	45 minutes
Ear piercing*	15 minutes

*excluding consultation and preparation

Outcome 2: Work effectively as part of a team

Being part of a team

You will at some time have experienced being in a team. This might have been in sport, in an orchestra or pop group, or as a member of the school play or local amateur dramatic society.

A team works to agreed aims or goals. A sports team aims to win a match, an orchestra or pop group aims to put together lots of different sounds from people playing different instruments, a drama group aims to take different characters and put together a play or musical. This will involve a team of not only the actors but also people to do make-up, costumes and lighting.

Many aspects of life involve working together as a team. This is particularly important in the workplace. Whatever the business, be it in the manufacturing, retail or service industry, it will rely on a team or teams of people working together to meet the aims of the company.

A beauty therapy salon is in the service sector of business, with the broad aim of providing a range of beauty therapy treatments to its clients. The salon owner will have a business plan in which the aims of the business are set out in more detail. The owner will require all the therapists to work together to achieve these aims.

As a team member in a beauty salon, you must be able to:

- demonstrate high standards regarding expected codes of conduct, (**professional ethics**) and appearance
- anticipate the needs of others and be willing to provide help and support when it is needed
- communicate effectively and share information
- get on with all members of the team
- accept responsibility from your supervisor and work within the limits of your authority
- resolve misunderstandings with colleagues.

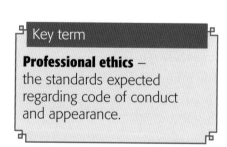

Key term

Professional ethics – the standards expected regarding code of conduct and appearance.

Providing help and support

When someone is very busy, they may become flustered and agitated. As a good team member you will recognise when a colleague is under pressure and needs help. This may be something as simple as checking the temperature of the wax or preparing a treatment room for the next client. Anticipating when a job needs to be done and keeping an eye on those tasks that need to be carried out throughout the day are important aspects of your role as a team member.

Treatment rooms or cubicles

Ensure that:

- equipment and materials from the previous client are cleared away
- the treatment couch is set up for the next client
- clean laundry is available
- products and equipment for the treatment are in place
- equipment is checked for safety and set up ready for the treatment
- the client's record card is available.

See Chapter 1 for further details.

Care of clients and reception duties

The duties of the receptionist are described in more detail in Chapter 2. However, in a busy salon everyone must play a part to ensure that the client is cared for.

Unplanned situations such as late arrival of clients, overbooking of clients or staff absence will require you to use your initiative by working together. You could look at the appointment schedule to ascertain, in the case of staff absence, whether another therapist could provide the treatment, or by ensuring that waiting clients are served with coffee, have a magazine to read and are kept informed. Clients who arrive without an appointment should be accommodated if at all possible.

Salon care

Ensure that the salon is clean, tidy and running smoothly. This will include seeing to the laundry, doing some cleaning, carrying out sterilising and hygiene procedures, and doing dispensary or stockroom duties such as stock checks, dispensing or mixing treatment products.

Chapter 3 deals with aspects of health and safety and salon care and maintenance. It also explains the importance of everyone taking responsibility for health and safety in the salon.

Communicating effectively

Communication is always important, not only between clients and staff, but also between staff and management and between the therapists themselves. Good communication is one of the key skills of a beauty therapist because of the demands of the job. Through effective

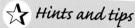

> ⭐ *Hints and tips*
> Support staff in the salon are as important as the therapists themselves. The smooth running of the salon depends on their behind-the-scenes work. Ensure that you give clear instructions on what you need.

Activity

While on work placement from your training establishment, look carefully at the reception area of the salon you are working in. What could you do to support the effective operation of the reception area?

 Remember...
Always be polite to your colleagues as well as to your clients.

communication, you should be able to develop a good relationship with clients, provide professional advice and be a good listener.

Good communication between staff will ensure that everyone is clear about the aims of the business and their individual part in achieving those aims, as well as their role as part of the team.

Team meetings

Team meetings are a very good way of ensuring that there is effective communication. If held on a regular basis, they can help to:

- encourage and motivate staff
- provide training opportunities
- allocate tasks in the salon through negotiation
- identify and help to resolve problems
- avoid misunderstandings, disagreements or mistrust within the team
- provide an opportunity for the exchange of ideas for the future development of the business.

A good team leader (your supervisor or manager) will ensure that everyone is involved in the meetings, allowing open discussion of views and problems.

Methods of communicating in the salon

- Written:
  - messages
  - fax
  - email
  - memorandum (memo)
  - appointment book
  - stock book
  - salon policies, rules and regulations.
- Verbal:
  - team meetings
  - telephone
  - oral instructions.
- Visual:
  - training videos
  - demonstrations
  - body language.

Body language

Body language is a method of communicating. The wrong impression can be given easily by gestures, posture, facial expression and manner. A poor attitude will be reflected in your appearance. Be aware of yourself and how you appear to others. A glum, stern face with the body posture in a slouching position with round shoulders will give totally the wrong impression. The therapist needs to be aware of their looks and posture. A bright, smiling face that is clean

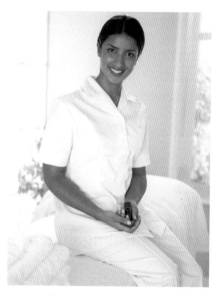

△ A professional appearance and attitude will inspire confidence

or well made-up reflects the skin care and appearance of the beauty industry that you wish to promote. An alert body stance with good posture will give the impression of being ready to help the client.

 Remember . . .

For the evidence to be valid for assessment it must relate to an activity that you have carried out. It must be signed and dated by your assessor before you can use it as evidence for your portfolio.

Activity

Put together a range of communication methods that you have used, for example a message, a fax or an extract from the appointment book.

Getting on with the team

Maintaining good relationships within the salon makes for a happy working environment. Clients can sense an atmosphere of discontent, and this may put them off coming back. Building good relationships will require you to be aware of others (their needs, temperament, moods) and will encourage you to treat them with respect. Never lose your temper, swear or raise your voice. This is a major difference for newly qualified therapists who will have been used to being part of a larger team at college. Working alongside friends is very different to working alongside colleagues!

Accepting responsibility

Accepting responsibility for your actions and how you may affect others is an important aspect of life at work. It is essential to maintain the aims of the business and to carry out your job effectively. An understanding of job roles and responsibilities within the business will help you to fit into the team by knowing what you are expected to do, who you should report to and who makes final decisions.

Activity

There are many examples of teamwork. Working together in a group, discuss your involvement in a team and what responsibilities you had as part of that team. You might discuss your role in a previous job or in a sports team, for example.

Test yourself

Test yourself on developing and maintaining your effectiveness at work by answering the following questions:

1. How long would you schedule for:
   a) an eyebrow tint, brow shape and eyelash tint?
   b) a facial, including a brow shape and eyelash tint?
2. Explain why it is important for the therapist to be polite at all times.
3. Give two methods of communicating in the salon.
4. Why is continuing professional development important?
5. Why is it important to have targets?

Are you ready for assessment?

The range of opportunities you must cover:

- Opportunities to learn
- Targets
- Assistance given

1. Practical observation

 Remember...

Your assessor will observe your performance on at least one occasion.

Your assessor will check that you can:

- improve your personal performance at work
- work effectively as part of a team.

 Remember...

The success of the salon relies on team work.

2. Knowledge and understanding

What you must understand:

Salon roles, procedures and targets

- Your job role and responsibilities.
- How to work as a member of a team.
- Where to find information about roles in the salon.
- Your responsibilities and what is expected of you.

Improving your performance

- How use of additional products and treatments will benefit the client and the business.
- How to introduce additional services or products to clients.
- How to give information to clients about services or products.

To ensure that you have the necessary knowledge and understanding of promoting services or products your assessor will:

- ask you questions before, during and after carrying out the procedure
- ensure that you have completed project work and written exercises relating to the unit
- check that you have recorded in a log/diary or the client record card sales you have made
- look at evidence of sales and promotion in your portfolio

 Remember...

Continuing professional development (CPD) is where people within a profession update their skills and knowledge on a regular basis.

 Remember...

Always keep your logbook handy.

3. **Sources of evidence**

- Certificates of achievement from commercial courses (manufacturers hold courses for new products and treatments).

- Following your attendance at a course ask your assessor to observe you showing your colleagues the skills you have learned.

- One-to-one tutorial with your assessor or salon supervisor to establish your progress and set targets. A copy of the tutorial report should be available for your portfolio.

- Observation by your assessor to establish your ability to work as part of a team during the salon day, for example salon duties at the end of the day.

- A written review of the number of treatments you have completed and how you can improve the number of clients the following week.

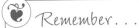

Remember . . .

Learning is a continuous process. It is said that we learn something new every day!

Part 4: Essential knowledge

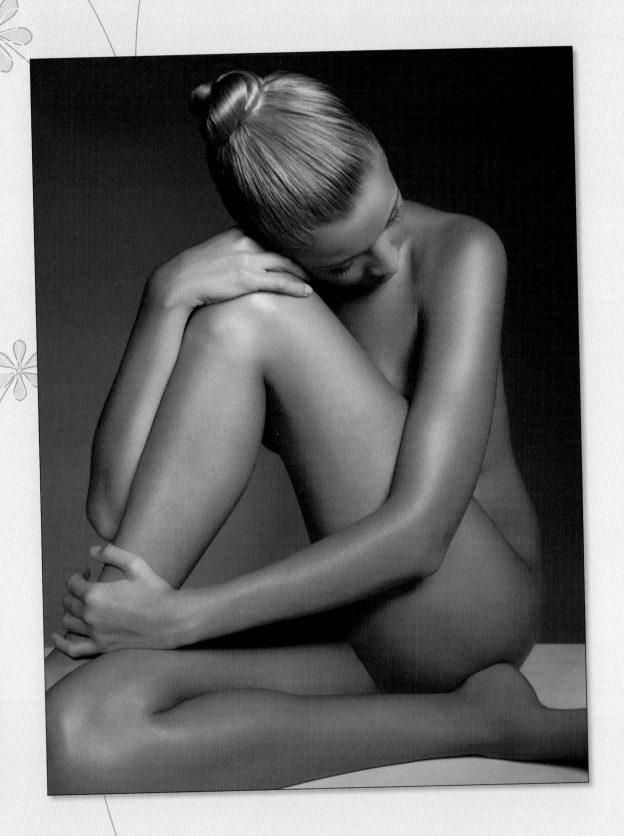

Chapter 19
Related anatomy and physiology

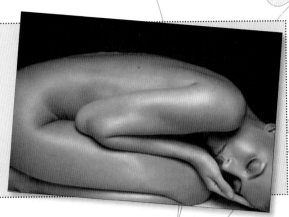

Learning objectives

In this chapter you will learn the relevant anatomy and physiology knowledge for the areas of the body on which you are performing treatments. Anatomy is the study of the structures of the body. Physiology is the study of how those structures work together. The relevant knowledge is:

- the structure of the skin
- function of the skin
- the structure of the hair
- types of hair growth
- principles of hair growth
- the structure of the nail unit
- the process of nail growth
- the bones of the head, neck, shoulder girdle, hand, lower arm, foot and lower leg and their position

- the position and action of the muscles of the head, face, neck, shoulder girdle, hand, lower arm, foot and lower leg
- the nervous system
- the composition and function of blood and lymph
- the blood circulation of the hand, lower arm, foot and lower leg
- the lymphatic drainage of the head, neck, arm, hand, leg and foot.

The knowledge contained within this chapter fulfils the requirements of the NVQ Beauty Therapy Level 2 units, as shown in the following table. Units that do not appear have no anatomy and physiology associated with them.

	B4 Provide facial skin care treatment	B6 Carry out waxing services	B8 Provide make-up services	B10 Enhance appearance using skin camouflage	B34 Provide threading services	N2 Provide manicure services	N3 Provide pedicure services	N4 Carry out nail art services	N5 Apply and maintain nail enhancements to create a natural finish
	Structure and function of the skin	Structure and function of the skin	Structure and function of the skin	Structure and function of the skin	Structure and function of the skin	Structure and function of the skin	Structure and function of the skin	Structure and function of the skin	Structure and function of the skin
	Bones of the head, neck and shoulder and their position					Bones of the hand and lower arm and their position	Bones of the foot and lower leg and their position		
	The position and action of the muscles of the head, face, neck and shoulder girdle					The position and action of the muscles of the lower arm and hand	The position and action of the muscles of the foot and lower leg		
	The composition of blood and lymph					Blood circulation to the lower arm and hand	Blood circulation to the foot and lower leg		
		The structure of the hair							
		Principles of hair growth			Principle of hair growth				
		Types of hair growth			Types of hair growth				
					Causes of hair growth				
						The structure of the nail unit	The structure of the nail unit	The structure of the nail unit	The structure of the nail unit
						The process of nail growth and different natural nail shapes	The process of nail growth and different natural nail shapes	The process of nail growth and different natural nail shapes	The process of nail growth and different natural nail shapes

The skin

The skin is the most important organ that a therapist needs to consider. All the beauty therapy treatments you will learn at Level 2 have an effect on the skin and its structures. A sound knowledge of the skin and its functions is required.

The structure of the skin

The skin is divided into three layers:

- the epidermis
- the dermis
- the subcutaneous layer.

The epidermis

The epidermis is the outermost layer of the skin nearest the surface and the one that is visible. As it is the most superficial layer it is greatly affected by beauty therapy treatments and the application of products.

It varies in thickness throughout the body, being thinnest on the lips and eyelids and thickest on the soles of the feet and the palms of the hands.

Although the epidermis consists mainly of dead cells, which are constantly being shed at the surface and replaced by new cells from underneath, under a microscope five distinct layers can be determined.

The **stratum germinativum** (basal layer) is the deepest layer consisting of 'live' cells that are cube-shaped, each with a nucleus. They are moist and obtain nutrients and oxygen from the tissue fluid that seeps from the blood vessels in the dermis and surrounds them. These nutrients are used for **mitosis**, where each cell divides to form two identical cells.

One in every 4–10 cells are specialised cells called **melanocytes** that produce a pigment called melanin giving the skin its colour. The more melanocytes the darker the skin is naturally.

Melanin darkens when exposed to ultraviolet light, either naturally from the sun or artificially from sun beds. This darkening protects the underlying structures within the **dermis** from the harmful effects of UV light.

As new cells are formed at the stratum germinativum, old ones are pushed towards the surface, undergoing change as they do so. The cells appear to grow spines or 'prickles', giving rise to the **stratum spinosum** or prickle layer. It is here in the epidermis that melanin is placed into the cells from the melanocytes. Not all cells of the stratum spinosum have nuclei and there is still some mitosis taking place.

As the cells move towards the surface they get impregnated with a protein called keratin to form the **stratum granulosum**, or granular layer. This process is called keratinisation and the cells begin to 'die', losing their moisture and harden. The nuclei and the cell wall break down as they work upwards towards the surface.

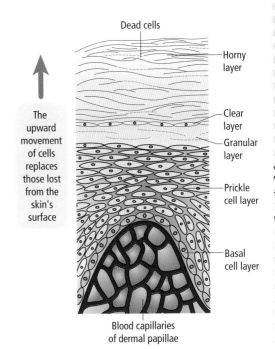

Dead cells

Horny layer

Clear layer

Granular layer

Prickle cell layer

Basal cell layer

The upward movement of cells replaces those lost from the skin's surface

Blood capillaries of dermal papillae

△ The epidermis

The absence of nuclei and cell walls in the **stratum lucidum** causes it to appear clear under a microscope. An enzyme has destroyed the melanin and the keratin has dried the cells causing them to flatten, giving the transparent appearance. There is also a thick mucus-like substance present at this area of the epidermis called the 'Rheims barrier', formed as the cells of the stratum granulosum expel water and mix with the fatty acids present in the skin. This barrier prevents water, products and micro-organisms from penetrating the epidermis into the dermis.

Eventually the cells appear as dry, flat, keratinised flakes of the **stratum corneum** or horny layer. These hardened cells are shed from the surface by natural rubbing (for example from clothing) and by special skin products containing granules that slough off the dead skin. This process is called **desquamation**.

The dermis

The dermis lies beneath the epidermis and is also known as the true skin, as all the living and functioning structures of the skin can be found here. It is approximately 3 mm thick all over the body and can be divided into two distinct areas.

1. The **papillary layer** is the uppermost portion of the dermis and lies directly under the epidermis. Its name is derived from the projections that point upwards into the epidermis, called **papillae**. Many of these papillae are supplied with blood vessels, providing nutrients and oxygen to the cells of the stratum germinativum, while others contain sensory nerve endings.

> ⭐ *Hints and tips*
> *The **stratum lucidum** is not present in the epidermis of skin in all areas of the body but is thickest on the palms of the hands and the soles of the feet.*

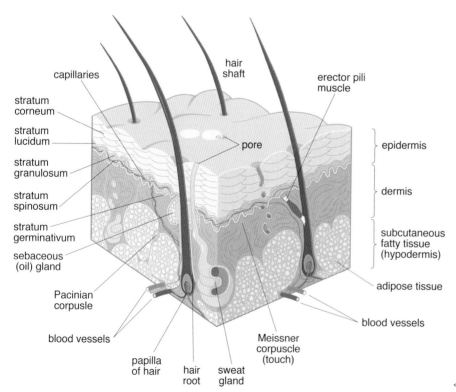

◁ Structure of the skin

2. The **reticular layer** lies beneath the papillary layer and contains a dense network of collagen and elastin fibres running parallel to the skin surface. Together, these fibres give the skin its elasticity and when damaged (for example by ultraviolet light) premature ageing results.

The dermis contains glands and other structures that enable the skin to perform its functions. These structures are described below.

The **blood supply** to the skin is a network of arteries that run parallel to the skin's surface under the dermis. Smaller vessels branch off upwards to form capillary networks around the hair follicles, sweat and sebaceous glands, arrector pili muscles and the dermal papillae in the papillary layer. The capillaries provide fresh blood containing nutrients and oxygen necessary for mitosis, muscle contraction and the formation of sweat and sebum. Deoxygenated blood passes downwards in small vessels to the main venous network in the dermis. The amount of blood flowing to the surface is controlled by the motor nerve supply in the artery walls, which bring about vasodilation or vasoconstriction.

The **lymph capillaries** form a fine network of vessels throughout the dermis, which act as a waste disposal system. The capillaries drain away excess tissue fluid containing waste products from cell activity and foreign bodies such as micro-organisms that may have entered through an opening in the epidermis.

The **nerve supply** of the skin provides the skin with sensations of **touch**, **pain**, **pressure** and **temperature**. This is possible due to the network of **sensory nerve endings** or **receptors** present. Most lie deep in the dermis, but others that register pain and temperature can be found in the lower epidermis. When stimulated by the external environment, an 'electrical message' is taken along sensory nerve fibres to the central nervous system (CNS) where the brain decides how to act upon the information. This usually results in the CNS sending another 'message' to a muscle or gland to bring about an action. **Motor nerve endings** found in the skin carry these messages to the arrector pili muscles, sweat glands and blood vessels to activate these structures.

The **sweat glands** are made up of a coiled tube deep in the dermis and a long tube or **duct** that reaches up through the epidermis to the skin surface. There are two types of gland but both produce sweat almost constantly to regulate the body temperature. The difference comes in the type of sweat they produce. The **eccrine glands** are found in abundance over the entire body and excrete water and body salts. The **apocrine glands** are found in the armpits and genital area and open out into hair follicles rather than the skin surface. They excrete water, salts, urea and fats. It is the breakdown of this type of sweat by bacteria that causes body odour.

The **hair follicle** is formed by a depression of epidermal cells downwards, deep into the dermis. It is responsible for the production of a keratinised structure called **hair** from the **bulb** at the base. The necessary nutrients and oxygen required for hair growth are supplied by blood vessels in the **dermal papilla**. Connected to the follicle is

Hints and tips

The skin plays an important part in maintaining 'homeostasis' within the body, which is the body's ability to regulate its internal environment by a system of feedback controls to maintain health and function regardless of the outside environment.

the arrector pili muscle, which, when it contracts, pulls the follicle and therefore the hair into an upright position causing 'goose bumps' and trapping an insulating layer of air next to the skin to keep the body warm.

The number of **sebaceous glands** found over the body varies greatly. They are more numerous on the scalp, face, chest and upper back, with few being found at the knees or elbows and none on the soles of the feet and the palms of the hands. They commonly open out into hair follicles but some open onto the skin surface. The glands produce an oil called sebum, which lubricates the skin, keeping it soft and pliable and preventing moisture loss from the dermis. If the glands are overactive the skin becomes oily or greasy and the formation of blocked pores, **comedones** or blackheads and **pustules** is likely. When underactive the skin is dry, rough to touch and may appear flaky.

The subcutaneous layer

The subcutaneous layer is made of fat cells held by a network of collagen and elastin fibres that form a protective and insulating structure and acts as an energy store for the body.

The functions of the skin

The skin performs important functions that contribute to the maintenance of the body's internal environment and general everyday functioning.

Sensation

The skin is equipped with many sensory nerve endings, making it sensitive to touch, differences in temperature, pain, itching and pressure. The skin acts as a receptor, informing the central nervous system (CNS) of the external environment and structures in the skin respond to this information under 'instruction' from the CNS.

Heat regulation

The body must maintain a temperature of 37°C in order to be healthy and function normally. The skin plays an important role in this.

When the body temperature rises, the **sweat glands** begin to produce **sweat**. This cools the body by using heat from the body to evaporate the sweat from the skin surface.

The blood vessels near the surface of the skin **dilate** or widen to allow more blood to come to the surface and the skin becomes red. This is known as **erythema**. The body heat in the blood is lost to the atmosphere, a little like a central heating system losing heat to a room through a radiator.

When the body is cold, the skin slows the sweating process and the blood vessels **constrict** or narrow to keep body warmth under instruction from the CNS.

The adipose tissue contained in the subcutaneous layer of the skin helps to keep us warm by insulating the body from the cold.

> ⭐ **Hints and tips**
>
> The many 'touch' receptors in the fingertips make them so sensitive that blind people can learn to read and write with a special communication system consisting of raised dots called 'Braille'.

> ⭐ **Hints and tips**
>
> 'Goose bumps' occur as a result of each **arrector pili muscle** contracting and lifting the hairs away from the skin to trap a layer of air next to it as insulation. As we have very little hair on our bodies this does not work well in humans but is effective in animals.

Absorption

The skin is able to absorb very little as its main job is to prevent the entry of external harmful substances. Certain substances, however, can pass through the epidermis. The epidermis can absorb cosmetic preparations containing natural oils, such as those obtained from plants, and sunlight can penetrate the epidermis to the dermis, destroying dermal structures such as collagen and elastin fibres. Other substances that are known to penetrate the skin are drugs (for example those used in hormone replacement therapy or nicotine patches), anaesthetics and essential oils.

Excretion

This is the removal of waste products and the skin is one of three excretory organs of the body, the lungs and kidneys being the others. The skin assists in this role by sweating, which removes excess water and salts from the body. The other 'waste product' the skin eliminates is heat and this is done as described earlier.

Secretion

Sebum, the natural oil produced by the sebaceous glands, flows from the glands onto the skin surface, lubricating and maintaining the skin's softness and pliability and rendering it waterproof. When sebum mixes with sweat on the skin surface the **acid mantle** is formed, which protects the skin from the growth of harmful micro-organisms.

Protection

The skin protects the body from injury and invasion by foreign bodies such as micro-organisms.

The uppermost layers of the epidermis thicken with pressure such as on the soles of the feet and are able to quickly replace themselves if damaged. The acid mantle inhibits micro-organism growth and makes the skin waterproof, controlling water loss through the epidermis.

Specialised cells called melanocytes present in the bottom-most layer of the epidermis produce melanin, a pigment that colours the skin to absorb sunlight and prevent its harmful rays from damaging the dermis and its structures.

Vitamin D production

Vitamin D is formed by the action of sunlight on a fatty substance present in the skin. It is absorbed into the blood vessels and used with calcium and phosphorus for the formation and maintenance of bones. Excess vitamin D is stored in the liver.

The hair

Hair is a dead keratinised structure protruding out of an indentation in the skin and consists of two parts:

1. The hair shaft – the portion extending above the skin surface.
2. The hair root – the portion below the surface of the skin.

Types of hair

There are three main classifications of hair:

1. **Lanugo hair** is the soft, downy hair seen on babies while in the womb and is shed before birth or becomes the terminal hair of the scalp, eyelashes and eyebrows.

2. **Vellus hair** is the soft, downy colourless hair found all over the body, except the eyelids, lips, palms of hands and soles of the feet. This type of hair often originates from a lobe of a sebaceous gland or a shallow follicle. When the follicle is stimulated by hormonal changes (for example during puberty) or by shaving it is possible for vellus hair to become coarse, dark terminal hair.

3. **Terminal hair** is deep-seated, strong hair that extends from a deep downward growth of epidermal cells into the dermis called **a follicle**. It is from the blood supply in the dermis that terminal hair gains the nutrients and oxygen required for growth. These hairs are found on the scalp, underarms, eyebrows, pubic regions, arms and legs. Naturally, terminal hair can be straight, wavy of curly and along with natural colour is a distinguishing feature used to describe ethnic origin. It is the shape of the follicle that moulds the hair and determines this distinguishing feature.

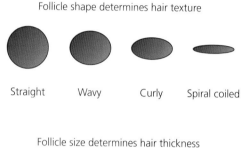

Follicle shape determines hair texture

Straight   Wavy   Curly   Spiral coiled

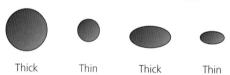

Follicle size determines hair thickness

Thick   Thin   Thick   Thin

△ Links between the shape of the hair and its features

Hair structure

The structure of each hair is divided into three layers:

1. the cuticle
2. the cortex
3. the medulla.

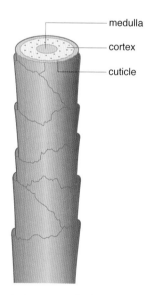

medulla

cortex

cuticle

△ Structure of a hair

The cuticle

This outermost layer is composed of overlapping transparent scales. The cuticle protects the layers that lie underneath. When substances such as lash tint come into contact with the cuticle, the scales become raised due to the alkalinity of the chemicals. This allows the chemicals to enter into the cortex of the hair.

The cortex

Made of many **micro-fibrils** arranged into bunches to form elongated cells, the cortex makes up the bulk of the hair and gives it strength and elasticity.

It is within the cells of this layer that granules of pigment can be found. This gives the hair its colour: melanin produces the brown-black shades and pheomelanin gives the red-yellow shades.

The medulla

This layer is not always present, particularly in fine hair. When seen it lies in the centre of the cortex. Its function is unclear.

The structure of the hair follicle

The hair follicle is formed by a depression of the epidermis downwards into the dermis to form a tube-like structure. It is from this that the hair grows. The lower portion of the follicle is called the **bulb** and approximately two-thirds up the follicle are the sebaceous glands, which produce sebum, a natural oil. This lubricates the neck of the follicle, the skin surface and the hair.

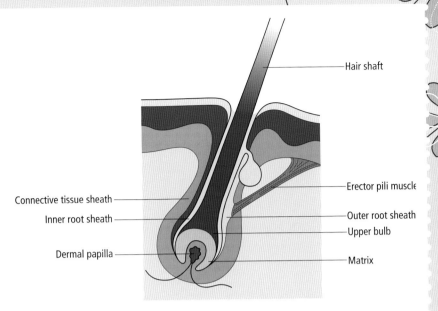

△ Structure of the hair follicle

The bulb

The hair bulb is the slightly swollen or 'bulbous' portion of the hair follicle and is the deepest part of the hair follicle into the dermis when the hair is actively growing.

The dermal papilla

There is an elevation into the base of the bulb, which contains a rich blood supply known as the dermal papilla. It is from here that the cells receive the nutrients and oxygen necessary for mitosis. While the follicle is in contact with the dermal papilla it will be active, in other words, capable of producing cells to form a growing hair.

The matrix

The matrix is situated at the top of the elevated part of the bulb and is in contact with the dermal papilla. It is a continuation of the germinating layer of the epidermis and is where the cells divide by mitosis and grow or mature. As the new cells mature they are impregnated with melanin from the melanocytes present and are pushed upwards by ones forming underneath. The cells change shape as they do so until they enter the upper bulb or **keratogenous zone** where they harden and die to form the layers of the hair or inner root sheath.

The inner root sheath

The inner root sheath is also formed in the matrix and grows up with the hair. It is made of similar cells to the cuticle of the hair, which allows them to 'interlock' to secure the hair in the follicle. This structure is continuous with the hair as it grows up the follicle but discontinues at the level of the sebaceous gland. It can only be seen when the hair is actively growing.

The outer root sheath

The outer root sheath forms part of the follicle wall and is continuous with the stratum germinativum of the epidermis. It therefore enables the follicle to grow and renew cells during its life cycle. The root sheath can be seen clearly, as a silver sheath on hairs when they are plucked from the follicle during the active growing stage. It also remains in contact with the dermal papilla during the resting stage of the hair growth cycle and takes an active part in the formation of a new follicle wall during early anagen.

The connective tissue sheath

The connective tissue sheath surrounds the hair follicle and sebaceous gland forming part of the follicle wall. It has a prolific blood and nerve supply providing the follicle with sensitivity.

The growth cycle of hair

A hair follicle actively produces hair for distinct periods of time, before going through stages of change and then rest. A follicle goes through three stages:

1. **Anagen** – the active, growing stage.
2. **Catagen** – the changing stage.
3. **Telogen** – the resting stage.

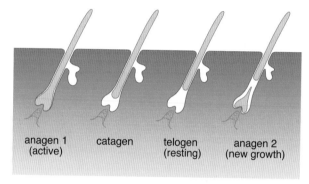

anagen 1 (active)   catagen   telogen (resting)   anagen 2 (new growth)

△ Three stages in the life cycle of a hair

Anagen

At the onset of anagen, the hair germ cells in the outer root sheath are stimulated into activity by hormones. This results in the formation of the **dermal cord**. The cells of the dermal cord undergo mitosis and a new follicle is produced. This grows in length and width, obtaining the food and oxygen for growth from the connective tissue sheath. The newly formed follicle extends downwards to the dermal papilla, which enlarges and the bulb is formed around it.

The bulb begins production of new hair cells, receiving the necessary nourishment from the dermal papilla. These new cells become the inner root sheath first and then a new hair. As the new hair grows up the follicle, it may push the old hair out if it has not fallen out already and eventually the new hair appears at the surface. The hair continues to grow while the follicle is active. The time varies according to the area of the body but can be as long as six years. Towards the end of anagen, melanin production begins to slow down and eventually ceases as the follicle enters the next stage.

Catagen

This stage is also known as the transitional stage, where the dermal papilla breaks down and the hair detaches itself from the base of the follicle and the bulb shrinks. The hair is now known as a **club hair** because of its appearance. Club hairs initially are only attached to the follicle by the inner root sheath but as the hair continues to rise up the follicle to a level just below the sebaceous gland it is no longer attached. The follicle below the hair shrinks and breaks away from the dermal papilla but the remaining cells are already organising themselves to form the new matrix and hair germ cells. All this takes place over a period of a few days.

Telogen

Known as the resting stage, the follicle remains at approximately half of its normal length for a few weeks before anagen begins again. At this time the hair can be removed from the follicle just by brushing. On removal the hair will appear dry and the root often appears rough giving rise to the name **'brush hair'**. Sometimes epidermal cells will grow around the end of the hair, anchoring it in the skin, but when removed appear as a small white ball of cells. The telogen stage may not happen, as the follicle can be stimulated to produce a new hair immediately.

The causes of hair growth

There are three main causes of hair growth:

1. Congenital causes refers to an inherited pattern of hair growth.
2. Topical causes refers to local areas of skin with increased hair growth.
3. Systemic causes refers to normal and abnormal activity of the endocrine system and the hormones they produce.

Congenital causes

Every child is born with a pre-determined pattern of hair growth, inherited from its parents, whose genetic structure shapes that of their child. A congenital pattern of hair growth is influenced by hereditary factors including areas such as eyebrows, eyelashes, nostrils, scalp and body hair.

Normal congenital patterns vary greatly from one ethnic group to another; for example those of Nordic or Scandinavian origin are less hairy than Mediterranean individuals; in general white skins are hairier than black skins.

Some individuals have a tendency to inherit unusually excessive hair growth known as 'congenital hypertrichosis', which can appear at birth or later on in life. In extreme cases the whole body can be covered. This is the result of an unusual genetic structure.

Topical causes

Localised areas of skin can develop hair growth, for a range of reasons:

- Irritation – if sustained in any area it may result in increased hair growth. Hair growth in the immediate area will become deeper and coarser to protect the epidermis from irritation. This occurs because the irritation causes increased blood supply to the follicle and the hair receives better nourishment.

Hints and tips
Knowledge of the hair growth cycle is important to a beauty therapist when giving advice and understanding the benefits of treatments. It can explain the premature appearance of hairs after waxing and the time periods between treatments as well as being able to judge the effectiveness of an epilation treatment.

Hints and tips
Someone whose leg has been broken and placed in plaster can develop hair growth from the constant rubbing of the plaster onto the skin. The hair growth will fall out naturally when the plaster is removed.

- Moles and birthmarks – hairs often protrude in moles and birthmarks because they have an unusual amount of blood capillaries near to the skin's surface, which provide extra nourishment.

- Physical Irritation – other irritations may increase hair growth including plasters, excessive scratching, x-rays, ultra-violet and sunburn.

- Tweezing – tweezing is capable of initiating hair growth from a resting follicle. When a club hair is lost there is a loosening of cells, which stimulate the new hair to be produced.

Systematic causes

Some of the hormones produced by the endocrine system are responsible for hair growth in both males and females. The endocrine system consists of a series of glands, which secrete hormones and are found throughout the body. Hormones are chemicals, which cause changes within the body. The endocrine glands secrete the hormones directly into the bloodstream. Under normal circumstances the endocrine system controls the correct amount of hormones in harmony with the body's needs. Endocrine hormones are responsible for influencing and stimulating growth at the follicle cells, which in turn determines the pattern, quantity, texture and distribution of body hair.

Normal hormonal stimulation of the hair follicles includes puberty in both males and females and pregnancy and menopause in females.

Abnormal hormonal stimulation is caused by disorders of the endocrine system such as polycystic ovarian syndrome; the development of ovarian cysts. There are many endocrine disorders that can result in hair growth where it did not grow before.

The structure of the nail

The nail is made of layers of dead cells containing a protein called **keratin**, also found in skin and hair. The layers are held together by a substance called **lamellae**. The nail is divided into three main parts:

1. the **free edge** – the part that protrudes over the fingertip

2. the **nail plate** – forming most of the visible portion of the nail

3. the **nail root** – the part of the nail buried into the skin.

The upper part of the nail root forms the **nail fold** and the lower part forms the **matrix**. This is part of the germinating layer (stratum germinativum) of the epidermis and is the region from which the nail grows. The matrix receives the nutrients and oxygen for growth from a network of blood vessels in the **nail bed**.

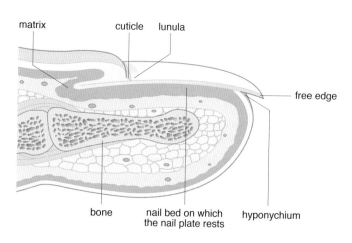

△ Cross section through the end of a finger and nail

▽ Nail structure

Part of nail	Description	Function
Free edge	The part of the nail plate that protrudes over the fingertip, likened to the claws of an animal	Protects the fingertips from physical harm; improves the appearance when manicured
Hyponychium	A layer of epidermis found under the free edge	Prevents bacteria and dirt from getting under the nail plate and infecting the nail bed
Nail plate	The main part of the nail, made up of layers of dead keratinised cells	Protects the tips of the fingers and toes, which have a network of sensory nerve endings
Lunula	Also known as the half-moon, it is the visible portion of the matrix and appears pale due to a reduced blood supply	As the upper part of the matrix, it is part of the growing area for the nail and the nail bed
Cuticle	A layer of epidermis that overlaps the base of the nail plate	Prevents bacteria and dirt from entering the nail fold
Eponychium	Part of the cuticle at the base of the nail over the lunula, which moves forward with the nail plate as it grows	Protects the growing part of the nail
Matrix	Lies beneath the nail fold – an injury to the matrix can cause deformity in the nail plate or the plate can be shed completely from the nail bed	The matrix has a rich blood supply, which enables it to produce the nail plate and bed
Nail bed	This is the portion on which the nail plate rests; it has a plentiful blood supply when healthy and so gives the nail its pink colour	The blood supply provides the food and oxygen to the matrix and the ridges anchor the nail plate to prevent lifting; it also has a nerve supply making the nail bed sensitive to pain and pressure
Nail wall	The folds of skin running up the sides of the nail plate	Forms the frame to the nail and provides protection from physical harm
Lateral nail fold	Either side of the nail plate the skin folds over to enclose the nail plate	Guides the nail to grow straight

Nail growth

The nail originates from the cells of the stratum germinativum within the nail fold and the matrix. As the cells divide they push old ones up towards the free edge. The cells keratinise, die and form the nail plate in layers held together by water from the cells and the fatty acids present called lamellae. The nail bed is formed at the same time but the keratinisation process is not completed so the cells remain living until they reach the hyponychium, where they dry out and die to form a protective strip under the free edge.

The skeleton

Introduction

The bones of the head, neck and shoulder, lower arm and hand, and lower leg and foot form part of the skeleton which is made up of two types of tissue: **cartilage** and **bone**.

Cartilage is less rigid than bone and is slightly flexible. It is found on the surfaces of bones for the protection of the articulating surfaces at movable joints, where flexibility is needed to allow limited movement such as in the ribcage, and also in the nose, ears, larynx and windpipe where some rigidity and flexibility is needed.

Bone is a rigid structure composed of a living tissue, mainly collagen fibres densely packed and impregnated with inorganic salts (namely calcium phosphate) to give it strength and rigidity. Bones are living structures with a blood and nerve supply and are influenced by changes in diet, hormone levels and the stresses they are exposed to, such as an injury or overuse.

Where two bones come together a **joint** is formed. There are three main types of joint:

1. **Fixed joints** – also known as immovable and fibrous joints. As the name suggests, no movement occurs, for example the sutures of the skull.

2. **Cartilaginous joints** – slightly movable and distinguished by the presence of a pad of cartilage between the bones, for example the bones of the vertebral column.

3. **Synovial joints** – freely movable to allow a wide range of movements, for example the knee, elbow and hip.

The functions of bones

1. **Shape and support** – there is a similarity between the shape of the skeleton and that of the external body, which can also be seen on other animals. The axial skeleton, that is the skull, vertebral column and ribs, supports the limbs of the appendicular skeleton. Together, the skeleton and muscles hold the body upright and give us our posture.

2. **Protection** – the cranium and vertebral column protect the brain and spinal cord respectively, the ribcage protects the heart and lungs, and the pelvis protects the reproductive organs in the female.

3. **Production of blood cells** – the blood brings the required nutrients and oxygen necessary for red blood cell formation, which occurs in the bone marrow of long bones, for example the femur.

4. **Calcium storage** – the blood supply of the bones provides nutrients that are stored and removed depending on the demands of the body, for example calcium, phosphorus and fat.

5. **Muscle and tendon attachment** – these are bony protrusions and rough surfaces of bones that allow for adhesion of muscles and tendons.

6. **Movement and locomotion** – by using joints and with the contraction of muscles, the body is able to move.

The bones of the head

The bones of the head are also known as the skull and are divided into two groups: the **cranium** and the **face**. Most of the bones of the skull form fixed joints called **sutures**. The only free-moving joint is that between the mandible – the lower jaw – and the temporal bones, which allow the lower jaw to move up and down when chewing.

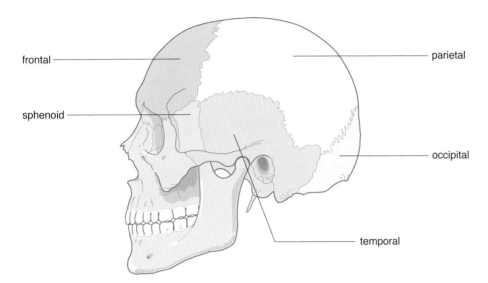

frontal

sphenoid

parietal

occipital

temporal

◁ Lateral view of the skull showing the bones of the cranium

The cranium

Eight bones form the cranium, a box-like structure that protects the brain.

▽ The cranium bones

Name of the bone	Position of the bone
Frontal	One bone forming the front of the cranium including the forehead and upper eye sockets
Parietal	Two bones forming the top and sides of the cranium
Occipital	One bone forming the back and floor of the cranium
Temporal	Two bones forming the sides of the cranium, above and around the ears
Sphenoid	One bone forming the floor and the sides of the cranium at the temple region and the back of the eye sockets
Ethmoid	One bone forming the front floor of the cranium, the roof of the nasal cavities and the inner sides of the eye sockets (not shown in illustration)

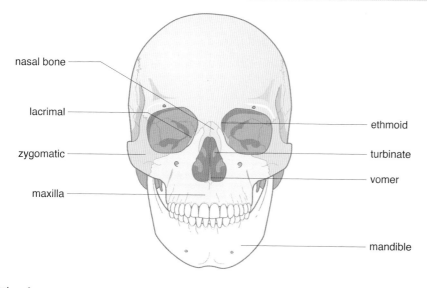

nasal bone

lacrimal

zygomatic

maxilla

ethmoid

turbinate

vomer

mandible

△ Anterior view of the skull, showing the bones of the face

The face

Fourteen bones form the facial structure and features.

▽ The face bones

Name of the bone	Position of the bone
Zygomatic	Two bones that form the cheekbones and the floor and side wall of the eye sockets
Maxilla(e)	Two bones forming the upper jaw, the front part of the roof of the mouth, the sides of the nose and the floor of the eye sockets. The upper teeth are embedded in the maxillae
Nasal	Two bones forming the bridge of the nose
Mandible	One bone forming the lower jaw in which the lower teeth are embedded
Lachrymal	Two bones forming the inner walls of the eye sockets
Palatine	Two bones forming the back part of the roof of the mouth and sides of the nasal cavities (not shown in illustration)
Vomer	One bone forming the central division of the nasal cavities
Turbinate	Two bones forming the side wall of the nasal cavities

The bones of the neck

The neck forms part of the **vertebral column**, which is a series of irregular-shaped bones stacked on top of each other to form a column. Each vertebra is separated from the one above and below it by a disc of cartilage, which prevents the bones from rubbing against each other and acts as a cushion or shock absorber for physical stress administered from the upper body to the lower or vice versa.

The bones are named after the area in which they are situated, hence the neck bones are called the **cervical vertebrae**. There are seven of them. The upper two vertebrae nearest the skull are specialised and have a different structure to the others. The top vertebra is attached to the underneath of the occipital

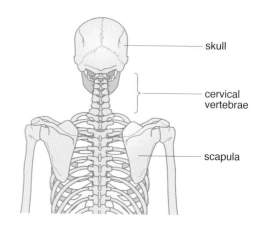

skull

cervical vertebrae

scapula

△ The relationship between the cervical vertebrae and the skull and shoulder

454

bone of the skull and has a hole through which passes a peg-like structure of the second vertebra. This arrangement forms a type of synovial joint called a **pivot joint**, which allows rotation of the head.

The bones of the shoulder girdle

The shoulder girdle is made up of the **clavicle**, **scapula** and **humerus bones**. The clavicle or collarbone is situated at the front of the body and forms a joint with the sternum or breastbone. The scapula is commonly called the shoulder blade and is situated at the back of the body, forming a ball-and-socket joint with the humerus, the upper bone of the arm.

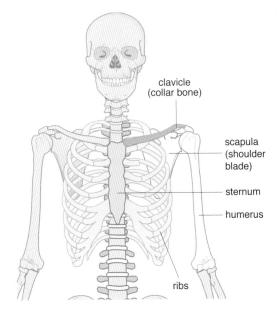

△ The shoulder girdle bones

Name of the bone	Position of the bone
Clavicle	Two long bones, a left and a right, found at the front of the body from the shoulder to the sternum
Scapula	Two flat bones, a left and a right, found in the upper back of the body at the shoulder
Humerus	Two long bones, a left and a right, forming the upper arm with joints at the shoulder at one end and the elbow at the other
Sternum	One flat bone found centrally at the front of the body in the chest forming joints with the clavicle at the top and the ribs along its length

The bones of the lower arm and hand

The humerus bone extends from the shoulder to form the upper arm. The lower end of the humerus forms a hinge joint at the elbow with the lower arm bones called the **ulna** and **radius**. The ulna is the stronger of the two bones and is weight bearing. It allows for the attachment of the muscles that move the wrist and hand. The radius carries little weight but is mainly for muscle attachment. These bones extend from the elbow to form the lower arm and at the lower end form joints with the wrist or **carpal** bones: eight irregular-shaped bones arranged loosely in two rows of four. The carpals form joints with the **metacarpals** of the hand or palm. These in turn articulate with the small bones of the fingers and thumb, known as the **phalanges**.

The ulna and radius articulate with each other to form pivot joints that allow the palm of the hand to turn forwards, a movement known as **supination** and backwards known as **pronation**.

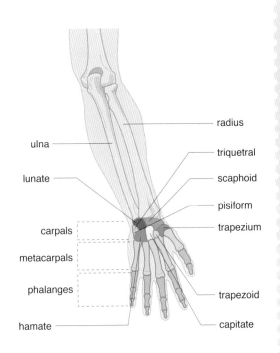

△ The forearm and hand bones

▽ The lower arm and hand bones

Name of the bone	Position of the bone
Ulna	Runs down the little finger side of the lower arm
Radius	Runs down the thumb side of the lower arm
Scaphoid	Found in the top row of carpals and articulates with the radius on the thumb side
Trapezium	Found in the lower row of carpals and articulates with the thumb metacarpal
Lunate	Top row, next to the scaphoid
Triquetral	Top row, next to the lunate
Pisiform	Top row of the carpals overlapping the triquetral on the little finger side
Trapezoid	Bottom row, next to the trapezium
Capitate	Bottom row, next to the trapezoid
Hamate	Bottom row, next to the capitate
Metacarpals	Five long bones of the palm of the hand, one for each of the digits
Phalanges	Fourteen small bones in each hand that make up the digits, arranged with three to each finger and two to the thumb

The trapezium and the metacarpal of the thumb form a 'saddle' joint which allows 'opposition of the thumb'; an important feature that gives us great dexterity and grip and separates us from other mammals.

The bones of the lower leg and foot

The **femur** extends down from the hip to the knee where it articulates with the **tibia** to form a hinge joint. 'Floating' over the knee is the kneecap or **patella**, which is embedded in the tendon of the front thigh muscles, the quadriceps.

The tibia forms the main bone of the lower leg and supports the weight of the body. Running parallel to it on the lateral side of the body is the **fibula**, which has largely a muscle attachment function.

The tibia and fibula form a hinge joint with the **talus** of the ankle. This arrangement allows for **dorsiflexion** and **plantarflexion** of the foot.

The seven bones making up the ankle are collectively known as the **tarsals**. These support and distribute the body weight from the feet throughout the body. The **calcaneus** forms the heel and attaches the strong muscles of the calf to the foot and enables walking and running, etc.

☆ *Hints and tips*

The bones of the feet are not flat but form transverse arches; one across the ball of the foot and another towards the heel and two longitudinal arches; one to the inside of the foot and the other to the outside. The four arches support the weight of the body, aid posture and fully utilise energy to propel the body forward when walking and running, etc.

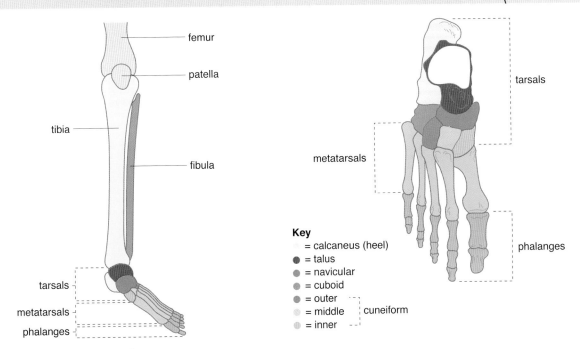

△ The lower leg and foot bones

▽ The lower leg and foot bones

Name of the bone	Position of the bone
Tibia	To the medial side of the lower leg, from knee to ankle
Fibula	To the lateral side of the lower leg, from knee to ankle
Patella	At the knee joint, commonly called the kneecap
Calcaneus	Forms the heel at the lower back of the ankle
Talus	Found at the top front of the ankle
Navicular	Forms part of the top of the foot at the ankle
Cuboid	Lies to the outside of the foot at the ankle
Outer cuneiform	Lies between the cuboid and the middle cuneiform
Middle cuneiform	Lies between the outer and inner cuneiform
Inner cuneiform	Lies next to the middle cuneiform to the medial side of the foot
Metatarsals	Five long bones making up the length of the foot one for each of the toes
Phalanges	Fourteen small bones of the toes in each foot. Two in the big toe and three in the other toes. Can be fused together in the little toe

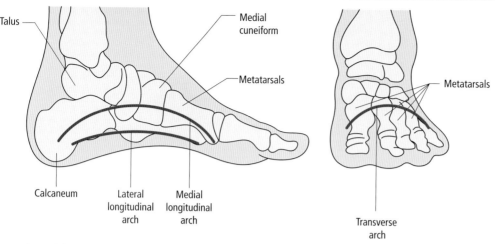

△ Arches of the foot

Muscles

Muscle is a special type of tissue that is able to contract. When it does so it usually becomes shorter, fatter and harder to the touch.

Muscle types and function

There are three types of muscle tissue:

1. **Voluntary muscle** brings about movement and locomotion. It is also called skeletal muscle as it is attached to and moves bones about the joints, or **striped** or **striated** muscle due to its appearance under a microscope. Voluntary muscle is under conscious control and the muscles discussed later are all of this type.

2. **Involuntary muscle**, also called **smooth** muscle, is under subconscious control and is found in organs and systems of the body such as the blood circulatory system.

3. **Cardiac muscle** is found only in the heart.

Voluntary muscle contraction is brought about by a series of events. First, the central nervous system, the brain and spinal cord, send a message in the form of an electrical impulse along a **motor nerve** to the muscle. When it reaches the muscle the nerve divides so that a nerve fibre serves each muscle fibre. This area is called the **motor point**. The message is passed from the nerve to the muscle fibres and the muscle contracts.

The ends of the muscles attached to bones across a joint bring about movement at that joint. In the face the muscles can be connected to bone at one end and skin or another muscle at the other. This allows the skin to move and create facial expressions.

To reverse a particular movement another muscle must contract. For example, the biceps muscle bends the elbow and the triceps straightens the elbow. These are known as antagonistic pairs and virtually all movements of the body are brought about in this way. The correct terminology used to describe muscle movements can be found in the glossary.

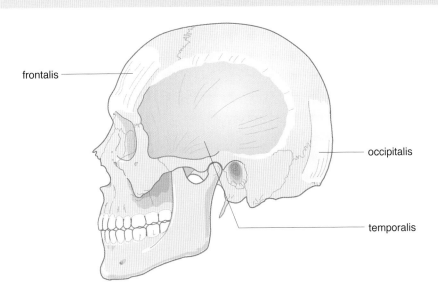

frontalis

occipitalis

temporalis

◁ Lateral view of muscles of the head

The muscles of the head and face

Name of the muscle	Position	Action of the muscle
Occipitalis	Found at the back of the head, attached to the occipital bone and the skin of the scalp	To move the scalp
Frontalis	At the forehead across its width, attached to the skin of the eyebrows and the skin of the scalp	Wrinkles the skin of the forehead and raises the eyebrows creating a surprised expression
Temporalis	Surrounds the ear and lies over the temporal bone, passing under the zygomatic arch to attach to the lower jaw	Raises the jaw when chewing
Corrugator	Between the eyebrows, attached to the frontalis muscle and the frontal bone	Brings the eyebrows together creating frowning
Procerus	Between the eyebrows, attached to the nasal bones and the frontalis muscle	Draws the eyebrows inwards creating a puzzled expression
Nasalis	At the sides of the nose attached to the maxillae bones and the nostrils	Dilates and compresses the nostrils
Orbicularis Oculi	Surrounds the opening of the eye socket attached to the bones at its outer edge and the skin of the eyelids at the inner	To close the eyes as in sleeping winking, squinting and blinking

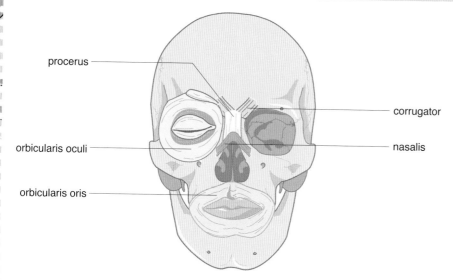

procerus

corrugator

orbicularis oculi

nasalis

orbicularis oris

◁ Anterior view of muscles of the face

▽ The face muscles

Name of the muscle	Position	Action of the muscle
Orbicularis oris	Surrounds the opening of the mouth occupying the entire width of the lips	Closes or narrows the lips, used to press the teeth against the teeth and to purse the lips as in whistling
Levator labitis of the upper lip	Towards the inner cheek beside the nose, attached to the maxillae and the skin of the corners of the mouth and upper lip	Raises the corner of the mouth to create a snarling expression
Buccinator	Main muscle of the cheek, attached to both the maxilla and mandible. Forms a muscular plate between the teeth	To keep the cheek stretched during all phases of opening and closing the mouth. Also to compress the cheeks when blowing
Depressors of the lower lip	Under the corners of the mouth and lower lip, from the mandible to the skin of the lip	Draws down the corners of the mouth to give a sad expression
Mentalis	Located at the point of the chin, attached to the mandible and the skin of the lower lip	Lifts and wrinkles the skin of the chin and turns the lower lip outwards creating a pouting expression
Masseter	Found at the outer cheek in front of the ear attached to the zygomatic arch and the mandible	Raises the lower jaw, exerting pressure on the teeth when chewing
Risorius	Lies above the buccinator, attached to the angle of the mandible and the skin at the corner of the mouth	Pulls the corner of the mouth sideways to create a grinning expression
Zygomaticus	Lies across the inner cheek, attached to the zygomatic bone and the corners of the mouth	Lifts the corners of the mouth upwards and sideways to create a smiling expression

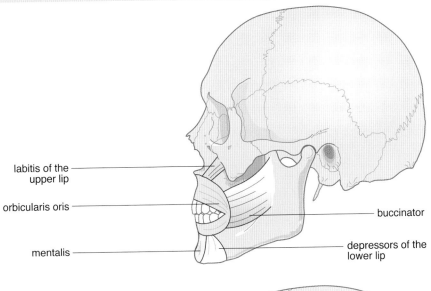

labitis of the upper lip

orbicularis oris

mentalis

buccinator

depressors of the lower lip

◁ Lateral view of muscles to the face 1

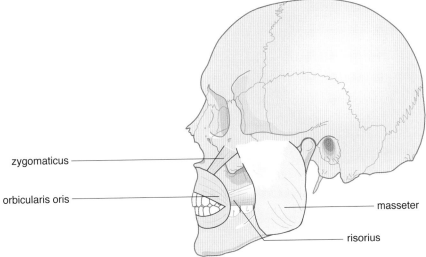

zygomaticus

orbicularis oris

masseter

risorius

◁ Lateral view of muscles to the face 2

The muscles of the neck and chest

▽ The neck and chest muscles

Name of the muscle	Position	Action of the muscle
Sternocleidomastoid	Lies across the side of the neck, attached to the clavicle and sternum and the mastoid process of the temporal bone	Contraction of one muscle turns the head in the opposite direction and when together the chin is pulled down towards the chest
Platysma	Extends down the front of the neck from the sides of the chin across the mandible to the clavicle, either side of the throat	Draws down the mandible and lower lip causing wrinkling in the skin of the neck
Pectoralis	In the chest, attached to the clavicle and sternum across the ribs to the humerus	Brings the arm forward and across the chest, used in pushing

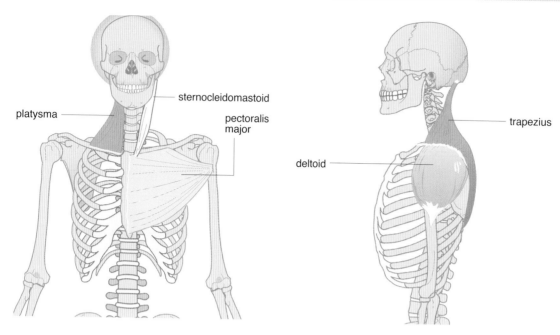

△ The neck and chest muscles   △ The neck and shoulder muscles

The muscles of the neck and shoulder

▽ The neck and shoulder muscles

Name of the muscle	Position	Action of the muscle
Trapezius	Diamond-shaped muscle at the upper back, neck and shoulder, attached to the occipital bone and the vertebrae of the neck and thorax to the scapula and outer end of the clavicle	Raises the shoulder to the ear, holds the scapula and shoulder still during arm movements and extends the neck
Deltoid	Forms a cap over the shoulder. The front is attached to the clavicle and the back to the scapula, and the two meet to attach to the humerus	The front brings the arm forward, the back takes it backwards and together they take the arm out to the side

The muscles of the lower arm and hand

The muscles that bring about movement of the lower arm at the elbow are situated in the upper arm and the wrist and hand in the forearm. The tendons that attach these muscles to the bones of the lower arm and hand are long and need to be held in place by ligaments at the wrist. This formation gives strength and power to the hands and wrist. The numerous muscles in the lower arm are grouped by the action they perform in the following table but the diagram shows them individually.

▽ The lower arm muscles 1

Name of the muscle	Position	Action of the muscle
Supinator	Lateral aspect of the lower humerus and the radius	Supinates the forearm and palm of the hand
Extensors	Lateral aspect of the forearm attached to the lower humerus, radius and ulna and the metacarpals and phalanges of the fingers	Extend the wrist, fingers and thumb
Brachio radialis	Lateral aspect of the forearm across the elbow, attached to the humerus and the radius bones	Flexes the elbow

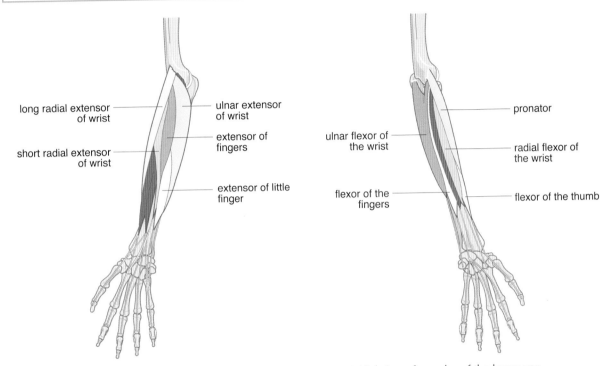

long radial extensor of wrist

short radial extensor of wrist

ulnar extensor of wrist

extensor of fingers

extensor of little finger

ulnar flexor of the wrist

flexor of the fingers

pronator

radial flexor of the wrist

flexor of the thumb

△ Lateral view of muscles of the lower arm

△ Medial view of muscles of the lower arm

▽ The lower arm muscles 2

Name of the muscle	Position	Action of the muscle
Pronators	Medial aspect of the lower humerus and the radius	Pronates the forearm and hand
Flexors	Medial aspect of the forearm, attached to the lower humerus, radius and ulna and the metacarpals and phalanges of the fingers	Flex the wrist, fingers and thumb

▽ The hand muscles

Name of the muscle	Position	Action of the muscle
Hypothenar eminence	In the palm of the hand below the little finger, attached to the carpals, metacarpals and phalanges of the little finger	Abducts, adducts and flexes the little finger
Thenar eminence	In the palm below the thumb, attached to the carpals, metacarpals and phalanges of the thumb	Abducts, adducts and flexes the thumb and draws it towards the palm
Mid-palm group	Centre of the palm below the middle three fingers, attached to the carpals, metacarpals and phalanges of those fingers	Abducts, adducts and flexes the middle three fingers

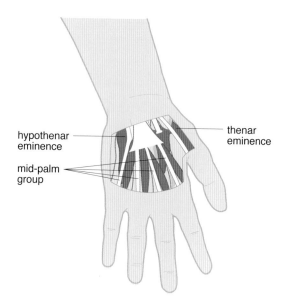

hypothenar eminence

thenar eminence

mid-palm group

△ Muscles of the hand

The muscles of the lower leg and foot

The muscles that bring about movement of the lower leg at the knee are situated in the thigh or upper leg and the ankle and toes in the lower leg, in a similar way to the lower arm. These muscles have long tendons that attach the muscles to the bones of the lower leg and foot. Some of the muscles have been grouped by their action in the table and on the diagrams, others are shown individually as they are large and the main muscle in the area.

▽ The lower leg and foot muscles

Name of the muscle	Position	Action of the muscle
Tibialis anterior	Anterior aspect of the lower leg, attached to the tibia and the middle cuneiform and first metatarsal	Dorsiflexes the ankle and inverts the foot
Extensors of the toes	Anterior and lateral aspect of the lower leg, attached to the tibia and fibula and the phalanges of the toes	Extend the toes and help dorsiflex the ankle
Gastrocnemius	Posterior aspect of the lower leg, main muscle forming the calf. Attached to the lower part of the femur across the back of the knee and ankle to the calcaneum	Flexes the knee and plantar-flexes the ankle
Soleus	Under the gastrocnemius, attached to the tibia and fibula across the ankle to the calcaneum	Plantar-flexes the ankle, an important action for propelling the body forward in walking and running
Tibialis posterior (not shown on diagram)	Very deep in the calf, attached to the tibia and fibula across the ankle to the navicular bone in the ankle	Inverts the foot
Peroneus	A group of three muscles found laterally and posterior in the calf, attached to the fibula across the ankle to the underneath of the first and fifth metatarsals	Everts the foot
Flexors of the toes	Muscles deep in the posterior aspect of the lower leg attached to the tibia and fibula and the phalanges of the toes	Flexes the toes and helps to plantar-flex the ankle

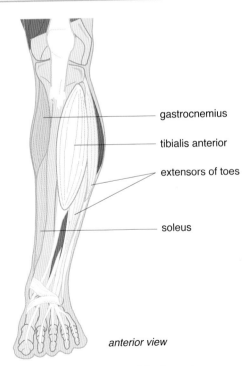

anterior view

△ Anterior view of muscles of the lower leg and foot

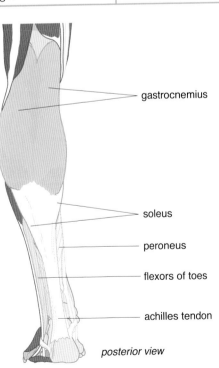

posterior view

△ Posterior view of muscles of the lower leg and foot

465

The nervous system

The nervous system consists of special cells called **neurones** that make up the brain, spinal cord and pairs of nerves. Its function is to receive and transmit impulses or messages to and from organs and muscles. In doing so the nervous system integrates and controls all the functions of the body. The nervous system is divided into two parts. These are the **central** and the **peripheral** systems.

The central nervous system (CNS)

The brain and the spinal cord make up the CNS. These important organs are protected by bone that completely surrounds them. In the case of the brain, it is the **cranium**. The spinal cord is protected by the **vertebrae** of the spine. From the brain and spinal cord come pairs of nerves that make up the peripheral nervous system.

The peripheral nervous system

There are 12 pairs of nerves from the brain called **cranial** nerves and 31 pairs from the spinal cord called **spinal nerves**. Each pair can contain either **motor** or **sensory** neurones or both.

- **Sensory neurones** take messages from the sense organs, such as those in the skin, to the central nervous system.
- **Motor neurones** take messages from the CNS to muscles or glands such as the sweat glands in the skin.

The autonomic nervous system

The autonomic nervous system is a specialised part of the peripheral nervous system and is **involuntary**, which means that it is under subconscious control. It is responsible for controlling involuntary actions of the body such as heartbeat, breathing rate, pupil dilation and the involuntary muscles that make up the blood vessels and digestive tract. The autonomic nervous system has two parts:

1. The **parasympathetic system** helps to create the conditions needed for rest, sleep and digestion.
2. The **sympathetic system** works antagonistically with the parasympathetic system to create the conditions needed for physical activity. It works with the hormone **adrenaline** to prepare the body for 'fight or flight' and is responsible for the conditions associated with 'stress' in modern-day living.

The effects of the autonomic system are summarised in the table below.

▽ The effects of the autonomic nervous system

Part of body affected	Sympathetic NS	Parasympathetic NS
Pupils	Dilate	Constrict
Blood vessels	Those in the digestive tract constrict giving the feeling of 'butterflies in the tummy'; those in skeletal muscles dilate and tone is increased in walls of large blood vessels leading to high blood pressure	Blood vessels supplying glands dilate
Heart	Beats quickly and more strongly	Beats slowly
Breathing	Quickens and deepens	Slowly and more shallow
Sweat gland	Activity increases	Activity decreases
Digestive tract	Action is decreased	Action is returned to normal

The 31 pairs of spinal nerves are numbered according to the section of the spinal column from which they arise. Each serves an area of the body according to its position, as follows:

8 pairs	**cervical** nerves (neck region)
12 pairs	**thoracic** nerves (chest region)
5 pairs	**lumbar** nerves (lower back region)
5 pairs	**sacral** nerves (bottom region)
1 pair	**coccygeal** nerves (tail region)

The nerves of the head and neck

The fifth and seventh cranial nerves are responsible for the sensations and movement of the facial muscles.

The fifth cranial nerve or trigeminal nerve

This has mainly a sensory function, carrying information to the brain from the skin of the face, the teeth and the membranes of the nose and mouth. There is also a motor branch to the muscles of mastication. The main branches are the mandibular, maxillary and ophthalmic branches.

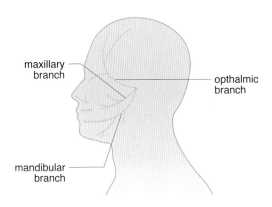

△ The branches of the fifth cranial or trigeminal nerve

The mandibular branch	**Sensory** for the teeth of the lower jaw, membranes of mouth and cheeks, and the skin of the lower part of the face
	Motor to the masseter and temporalis muscles; those involved with chewing food
The maxillary branch	**Sensory** for the upper jaw, the skin on the temples, sides of forehead and upper cheeks
The ophthalmic branch	**Sensory** for tear glands and the skin of forehead, nose and upper eyelids

The seventh cranial nerve or facial nerve

This is mainly a motor nerve serving the muscles of facial expression, but has a small sensory branch for the sensation of taste from the front of the tongue. There are five main branches.

The sternomastoid and the trapezius muscles are served by the eleventh cranial nerve or accessory nerve.

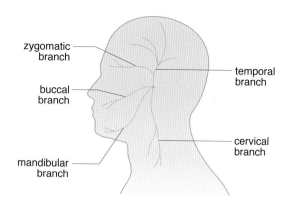

△ The branches of the seventh cranial or facial nerve

The temporal branch	**Motor** serves the muscles of the ear, the orbicularis oculi and the frontalis
The zygomatic branch	**Motor** serves the orbicularis oculi
The buccal branch	**Motor** serves the buccinator, the upper lip, and sides of the nose
The mandibular branch	**Motor** serves to the lower lip and the mentalis muscle
	Sensory from the front of the tongue
The cervical branch	**Motor** serves to the platysma muscle in the neck

Blood

Blood is a liquid that travels inside vessels of varying thickness. The vessels are called:

- arteries
- arterioles
- capliaries
- venules
- veins.

It moves along arteries due to the pumping action of the heart and the muscular arterial walls. In veins the blood is under less pressure and flow is controlled by a series of valves along the length of the veins.

Composition of blood

Blood is made up of the following:

Plasma	A fluid that is 90 per cent water, in which salts, nutrients and waste products are dissolved
Erythrocytes	Red blood cells which carry oxygen to the tissues and give blood its red colour
Leucocytes	White blood cells fight disease and prevent infection by destroying foreign bodies such as bacteria
Thrombocytes	Platelets and **blood proteins** such as **fibrinogen** help the blood to clot, preventing micro-organism invasion and blood loss
Other chemicals	For example, hormones (chemical messages that are transported round the body.)

Functions of blood

The functions of the blood are transport, defence and heat distribution and regulation.

Transport

Transport is the main and most important function of the blood:

- Oxygen is carried from the lungs to all living tissues.
- Carbon dioxide is carried from the tissues to the lungs to be exhaled.
- Nutrients from the digestive system are carried to the tissues.
- Excess water is taken from the tissues to the kidneys for excretion.
- Waste products from cell activity are taken to the kidneys or skin for excretion.
- Hormones released from endocrine glands are carried to their target organs.

Defence

The blood also performs an important function in the defence of the body against disease and injury:

- White blood cells are taken to a site of injury to fight invading bacteria and so stop infection.
- Other white blood cells produce **antibodies** that fight diseases that have entered the bloodstream.
- Blood proteins and platelets combine at the site of injury or damage to form a clot that plugs the wound, preventing blood loss and the invasion of bacteria. The clot hardens to form a scab which protects the area while new tissue grows underneath.

Heat distribution and regulation

As the blood flows around the body it is able to maintain the body temperature at 37°C:

- Body heat produced in the organs and muscles of the body is distributed around the body to the skin surface.
- The dilation of the blood capillaries in the skin allows excess heat to be lost to the atmosphere.
- When the temperature of the body needs to be maintained, the blood capillaries constrict, preventing blood from nearing the surface of the skin.

Blood circulation

As mentioned previously, blood is moved along the vessels by the pumping action of the heart. The heart has four chambers: **right atrium**, **right ventricle**, **left atrium** and **left ventricle**. A wall separates the left and right sides and valves that open and close separate the top chambers from the bottom.

The valves allow blood to flow from the top atria into the bottom ventricles. When the heart contracts or beats, the right side beats just before the left and this pushes blood out of the **ventricles** into the blood vessels. Other valves in the vessels prevent the blood from reversing back into the heart so that when it relaxes blood is drawn into the **atrium**. The vessels from the lower right ventricle carry blood to the lungs where it gives up carbon dioxide and takes on fresh oxygen. It then returns to the heart, entering the top left atrium. The blood passes through the valve into the bottom left ventricle where it is pumped out along a large vessel called the **aorta**, which supplies the whole body with blood. To complete the journey, blood returns from the areas of the body through the inferior and superior vena cava to the top right chamber to begin the cycle again.

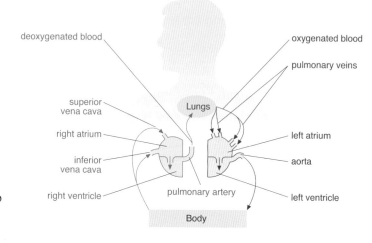

Blood supply to the head and neck

△ A simplified diagram to show blood circulation

Oxygenated blood leaves the heart through the aorta. This large vessel stretches upwards in front of the heart and then arches over to run down behind it. Two smaller arteries branch off and travel upwards on either side of the neck. Once in the neck area, they are called the **common carotid arteries**. As they near the head they divide to form the **external** and **internal carotid arteries**. At the level of the ear, the internal carotid disappears through a hole in the skull to supply blood to the brain and eyes. The external carotid artery divides further to supply blood to the skin and muscles of the face and scalp. There are three main branches, called the **facial artery**, the **temporal artery** and the **occipital artery** and they supply blood to the areas after which they are named.

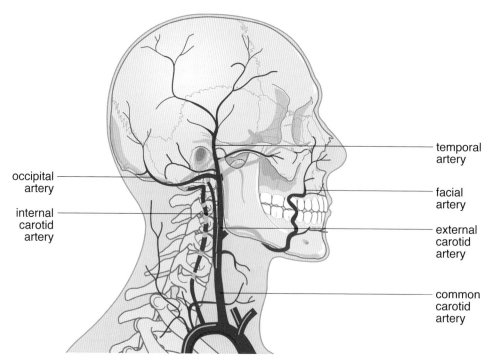

△ Arteries of the head and neck

As arteries become smaller they are known as **arterioles**. These become smaller still until they are the thickness of a hair, when they are known as **capillaries**. The walls of a capillary are very thin; just one cell thick. This allows the food and oxygen contained within the blood to be lost to the surrounding tissues and the waste products of cell activity to be collected by the blood. This process is called **capillary exchange**. Once this has happened the blood begins its journey back to the heart. The capillaries join to form small vessels called **venules**, which in turn join up to form **veins**. The veins returning the blood back to the heart from the head and neck are called the **internal** and **external jugular veins**. The former exits the skull through a hole near the ear as before and the external jugular vein drains blood from the **facial**, **temporal** and **occipital veins**.

The internal and external jugular veins do not join together. They run down the neck independently to join a large vein called the superior vena cava, which eventually returns the blood to the heart.

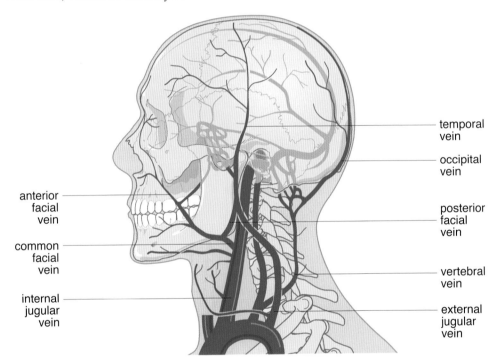

temporal vein

occipital vein

anterior facial vein

posterior facial vein

common facial vein

vertebral vein

internal jugular vein

external jugular vein

△ The veins of the head and neck

Blood supply to the arm and hand

The blood supply to the arm begins with the **subclavian artery**, which has branched off the **aorta**. The subclavian artery becomes the **axillary artery** and then the **brachial artery**, which runs down the inner aspect of the upper arm to about 1 cm below the elbow, where it divides into the **radial** and **ulnar arteries**. The radial artery runs down the forearm next to the radius bone to the wrist where it nears the surface and can be felt as the **radial pulse**. It continues over the carpals to pass between the first and second metacarpals into the palm. The ulnar artery runs down the forearm next to the ulna bone, across the carpals into the palm of the hand. Together they form two arches in the hand, the **deep** and **superficial palmer arches**. From all these arteries branch others to supply blood to the structures of the upper arm, forearm, hand and fingers.

The venous return of blood from the hand begins with the **palmer arch** and **plexus**, which is a network of capillaries present in the palm. Three veins carry the deoxygenated blood up the forearm: the **radial vein**, the **ulnar vein** and the **median vein**. The former two run parallel to the bones of the same name, the latter runs up the middle. Just above the elbow, the radial and ulnar veins join to become the **brachial vein**, and the median vein joins the **basilic vein**, which originated just below the elbow along with the **cephalic vein**. As the veins continue over the elbow they link to form a network that eventually divides, with the basilic vein joining the brachial vein, which then becomes the **axillary vein**. The cephalic vein travels up the arm separately and becomes the **subclavian vein** in the upper chest.

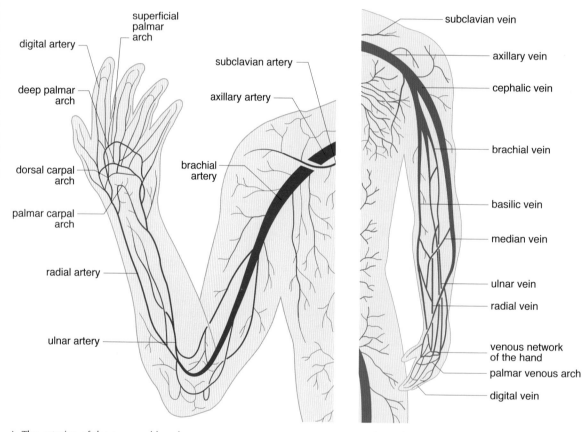

△ The arteries of the arm and hand   △ The veins of the arm and hand

Blood supply to the leg and foot

The aorta travels down the length of the trunk to the lower abdomen where it divides into two arteries which supply either leg. The artery in the thigh is called the **femoral artery**, named after the bone of the thigh. At the knee the femoral artery becomes the **popliteal**

artery, which divides into two below the knee. One of these arteries runs down the front of the lower leg and is called the **anterior tibial artery**, while the other runs down the back and is known as the **posterior tibial artery**. This artery divides at the inside of the ankle becoming the **medial plantar artery** on the inside of the foot and the **plantar arch** on the sole of the foot. The anterior tibial artery becomes the **dorsal metatarsal artery** on top of the foot.

There is a network of veins in the foot that become the **dorsal venous arch** on top of the foot. This travels the inside of the foot to the ankle where it becomes the **small saphenous vein**. It continues up the back of the whole leg to the thigh where it is known as the **great saphenous vein**. Two small veins called the **anterior tibial veins** travel up the front of the lower leg while two veins, the **posterior tibial veins**, run up the back. These four veins converge just below the knee to become the **popliteal vein** at the back of the knee and then eventually the **femoral vein** in the thigh. The great saphenous vein and the femoral vein join at the groin and return to the heart via the inferior vena cava.

The effects of blood circulation on skin and muscle tissue

When an area of the body has good blood circulation the skin feels soft and warm to the touch and it is a pink healthy colour. It is healthy due to the food and oxygen it receives and because waste products are not allowed to accumulate. Consequently, the skin has a medium texture with good elasticity. In areas of poor blood circulation the skin appears pale or bluish in colour and is cold to the touch. The skin's functions are impaired due to the lack of food and oxygen and/or the build up of waste products in the area.

Muscles require energy to perform their function of contraction. The food and oxygen contained within blood provides that energy. Without it the muscles perform 'anaerobically' which produces a waste product called lactic acid. When allowed to accumulate lactic acid causes muscle fatigue where the muscle becomes weak and tired and contracts erratically causing shakes and spasms called cramp. When blood returns to the muscle the lactic acid is exposed to oxygen and reverts back to a usable source of energy again.

The lymphatic system

The lymphatic system defends the body from infection and works as a waste disposal system through the removal of waste products and toxins from the tissues by a network of fine tubes and larger vessels.

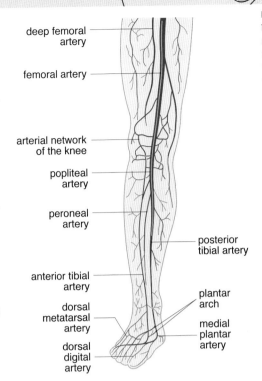

deep femoral artery
femoral artery
arterial network of the knee
popliteal artery
peroneal artery
posterior tibial artery
anterior tibial artery
dorsal metatarsal artery
dorsal digital artery
plantar arch
medial plantar artery

△ The arteries of the leg and foot

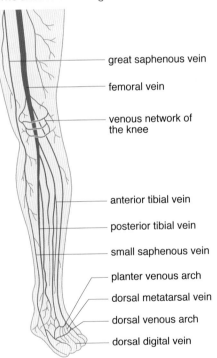

great saphenous vein
femoral vein
venous network of the knee
anterior tibial vein
posterior tibial vein
small saphenous vein
planter venous arch
dorsal metatarsal vein
dorsal venous arch
dorsal digital vein

△ The veins of the leg and foot

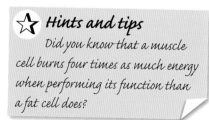

☆ *Hints and tips*
Did you know that a muscle cell burns four times as much energy when performing its function than a fat cell does?

The functions of lymph

The functions of lymph are to:

- fight infection
- return nutrients and blood proteins from the tissues to the blood circulatory system
- transport white blood cells to the blood circulatory system
- transport fats from the small intestine to the liver
- prevent oedema (swelling) by draining excess tissue fluid from the tissues
- produce lymphocytes (a type of white blood cell).

Composition of lymph

Lymph is a liquid very similar in composition to that of blood plasma, except it contains no erythrocytes. Because of this it appears straw-coloured instead of red. It also contains fewer blood proteins and nutrients but has a larger number of white blood cells, fats and waste materials.

The structures of the lymphatic system

The liquid lymph is transported in the body by a series of vessels called lymph capillaries, lymph vessels, lymph nodes and lymph ducts.

Lymph capillaries

These are fine, blind-ended tubes about the size of a human hair. They are present between the cells of all tissues but are found in large numbers in the areas of the body that are most likely to become infected or where micro-organisms can enter easily, such as the toes, fingers, around the stomach and small intestine, the mouth, ears, eyes and nose.

Lymph vessels

The lymph capillaries form a network that join to form larger **lymph vessels**. These are similar to veins in structure and they also follow the venous return of blood to the heart. They have thin, weak muscular walls and valves to prevent the backflow of lymph, again similar to veins.

The lymphatic system relies on the pumping action of surrounding muscles to move the lymph along these vessels. As the muscles contract they become shorter and fatter, which squeezes the lymph vessels and pushes the lymph along, the valves preventing its return. This causes a vacuum below the valve, which is filled from lymph further down the vessel and this causes more tissue fluid to be drawn into the lymph capillaries.

Lymph nodes

Lymph nodes are swellings along the lymph vessels where the lymph is cleansed by first being filtered and then by the action of special white blood cells. These cells destroy micro-organisms and other unwanted material so that when the lymph leaves the node it consists of mainly white blood cells and food materials. The nodes are found in groups so the lymph is forced to pass through several nodes to be cleansed before being deposited back in the bloodstream at the chest.

Lymph ducts

Once the lymph has been cleansed it travels along vessels to the chest area where it is deposited back into the bloodstream through large vessels called **lymph ducts**. Lymph collected from the right side of the head, chest and the right arm drains into the **right lymphatic duct** while lymph from the rest of the body drains into the **thoracic duct**. These ducts deposit the lymph into the subclavian veins.

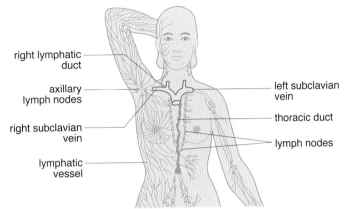

△ The position of the the lymph ducts

Lymph drainage

These structures together are responsible for **lymph drainage** where fluid within the body tissues is removed, cleansed and deposited back into the blood stream at the subclavian veins.

▽ Factors affecting lymph drainage

General blood circulation	If the heart works well there will be good lymph drainage due to capillary exchange in the tissues; if not oedema (swelling) will occur
Exercise	The action of the muscles on the lymph vessels speeds up lymph drainage and improves the performance of the heart
Massage	Deep movements press on the lymph vessels forcing the lymph along them. These movements are always performed towards the heart, which is in the direction of lymph flow

The effects of lymph drainage on skin and muscle tissue

Good lymph drainage benefits the function and appearance of the skin and enhances the performance of muscle tissue by improving the internal environment through the removal of waste material. The removal of the waste allows further capillary exchange to occur with the local blood capillaries, hence more food and oxygen is provided for the cells.

Lymph drainage from the head and neck

The lymph capillaries collect the fluid from the tissues of all the organs and structures within the head and neck. It flows downwards towards the chest, passing through the lymph nodes shown in the diagram on p. 478. Numerous nodes are present due to the large number of openings i.e. the ears, nose and mouth, through which micro-organisms could potentially enter the body. Swelling is unlikely in this area due to the effect of gravity assisting lymph flow, although 'puffiness' around the eyes caused by blocked sinuses can be improved by lymph drainage massage techniques. The right lymphatic duct collects lymph from the head and neck into the blood circulatory system.

Lymph drainage from the arm and hand

The lymph drainage from the arm and hand follows the venous blood flow up the arm towards the chest. The major lymph nodes are found in the inner part of the elbow and the armpit (axillary). The cleansed lymph from the right arm and hand is collected by the right lymphatic duct. The cleansed lymph from the left arm and hand is collected by the thoracic duct.

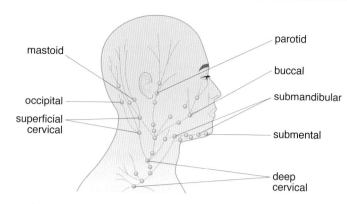

△ The lymph nodes of the head and neck

Lymph drainage from the leg and foot

Lymph drainage in the leg works against gravity. Tissue fluid can collect in the feet and ankles causing **oedema** (swelling). This is more likely in someone who stands still for long periods of time. The major lymph nodes are found at the back of the knee and in the front of the groin. The lymph from both legs and feet are collected by the thoracic duct to be emptied into the blood circulatory system at the chest.

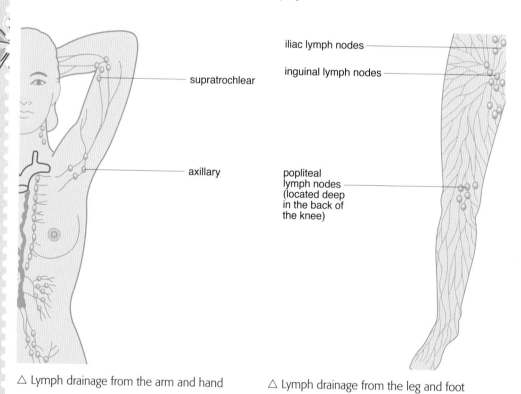

△ Lymph drainage from the arm and hand   △ Lymph drainage from the leg and foot

Test yourself

Test your knowledge of anatomy and physiology by answering the following questions.

Skin

1. The process by which epidermal cells are shed from the surface of the skin is called:

    a) mitosis

    b) pigmentation

    c) desquamation

    d) oxidation.

2. Sweat is produced by:

    a) the sebaceous gland

    b) the endocrine gland

    c) hair follicles

    d) the sudoriferous gland.

3. Give four functions of the skin.

4. The function of sebum is to:

    a) lubricate

    b) stimulate

    c) irritate

    d) desquamate.

5. Cell division is called:

    a) mitosis

    b) lordosis

    c) kyphosis

    d) cellosis.

6. A healthy skin is slightly acid. Is this statement true or false?

Hair

7. The papilla at the base of the hair follicle is:

    a) nerve fibres

    b) growing cells

    c) a type of hair

    d) blood vessels.

8. What are the two types of hair found over the body in adults called?

9. What areas of the body is hair NOT found?

10. What are the layers making up the structure of a terminal hair called?

11. The active stage of growth of the hair follicle is called:

    a) Telogen

    b) Catagen

    c) Anagen

Nails

12. What structure of the nail unit forms the frame to the nail?

13. Where on the nail unit is the hyponychium found?

14. What is the correct name for the half-moon?

15. What is the function of the matrix?

16. Describe the appearance of a healthy nail.

17. From which layer of the skin does the nail originate?

Skeletal

18. Name the two bones of the forearm.

19. What is the difference between a ligament and a tendon?

20. The metacarpals are found in the:

    a) foot

    b) knee

    c) hand

    d) neck.

21. Name three bones of the cranium.

22. Name the bone that forms the cheekbone.

23. The bone of the lower jaw is called the:

    a) lacrimal

    b) turbinate

    c) mandible

    d) vomer.

24. How many bones make up the ankle?

25. What is the correct name for the knee cap?

Muscles

26. The buccinator is found in:

    a) the forehead

    b) the cheek

    c) the neck

    d) around the mouth.

27. The action of the orbicularis occuli is to:

    a) open the mouth

    b) close the eyes

    c) wrinkle the nose

    d) chew.

28. The sternocleidomastoid is found in the:

    a) face

    b) arm

    c) shoulder

    d) neck.

29. The gastrocnemius is found in the:

    a) calf

    b) ankle

    c) upper leg

    d) arm.

Nerves

30. The central nervous system is made up of the:

    a) brain and spinal cord

    b) brain

    c) cranium and spine

    d) nerves.

31. The autonomic nervous system controls:

    a) moving the arms

    b) nodding the head

    c) the heartbeat

    d) rubbing the hands.

Blood

32. Give two functions of the blood.

33. The main artery of the body is:

    a) pulmonary

    b) carotid

    c) temporal

    d) aorta.

34. Name the vessel that carries oxygenated blood away from the heart.

35. Oxygenated blood is carried through the veins. Is this statement true or false?

Lymph

36. The function of the lymph nodes is to:

    a) fight infection

    b) produce white blood cells

    c) drain tissue fluids

    d) all of the above.

37. The main lymph nodes in the neck are the:

    a) carotid nodes

    b) cervical nodes

    c) occipital nodes

    d) thoracic nodes.

Index

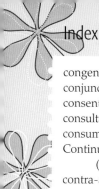